Atlas of Cancer Incidence in England and Wales 1968–85

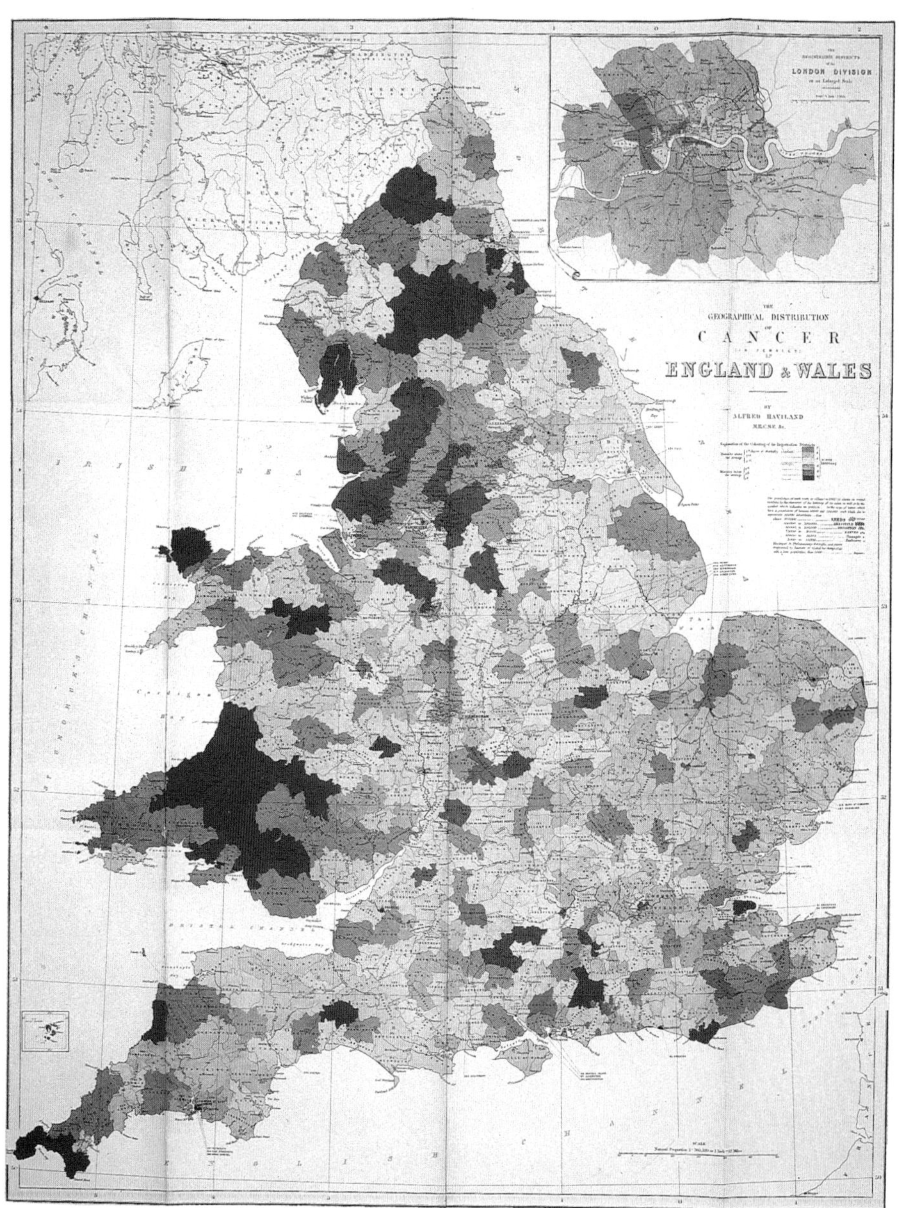

The geographical distribution of cancer in females in England and Wales, 1851–60. From Haviland (1878).

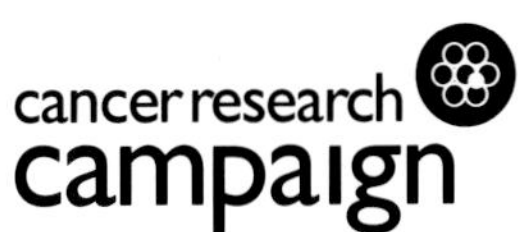

Atlas of Cancer Incidence in England and Wales 1968–85

(Based on data from the cancer registries of England and Wales, with the cooperation of the Office of Population Censuses and Surveys)

Anthony Swerdlow
and
Isabel dos Santos Silva

Epidemiological Monitoring Unit, Department of Epidemiology and Population Sciences, London School of Hygiene and Tropical Medicine

Oxford New York Tokyo
OXFORD UNIVERSITY PRESS
1993

Oxford University Press, Walton Street, Oxford OX2 6DP
Oxford New York Toronto
Delhi Bombay Calcutta Madras Karachi
Kuala Lumpur Singapore Hong Kong Tokyo
Nairobi Dar es Salaam Cape Town
Melbourne Auckland Madrid
and associated companies in
Berlin Ibadan

Oxford is a trade mark of Oxford University Press

Published in the United States
by Oxford University Press, New York

A catalogue record for this book is available from the British Library

Library of Congress Cataloging in Publication Data
(Data available)

ISBN 0 19 261993 4

Set by Graphicraft Typesetters Ltd, Hong Kong
Printed in Hong Kong

Foreword

Sir RICHARD DOLL

Emeritus Professor of Medicine, University of Oxford.

Until about thirty years ago, cancer mortality rates in the developed countries were an essential stock in trade of the cancer epidemiologist. There was little call for the more elusive incidence rates that were both more difficult to obtain and more subject to artificial distortion. For the diagnosis of cancer on death certificates was reasonably reliable and had been so for many years (at least for people under 70 years of age) and the efficacy of treatment had altered so little and was, for many types of cancer, so poor that variations in mortality from time to time and from place to place provided an adequate indication of underlying variations in incidence.

The situation now is very different. Childhood cancers, some of which were almost uniformly fatal, have cure rates of up to 80 per cent, which continue to improve, and every few years major advances are made in the control of one or other of the cancers of adult life. For some, control is improved by means of new and more effective treatments, for others by the spread of screening techniques that permit the recognition of disease at a stage when it is relatively easily cured. Now, also, the need for more precise information about variations in incidence has become more acute. For not only is there heightened public concern about the carcinogenic hazards that may be associated with changes in personal behaviour and in industrial development that may cause (or be thought to cause) local epidemics of cancer, but the increase in knowledge about practical ways of preventing the disease has created the need to monitor the extent to which the knowledge is applied.

With present knowledge it is possible to prevent about half of all cancers; or rather it is possible to halve the age-specific incidence rates, which is not the same thing because the incidence of cancers increases rapidly with age and may eventually return to much the same level, despite a reduction in the prevalence of carcinogenic agents, if life is sufficiently prolonged. For these 'preventable' cancers, such as cancer of the lung, the geographical distribution highlights the areas where further education or (as the case may be) further provision of services or further attention to the environment is needed. For other cancers, the causes of which are still unknown, the geographical variation, small though it is in the UK compared to that in the world as a whole, continues to challenge the cancer research worker to find a behavioural, or environmental, or (perhaps) genetic factor that varies in a similar way and offers him (or her) useful evidence to check the validity of hypotheses derived in other ways. For all these reasons the publication of an atlas of cancer incidence to supplement the atlas of mortality is timely and welcome.

Acknowledgements

We have received help from many sources in preparing this Atlas. Any errors and omissions, of course, remain ours. We thank particularly the Cancer Research Campaign who funded the work, the directors and staff of the regional cancer registries of England and Wales, without whose patient and careful data collection over many years the analyses would not have been possible, the Office of Population Censuses and Surveys who supplied the magnetic tapes of the aggregated national data set, and the Childhood Cancer Research Group who kindly provided data on childhood leukaemia and populations. We are also grateful to Chris Wale, who helped us to download the National Registry data from mainframe to microcomputer, Bill Nicholson who advised and instructed us on use of the Mapics package, which has more than lived up to the billing he gave it, and the staff of Oxford University Press who have given us friendly, patient, and professional guidance through the complexities of colour map publishing. We also thank for their valuable advice and support, Dr Nigel Kemp, Professor Gordon McVie, Jane Toms, and Sue Foden at the Cancer Research Campaign, Professor John Fox and staff in his Department at the Office of Population Censuses and Surveys, and staff in the Epidemiological Monitoring Unit at the London School of Hygiene and Tropical Medicine. The Epidemiological Monitoring Unit is funded by the Medical Research Council.

We thank the Ordnance Survey for permission to show county boundaries in the maps, and note that display of the boundaries is Crown copyright. The following gave kind permission for use of published material in tables and maps: the Cancer Research Campaign, the Central Statistical Office, Dr Paula Cook-Mozaffari, the Department of Education and Science, the Department of Health, the Controller of HMSO, the Home Office, the Inland Revenue, the Editor of the *Journal of Epidemiology and Community Health*, the Editors of the *Journal of the Royal Statistical Society*, the Meteorological Office, the Ministry of Agriculture, Fisheries and Food, the National Radiological Protection Board, the Office of Population Censuses and Surveys, and Dr M. Wadsworth. The sources, and whether the data have been modified, are indicated below the tables and maps.

We are grateful for unpublished data on 'exposure' variables to Professor Jocelyn Chamberlain for information about screening programmes, Professor Jean Golding and Dr Clive Osmond for data on height, Dr Julia Heptonstall for hepatitis B data, Dr John Osman for Asbestos Survey data, the Department of Health for data on attendances at venereal disease clinics, and the Office of Population Censuses and Surveys for medical, survey, and Census data.

We are particularly grateful to Sir Richard Doll for his kind foreword. We are also much indebted to Drs Lucy Carpenter, Sarah Darby, and Leo Kinlen, who generously gave many hours of their time to read through the manuscript and give detailed comments upon it. We are fortunate to have such colleagues. Lastly, we thank our families for their toleration of our time spent working on this Atlas, and for their encouragement.

Contents

Abbreviations

General

AIDS	acquired immunodeficiency syndrome
Bq	becquerel
CCRG	Childhood Cancer Research Group
CDSC	Communicable Disease Surveillance Centre
Cs	Caesium
DHSS	Department of Health and Social Security
GRO	General Register Office
Gy	gray
HIPE	Hospital In-patient Enquiry
HIV	human immunodeficiency virus
HLA	human leucocyte group A (antigen)
HMSO	His/Her Majesty's Stationery Office
HTLV1	human T-lymphotropic virus type 1
ICD (7, 8, and 9)	International Classification of Diseases (Seventh, Eighth, and Ninth Revisions)
MAFF	Ministry of Agriculture, Fisheries and Food
NHL	Non-Hodgkin's lymphoma
NRPB	National Radiological Protection Board
NS	Not statistically significant ($p \geq 0{\cdot}05$)
OPCS	Office of Population Censuses and Surveys
PIR	Proportional Incidence Ratio
Pu	Plutonium
RHA	Regional Health Authority
RHB	Regional Hospital Board
SAS	Statistical Analysis System
UV	Ultraviolet
WHO	World Health Organization
IIIN	III non-manual (social class)

County names (in maps)

England

Beds	Bedfordshire
Berks	Berkshire
Bucks	Buckinghamshire
Cambs	Cambridgeshire
Ches	Cheshire
Cleve	Cleveland
Derbys	Derbyshire
Glos	Gloucestershire
Hants	Hampshire
Hereford	Herefordshire
Heref & Worcs	Hereford and Worcester
Herts	Hertfordshire

Hunt	Huntingdonshire
IOW	Isle of Wight
Lancs	Lancashire
Leics	Leicestershire
Lincs H	Lincolnshire Holland
Lincs K	Lincolnshire Kesteven
Lincs L	Lincolnshire Lindsey
M/C	Greater Manchester
Mers	Merseyside
Northants	Northamptonshire
Northd	Northumberland
Notts	Nottinghamshire
Oxon	Oxfordshire
Rut	Rutland
Salop	Shropshire
Staffs	Staffordshire
E Suff	East Suffolk
W Suff	West Suffolk
E Sussex	East Sussex
W Sussex	West Sussex
Tyne	Tyne and Wear
Warwicks	Warwickshire
Westd	Westmorland
Wilts	Wiltshire
W Mids	West Midlands
Worcs	Worcestershire
E Yorks	East Yorkshire
N Yorks	North Yorkshire
S Yorks	South Yorkshire
W Yorks	West Yorkshire

Wales

Ang	Anglesey
Brec	Breconshire
Caer	Caernarvonshire
Card	Cardiganshire
Carm	Carmarthenshire
Den	Denbighshire
Fli	Flintshire
Glam	Glamorgan
M Gl	Mid-Glamorgan
S Gl	South Glamorgan
W Gl	West Glamorgan
Meri	Merionethshire
Monm	Monmouthshire
Mont	Montgomeryshire
Pemb	Pembrokeshire
Rad	Radnorshire

Tables

Maps

Maps of physical geography, population density, and geographical distribution of 'exposures'

Maps of cancer mortality in England and Wales, 1921–30. From Stocks (1936, 1937, 1939)

Maps of cancer incidence in England and Wales, 1968–85[1]

1 Childhood leukaemia (Maps 74, 75), 1966–83

Appendix 1

1

Introduction

'I feel convinced that by studying the geographical laws of disease we shall know where to find its exciting as well as its predisposing cause, and how to avoid it.' — Alfred Haviland, 1875

England and Wales have a long tradition of national data collection concerning cancer mortality and incidence. The former has been tabulated since 1868 on a site-specific basis (General Register Office 1890), and the latter has been collected in a national scheme since 1945 (Stocks 1950). There is also a long tradition of use of these data for description of cancer risks and in the search for causation. Cancer is a major cause of morbidity and death in England and Wales: during the period covered by this Atlas (1968–85) there were, on average, 180 000 malignancies occurring per year, and cancer was responsible for 67 000 deaths in men and 58 000 in women annually. Nevertheless, in geographical subdivisions of the country the number of cases of a particular site of cancer occurring in a year can be small, and many years of data may be needed to provide sufficient cases for underlying patterns of geographical distribution to become clear, and chance factors unimportant. Therefore we have assembled here cancer incidence data for 18 years from the files of the England and Wales national registry, in order to examine cancer distribution within these countries, based on 1·62 million registrations in men, and 1·56 million in women. This gave us an opportunity to map the distribution of cancers not previously examined, and also to investigate the recent distribution of others for which data have been published in the past, and therefore the development of the present pattern can be assessed. Some of the resulting distributions were unexpected and appear worthy of further investigation — for instance, a substantially raised risk of lip cancer in East Anglia, high risks of both cervical and penile cancer on the Island of Anglesey, and a focus of thyroid cancer risk in north Wales corresponding with patterns of non-malignant thyroid disease present for over half a century.

In the first report of the Registrar General, William Farr (1839) commented on the geographical mortality data that: 'In recommending a residence to patients the physician will find the registered causes of death an indispensable directory; and the utility of a sanatory map of the country, such as the returns will furnish, cannot fail to be felt in England, where a part of the population is constantly migrating from place to place in search of health'. While we do not expect the present maps to provide a guide for migration, we have enjoyed preparing them, and hope that they may be of interest to others and may assist in research into the causes of cancer in England and Wales and the reasons for its geographical variation.

2

History

Historically, examination of the geographical distribution of disease has had a central role in epidemiological efforts to discover aetiology. For example, Snow, in 1855, showed by his classical examination of cholera death rates in London houses supplied with polluted water by the Southwark and Vauxhall company, and in those supplied with unpolluted water by the Lambeth company, that cholera could be spread by faecal contamination of drinking water. Mapping of cancers in England and Wales also dates back to the nineteenth century. The earliest known cancer map is that of female cancer mortality published by Haviland in 1875, which we have reproduced as the frontispiece of this book. Haviland, of course, had no powerful computing facilities or mechanical pen-plotter: it is a comment on progress that his map is more elegant visually than any published in recent years.

Owen in 1889 produced further cancer maps, based on over 3000 replies to an enquiry sent to every registered medical practitioner in the United Kingdom asking whether cancer was common in their district. Since then, a range of geographical data have been published on cancer mortality in England and Wales. The first maps for specific cancer sites in these countries were produced by Greenwood in 1925, showing the county distribution of mortality from breast and uterine cancers in 1911–20. The major series of early maps, however, were those published by Dr Percy Stocks. Initially Stocks had published maps of cancer mortality by county in 1919–23 (Stocks 1928) and 1921–6 (Stocks and Karn 1930–31), not subdivided by site. During 1936–9 he published a series of 28 site-specific maps of cancer mortality in 1921–30 by county (Stocks 1936, 1937, 1939), whose production must have required a vast clerical effort. Comparison of these maps with the present ones allows some assessment of the evolution of the geographical distribution of cancer in England and Wales over a period of 50 years, and therefore we have reproduced several of them here (see Maps S1–S9). It should be kept in mind when making such comparisons, however, that Stocks's maps differed in several ways from the present ones. For example, they concerned mortality, not incidence; unlike ours they were standardized for degree of urbanization; and over time there have been changes in many aspects of diagnostic practice[1].

The other principal sources of early (but unmapped) geographical data on cancer mortality in England and Wales, are the Registrar General's Decennial Supplements, which have included site-specific cancer statistics for geographical subdivisions of the country since 1911–20 (General Register Office 1933).

In more recent times, Howe (1970) published mortality maps for four cancer sites for 1954–63, and more extensive cancer mortality maps have been published for England and Wales in the atlas by Gardner *et al.* (1983), which showed mortality during 1968–78, and in a Registrar General's Decennial Supplement (OPCS 1981) showing maps of deaths in 1969–73. Some of Gardner's maps were by county and others bv local authority, whereas the Registrar General's Decennial Supplement maps were by region. The forthcoming European Cancer Mortality Atlas (Smans *et*

1 There were also a few differences in the counties presented; see Appendix 1.

al., in press) will show risks in England and Wales in 1976–80 by new county,[1] for about 25 cancer sites or site groupings.

These maps have all been of cancer mortality rather than incidence[2]. For several purposes, including health-care planning and consideration of aetiology, incidence is, however, the measure of primary interest. The geographical distribution of mortality reflects the influence of incidence (new cases), but also that of survival (case-fatality). For cancers with good survival rates, therefore, mortality maps may poorly reflect incidence patterns.[3] Also the maps have been published for only a fairly limited range of cancer sites, mainly those causing large numbers of deaths.

Although cancer incidence data have been collected in England and Wales on a national basis since 1945, national maps of cancer incidence have not been published previously. Indeed, the only published national geographical data (in the National Registry annual publications) have been at regional level, and for single years of incidence, with corresponding instability of small numbers for many sites.

1 i.e. for counties as demarcated in the 1974 boundary reorganization (see Appendix 1).

2 Except for the maps by Owen in 1889, referred to above, which are of reported commonness (i.e. either incidence or prevalence), of all cancer sites combined.

3 There are merits and disadvantages to both incidence and mortality data for these purposes. For instance, mortality data are complete for the fact of death, but may omit cancers not deemed to be the underlying cause of death. Incidence data, on the other hand, may be incomplete because of failures in cancer registration, but are not generally dependent on the certification practice of doctors. In general, the advantages of mortality data will be greater for rapidly fatal tumours, and of registration data will be greater for tumours which are more slowly, or less often, fatal. Therefore in the text we have compared the findings in the present maps with those from mortality maps, where these exist.

3

Scope of the Atlas

This atlas presents maps of cancer incidence in England and Wales in 1968–85 by county of residence. The year 1968 was the first to be included, because it was the first year of data for which the Eighth Revision of the International Classification of Diseases (ICD) (WHO 1967) was used in England and Wales for coding the site of origin of cancer (in the body). The year 1985 was the most recent for which data were reasonably complete when we extracted data from the National Cancer Registry computer files to plot the maps.

Results are also presented, for each cancer site, on the comparative risk of cancer in rural, urban, and metropolitan areas of England and Wales, and in the text the geographical (county) distribution is considered separately within rural, urban, and metropolitan strata (although maps for these are not shown, because of space constraints). The data and maps relating to urbanization strata were for 1968–81, because the data for 1982–5 in the National Cancer Registry files were not coded by degree of urbanization. Where it would be of interest, we conducted analyses of geographical distribution of the cancers by age subdivision as well as for all ages.

For childhood leukaemia, we obtained data from the National Registry of Childhood Tumours at the Childhood Cancer Research Group, which are more accurate and complete than those available in the National Cancer Registry (OPCS) files. These data were for cases incident 1966–83, and could only be analysed overall, not by degree of urbanization.

In preparing the Atlas, we generated a large number of maps: for each cancer in each sex overall, for urban, rural, and metropolitan areas separately for most cancers,[1] and by age group for certain cancers. We have selected for publication those which seemed to be of greatest general interest; the others are commented upon in the text, and copies can be obtained on application to the authors. A full set of the odds ratios and confidence limits for the maps can also be obtained from this source.

As well as mapping cancer distribution, we also sought to examine the geographical distribution of environmental and behavioural factors which may have relevance to the aetiology of certain of these neoplasms. This involved seeking published sources of risk factor data, but also for certain variables we used unpublished tabulations or tabulations made specially from the 1971 Census. Again, this produced far more material than can be published here, so we have given references to the sources of much of the geographical data on risk factors, and have only published a few maps and several tables of factors which we thought to be of particular interest or which show unpublished material not available otherwise.

We have written the text mainly with reference uses in mind, or to dip into, rather than to be read sequentially from end to end.

1 Conducted for all tumours except childhood leukaemia, cancer of the placenta, and some age subdivisions of the data, where small numbers precluded it.

4

Materials

Cancer registrations

The cancer registration data on which the maps in this Atlas are based come from the files of the England and Wales National Cancer Registry at the Office of Population Censuses and Surveys (OPCS). Cancer registration began in England and Wales in the 1920s, and since 1945 there has been a national registry, located initially at the Radium Commission, but since 1947 at the General Register Office, which subsequently became OPCS. Complete national coverage by registration was achieved in 1962. Cancers are registered by regional registries; in the 1950s there were 75 of these, but subsequently they have been amalgamated into 12. These registries collect data on cancers in residents of their region, and send a standard data set to OPCS, who conduct some validation and checks for duplicates and then amalgamate the data set. The regions covered by each registry are described in Appendix 1. The populations and numbers of cancers from each county included in this atlas are shown in Appendix 2.

Cancer registration in England and Wales is voluntary. Many different sources are used by the registries in an attempt to gain complete ascertainment of cancers. From OPCS each registry receives information from all death certificates in England and Wales on which cancer is mentioned. Other sources (for instance, pathology records, and hospital in-patient records) vary between regions. Completeness of registration has varied between registries and over time: in the best registries it has probably been over 95 per cent, but nationally for the period covered here it has probably been around 90 per cent.

Further details on data collection and validity can be found in Swerdlow (1986) and OPCS (1990), which also give references to publications from the national system since the 1950s. For certain of the regional registries, further background information and data quality measures are published in Cancer Incidence in Five Continents (Muir *et al.* 1987).

The childhood leukaemia data come from a different source from the other maps in the volume — the Childhood Cancer Research Group (CCRG) in Oxford. The Group hold data on childhood cancer deaths in England and Wales since 1953, and incident cancers in children since 1962. They receive data from the OPCS National Cancer Registry, and from all death certificates with cancer mentioned in persons under age 20, but also from several other sources, including specialist childhood cancer registries in some regions of the country, clinical trials, and paediatric oncologists. As a result, the Group's register is particularly complete and accurate.

Populations

For analyses of cancers other than childhood leukaemia, risks were estimated by odds ratios, and population denominators were not used (see statistical methods). For childhood leukaemia analyses, incidence rates were calculated, based on annual age- and sex-specific population estimates by county district calculated by OPCS for 1971 onwards, and extrapolated annual estimates calculated by the CCRG for 1966–70.

5

Methods

Coding and definitions

Site of cancers

Cancer site was coded in the national registration files to the Eighth Revision of the International Classification of Diseases (ICD8) (WHO 1967) for 1968–78 data, and to ICD9 (WHO 1978) for 1979–85. To give consistent categories for analysis throughout the period, we bridge-coded the data as shown in Table 1. In general, this bridge-coding gave three-digit ICD9 categories, but for male genital cancers, for which we particularly wanted to examine scrotal cancer separately from penile cancer, we deliberately analysed four-digit ICD9 categories.

Certain sites were grouped in analysis for a different reason: because they have particular potential for diagnostic or coding confusion or overlap. For this reason we grouped together, for instance, brain with other nervous system cancers, all non-Hodgkin's lymphomas, and all leukaemias regardless of histological subtype.

Date of incidence of cancer, and age at incidence

The date of 'incidence' of cancer is generally taken by the England and Wales cancer registration system as the date of first treatment, but for those not treated it is the date of first hospital admission or, failing that, first out-patient attendance, and, for those diagnosed only at post-mortem, the date of death. The age of patients in the analyses is their age at cancer incidence.

Geography

Place of usual residence of patients at incidence[1] of cancer was coded in the national registration files to various administrative and health service geographical units, whose boundaries and basis have changed periodically. The chosen unit of subdivision of England and Wales for this Atlas was the county, for several reasons. Counties have the advantage that they generally provide the stability of reasonably large numbers of cases over the study period, even for relatively uncommon cancers.[2] They are generally of fairly similar geographical size (although this has the associated disadvantage of considerable variation in population size and hence disparity in precision of risk estimation between the geographical units). Unlike several other areal units, it was possible to obtain data for the entire study period which was coded to, or could be recoded to, county level. Counties also have the merit that in aggregation they form other commonly used geographic subdivisions of England and Wales — 'Standard' regions, and Regional Health Authority/Board regions. The compositions of these regions and their relationships to county boundaries are shown in Appendix 1. Finally, and unlike other areal units available, county boundaries have remained almost unchanged for a long period (indeed for

1 Incidence defined as above. Place of usual residence as stated by the patient — for discussion see Swerdlow (1986).

2 It should be noted, however, that mapping at this scale is neither intended nor suitable for detection of local clusters of small numbers of cases, for instance around a particular industrial site.

Table 1 The cancer sites presented: ICD codes, numbers of cases incident, and numbers of deaths, England and Wales, 1968–85

Site of cancer	ICD8*	ICD9*	No (%) of incident cancers: Males		No (%) of incident cancers: Females		No (%) of cancer deaths: Males		No (%) of cancer deaths: Females	
Lip	140	140	5 628	(0·3)	999	(0·1)	719	(0·1)	162	(0·0)
Tongue	141	141	5 723	(0·4)	4 051	(0·3)	3 865	(0·3)	2 598	(0·2)
Salivary glands	142	142	3 847	(0·2)	3 925	(0·3)	1 588	(0·1)	1 183	(0·1)
Mouth	143–5	143–5	7 774	(0·5)	4 561	(0·3)	3 803	(0·3)	2 181	(0·2)
Gum	143	143	1 496	(0·1)	1 224	(0·1)	694	(0·1)	554	(0·1)
Floor of mouth	144	144	3 156	(0·2)	1 109	(0·1)	1 442	(0·1)	559	(0·1)
Mouth, other	145	145	3 122	(0·2)	2 228	(0·1)	1 667	(0·1)	1 068	(0·1)
Pharynx	146; 148	146; 148	7 686	(0·5)	5 339	(0·3)	4 962	(0·4)	3 756	(0·4)
Oropharynx	146	146	3 991	(0·2)	1 786	(0·1)	2 281	(0·2)	923	(0·1)
Hypopharynx	148	148	3 695	(0·2)	3 553	(0·2)	2 681	(0·2)	2 833	(0·3)
Tongue, mouth, and pharynx	141; 143–6; 148–9	141; 143–6; 148–9	22 613	(1·4)	14 908	(1·0)	13 857	(1·2)	9 278	(0·9)
Nasopharynx	147	147	2 102	(0·1)	1 168	(0·1)	1 579	(0·1)	847	(0·1)
Oesophagus	150	150	36 045	(2·2)	28 716	(1·8)	36 342	(3·0)	27 640	(2·6)
Stomach	151	151	126 226	(7·8)	86 291	(5·5)	121 341	(10·1)	86 530	(8·3)
Colon and rectum	153·0–153·8; 154	153; 154	189 514	(11·7)	208 393	(13·4)	135 875	(11·3)	158 118	(15·2)
Colon	153·0–153·8	153	103 279	(6·4)	136 888	(8·8)	77 929	(6·5)	108 083	(10·4)
Rectum	154	154	86 235	(5·3)	71 505	(4·6)	57 946	(4·8)	50 035	(4·8)
Liver	155; 197·8	155	9 139	(0·6)	6 043	(0·4)	10 925	(0·9)	7 756	(0·7)
Gallbladder	156	156	8 096	(0·5)	12 898	(0·8)	7 076	(0·6)	11 907	(1·1)
Pancreas	157	157	49 675	(3·1)	45 402	(2·9)	51 963	(4·3)	48 024	(4·6)
Nasal cavities	160	160	4 215	(0·3)	3 245	(0·2)	2 355	(0·2)	1 861	(0·2)
Larynx	161	161	24 731	(1·5)	5 043	(0·3)	11 082	(0·9)	2 787	(0·3)
Lung	162	162	471 433	(29·1)	133 581	(8·6)	467 452	(38·9)	130 409	(12·5)
Pleura	163·0	163	4 266	(0·3)	1 345	(0·1)	3 144	(0·3)	873	(0·1)
Bone	170	170	4 493	(0·3)	3 653	(0·2)	4 170	(0·3)	3 272	(0·3)
Soft tissue	171·0; 171·2–171·9; 192·4; 192·5	171	7 507	(0·5)	7 356	(0·5)	3 525	(0·3)	3 267	(0·3)
Skin (melanoma)	172·0–172·4; 172·6–172·9	172	10 376	(0·6)	20 135	(1·3)	5 875	(0·5)	7 416	(0·7)
Skin (non-melanoma)	173·0–173·4; 173·6–173·9	173	178 968	(11·0)	157 661	(10·1)	4 037	(0·3)	3 683	(0·4)
Breast (female)	174	174	—		369 254	(23·7)	—		212 307	(20·4)

Site of cancer	ICD8*	ICD9*	No (%) of incident cancers: Males		Females		No (%) of cancer deaths: Males		Females	
Breast (male)	174	175	3 110	(0·2)	—		1 471	(0·1)	—	
Cervix uteri	180	180	—		71 890	(4·6)	—		38 610	(3·7)
Placenta	181	181	—		352	(0·0)	—		111	(0·0)
Corpus uteri	182	179; 182	—		67 432	(4·3)	—		27 418	(2·6)
Uterus, unspecified	182·9	179	—		6 614	(0·4)	—		6 859	(0·7)
Body of uterus	182·0	182	—		60 818	(3·9)	—		20 559	(2·0)
Ovary	183	183	—		75 833	(4·9)	—		65 916	(6·3)
Vulva and vagina	184	184	—		17 859	(1·1)	—		9 662	(0·9)
Prostate	185	185	133 840	(8·3)	—		85 781	(7·1)	—	
Testis	186	186	13 717	(0·8)	—		3 894	(0·3)	—	
Penis	187	187·1–187·6; 187·8; 187·9	4 613	(0·2)	—		1 699	(0·1)	—	
Scrotum	172·5; 173·5	187·7	997	(0·1)	—		209	(0·0)	—	
Bladder	188	188	105 963	(6·5)	38 961	(2·5)	52 162	(4·3)	22 591	(2·2)
Kidney	189	189	28 841	(1·8)	17 391	(1·1)	19 661	(1·6)	12 280	(1·2)
Eye	190	190	3 031	(0·2)	2 937	(0·2)	1 341	(0·1)	1 503	(0·1)
Nervous system	191; 192·0–192·3; 192·9	191; 192	27 609	(1·7)	21 460	(1·4)	22 500	(1·9)	16 588	(1·6)
Brain	191	191	25 064	(1·5)	18 530	(1·2)	21 253	(1·8)	15 552	(1·5)
Nervous system, other	192·0–192·3; 192·9	192	2 545	(0·2)	2 930	(0·2)	1 247	(0·1)	1 036	(0·1)
Thyroid	193	193	3 441	(0·2)	9 585	(0·6)	1 968	(0·2)	5 005	(0·5)
Hodgkin's disease	201	201	14 314	(0·9)	9 408	(0·6)	7 384	(0·8)	4 841	(0·5)
Non-Hodgkin's lymphoma	200; 202	200; 202	29 769	(1·7)	26 049	(1·7)	19 576	(1·6)	17 125	(1·6)
Lymphosarcoma, etc	200	200	13 882	(0·9)	12 027	(0·8)	9 345	(0·8)	8 039	(0·8)
Lymphoma, other	202	202	15 887	(1·0)	14 022	(0·9)	10 231	(0·9)	9 086	(0·9)
Multiple myeloma	203	203	15 258	(0·9)	15 293	(1·0)	12 551	(1·0)	12 924	(1·2)
Leukaemia	204–207	204–208	37 134	(2·3)	30 647	(2·0)	31 632	(2·6)	26 979	(2·6)
Lymphoid leukaemia	204	204	16 559	(1·0)	12 022	(0·8)	11 821	(1·0)	8 463	(0·8)
Myeloid leukaemia	205	205	15 489	(1·0)	14 190	(0·9)	15 798	(1·3)	14 980	(1·4)
Monocytic leukaemia	206	206	1 230	(0·1)	1 063	(0·1)	1 082	(0·1)	932	(0·1)
Leukaemia, other	207	207; 208	3 856	(0·2)	3 372	(0·2)	2 931	(0·2)	2 604	(0·2)
All primary malignant neoplasms	140–195; 199–207	140–195; 199–208	1 620 732	(100·0)	1 559 664	(100·0)	1 198 134	(100·0)	1 038 577	(100·0)

* ICD8 for 1968–78, and ICD9 for 1979–85

several hundred years). This enables comparisons to be made between the present maps and previous cancer maps, for instance those of Stocks for 1921–30, and also enables comparison of the present cancer distributions with geographical data reflecting past exposures — for instance, census-based data on past socio-economic conditions, and disease-specific mortality data from many years ago. This is important because the aetiology of most cancers is a long process, with causal events often taking place many decades before the cancer becomes apparent. The long history of counties is also associated with a cultural identity, and hence probably with a degree of common behaviour within them (for instance, in dietary customs), not likely to be seen for administrative areas of recent definition.

Map E1 shows the physical geography of England and Wales in relation to the county boundaries, and Map E2 shows population density in 1971 by county.

In the OPCS files, the data for 1968–81 were coded to county, but those for 1982–5 were not, and therefore we recoded them. Local authority of residence had been coded for these years, and we aggregated registrations for appropriate local authorities to re-create data by county. For 28 of the 403 local authorities (county districts), the authority boundary crossed county boundaries. In these instances we obtained data on the 1971 Census population of the local authority according to county (these are not available for the 1981 Census), and allocated the authority to the county in which the majority of its population lay. In all but 21 (5 per cent) of the local authorities, over 90 per cent of the authority population were in one county. For this reason, and also because the allocation procedure was only needed for four of the eighteen years of data, the misclassification of determination of counties for the maps will have been negligible.[1]

As well as mapping data by county, we conducted analyses of risk in relation to degree of urbanization, and also of geographical risks within urbanization strata, for 1968–81 — the years for which data by degree of urbanization were available (see Appendix 3). The basis for categorizing urbanization, like that for counties, was essentially the same as that used by Stocks and in the Registrar General's publications over the last 50 years. The local government authorities within England and Wales had long been categorized as rural districts, urban districts, metropolitan boroughs, county boroughs, and London boroughs. In the analyses, rural districts constituted the 'rural' stratum, urban districts and metropolitan boroughs the 'urban' stratum, and county boroughs and London boroughs the 'metropolitan' stratum. The basis of demarcating each local authority district are laid down in the Local Government Acts. The allocation of each town and village within this scheme has been published by the General Register Office (1965*a*).

In general there are numerous local authority districts in the rural and urban strata of each county, but often the metropolitan stratum is composed of only one or two county districts within a county,[2] for which risk is effectively given when the county metropolitan risk is cited. The metropolitan districts within each county are therefore listed in Appendix 1.

Persons with variables unknown

A small number of registrations (less than 0·03 per cent) were excluded from the present analyses because their county of residence was unknown or not known in sufficient detail to code at county level.

1 The slight misclassification should anyway not have led to bias, because the geographical aggregation was on the same basis for the cases as for the controls in the odds-ratio calculations for cancers other than childhood leukaemia (see Statistical methods), and on the same basis for the numerators as for the denominators used to calculate childhood leukaemia rates.

2 Or in most of Wales, there are no metropolitan areas.

The extent to which cancer site is deemed 'not known' in the present data set depends on the way in which 'not known' is defined. For instance, tumours may be of completely unknown primary site, or the general area of the body involved may be known but not the specific organ, or the functional system of the body affected may be known but not the part of this system. As some indication of the extent of the problem, we note that 1·9 per cent of tumours in males, and 2·1 per cent in females in the study period were coded to unknown primary sites (i.e. ICD9 195 and 199) and a similar number of tumours were coded to stated secondary sites of malignancy (ICD9 196–8).

The national registry does not accept registrations from the regional registries until sex and year of birth, and hence age, are known. Therefore there were no registrations with these variables unknown in the files used for the present analyses.

Statistical

The maps in this volume[1] show the relative risk of cancer in each county of England and Wales compared with all other counties, as estimated by means of age-adjusted odds ratios. Cancer incidence rates were not calculated because there was some degree of incompleteness of cancer registration in England and Wales during the study period,[2] varying in degree between areas, and hence calculation of incidence rates would have been biased, i.e. rates would have tended to appear lower in counties with poorer registration. Odds ratios were calculated in preference to cancer incidence rates because, unlike the incidence rates, they are not dependent on equal completeness of registration of cancers overall in the different counties: unequal completeness between counties will only affect the odds ratio to the extent that the incompleteness varies in degree for different tumours. We have used odds ratios in preference to proportional incidence ratios (PIRs) for reasons discussed elsewhere (Miettinen and Wang 1981).

The odds ratios were obtained by considering the registration data as a series of case-control analyses, comparing risk of the cancer under analysis in a particular county with the risk of the same cancer in all other counties. The cases in the analysis were the registrations on the file for the cancer under study, and the controls were a weighted sample of the registrations of all other cancer sites. The weightings used for each control site were chosen to ensure that in each five-year age group, no single site contributed more than 7 per cent to the control data. This was done so that the controls were not dominated by a few common tumours; such domination would tend to have the effect that in counties in which risks of these few cancers were raised, odds ratios for all other sites would tend to be low, since in each county the total of all cancers must be 100 per cent. Details of this method, and of the similar methodology used for calculation of odds ratios in relation to degree of urbanization, are given in Appendix 3.

The odds ratios were age-adjusted using five-year age-groups, by the method of Mantel and Haenszel (1959). Test-based 95 per cent confidence intervals were calculated (Miettinen 1976) and are presented in tables at the end of this volume. Odds ratios whose confidence interval did not include 1·00 were deemed 'statistically significant' (at the 5 per cent level). In the text, non-significant risk is abbreviated as 'NS'.

It should be emphasized, however, that statistical significance is not synonymous with importance. Particularly in the present volume, where very large numbers of registrations have been analysed, slightly raised or decreased relative risks can be

1 Except those for childhood leukaemia — see p. 14.

2 Probably about 10% nationally.

statistically significant, while being of little aetiological or public health importance. The larger the population of the county and the more common the cancer, the more that this occurs; it is therefore especially notable for London, Lancashire, and the West Riding of Yorkshire, and for cancers of the lung in males and breast in females. Conversely, a pattern of much raised relative risks of a less-common cancer in several contiguous counties in a less-populated part of the country may be of importance even if not all of the odds ratios are statistically significant. The magnitude of odds ratios, their statistical significance (and confidence intervals), and the pattern of risks in adjacent counties, all need to be considered to form a balanced assessment.[1] Similarly, when assessing the risk in a particular county, the stability of the risk estimate should be considered: the smaller the population and the rarer the tumour, the wider will tend to be the confidence limits for the odds ratio and hence there can be less confidence that the underlying 'true' risk is close to the observed risk.

We have not presented statistical tests of the significance of the pattern of distribution of risks across different counties, because the appropriate test will depend on the question posed by the reader — for instance, whether the interest is in comparing risk in a particular region with that in other regions, or in deciding whether a particular aggregate of contiguous counties constitutes a high-risk area, or in determining whether a north–south gradient of risk exists. Tests of hétero-geneity of risks by county could be applied universally, but would not be very helpful since this is not usually the main question of interest.

Age-adjustment gives a summary measure across all ages at the possible expense of missing different effects at different ages. Therefore we also mapped risks for specific age groups, age-adjusted in five-year bands within these groups, where there was reason from the previous literature to believe that a tumour may have different epidemiology (and aetiology) at different ages.

For childhood leukaemia we adopted a different analytical method because the data received from the Childhood Cancer Research Group are believed to be 99 per cent complete (Stiller *et al.* 1991). It was therefore appropriate to calculate rates rather than odds ratios for these data, and we did so using population denominators produced for each county by aggregation of local authority populations, with leukaemia data likewise aggregated. These rates were used to calculate age-standardized incidence ratios (SIRs) using the overall age-specific rates for England and Wales as the standard (Breslow and Day 1987). The SIRs are presented as ratios rather than percentages, to facilitate comparison with the odds ratios in the other maps.

Mapping

For display of the data, the odds ratios for each site were divided into seven intervals of equal size on a logarithmic scale between the highest and lowest values found for the site, after excluding zero values and obvious outliers. The ratio of the upper limit of a category to the lower limit is therefore the same for each category. This method of division, unlike divisions based on fixed-percentage cut-offs, ensures that each map displays the full spread of actual results for the tumour involved[2]. Each category was then represented by a colour ranging from red for the

1 An alternative presentation, which we chose not to use, is to calculate Empirical Bayes estimates of risk. These estimates combine information on magnitude and significance in a single summary measure, but do so by 'shrinking' the point estimate of risk. We preferred to display the actual point estimates and their significance separately.

2 It should be noted, however, that the cut-offs are specific to each particular map, and this should be taken into account when making comparisons between maps.

highest-risk group, through yellow for the middle category, to green for the lowest.[1] The zero values in the maps were coloured white since there are effectively no risk data for them. The non-zero outliers, while not used in subdividing the mapping categories, are included in the key and coloured as indicated in it. They are detailed in the tables in Appendix 5. Statistically significant odds ratios (at $p < 0{\cdot}05$) are indicated in the maps by the symbol '*' plotted just below the county name.

Computing hardware and software, and printing

The analyses for this Atlas were conducted on an IBM PS/2 model 70 computer with a hard disk of 120 megabytes, and with data storage in cartridges using a Bernoulli box. The statistical procedures were carried out in SAS (SAS Institute 1988). The maps were drawn using the 'Mapics' computer package developed by Campbell and Nicholson (1989). The maps were drawn on a Hewlett Packard 7550A graphics plotter. A3-sized separate black-and-white images were produced for each of the seven colour categories, with a further black-and-white image for the boundaries and text, and another for the key and significance stars. The maps were then printed in four colours.

1 This seems a natural ordering to us now, but it is of interest to note that to Haviland, preparing the first cancer map in Victorian times, the opposite use of colours appears to have been more natural — in his map red areas represented the lowest rates and blue the highest.

6

Possible explanations of differences in cancer risk between counties

It is both a merit and a difficulty of maps that they are readily assimilable. Atlases are easy to understand, but it is also easy to jump to false or oversimplified conclusions without noticing the caveats which otherwise would be read in a non-pictorial presentation. Not all of the variations in cancer risk apparent in the present maps necessarily reflect real differences in incidence; there are many potential artefacts which might be responsible. The different potential explanations of geographical patterns are discussed in general terms here, since it is not practical to comment on them all separately in the discussion of each map.

Chance

All data on disease occurrence include an element of random variation, and thus chance is always a possible explanation of differences in apparent risks. 'Statistically significant' differences are less likely than others to be due to chance, but it is still possible that they may be. For instance, although a particular relative risk found to be significant at $p < 0{\cdot}05$ is unlikely to be due to chance, nevertheless a result reaching this level of significance is *to be expected* on the basis of chance alone in 5 per cent of values examined. The extremely large numbers of cancers in the present analyses, however, ensure that in general the confidence intervals around the risk estimates are narrow, i.e. the 'true' relative risks are likely to be close to the risks shown in the maps. Nevertheless, risks in small counties, particularly for less-common tumours (i.e. based on small numbers), require a cautious interpretation, and account should be taken of the patterns of risk as well as the individual findings.

Medical care use and diagnostic artefacts

Before a cancer can be registered, the patient with cancer must present to medical care, and the cancer must be diagnosed. Both of these stages can give rise to artefacts in the geographical distribution of registered cases. Thus, apparently low risks of cancer may occur in areas where individuals with a tumour tend not to present to medical care. Obviously, when a tumour is fatal the patient will be seen by a doctor (although the cancer will not necessarily be diagnosed) at death if not earlier. Therefore artefacts of medical care tend to occur particularly for those cancers which are least-often fatal, notably non-melanoma skin cancers.

Once the patient has presented to a doctor, the likelihood that cancer will be diagnosed depends upon the site of cancer, the intensity of investigation, the diagnostic practices and availability of diagnostic technology, and the diagnostic acumen of, and categorization used by, the clinicians and pathologists concerned. In fatal cases it will also be influenced by the extent of use of post-mortem investigations. Variation in any of these factors between areas could cause artefactual differences in apparent risks.

Completeness and accuracy of registration

For diagnosed cancers, geographical artefacts can still occur if cancer registration is incomplete or inadvertently duplicated. It is to avoid the effects of under-registration and duplicate registration as far as possible, that odds ratios rather than rates were calculated for this Atlas. Odds ratios will not be affected by incompleteness — or duplication — unless it is of substantially different magnitude for different tumours (see p. 13).

Accuracy of registration will also affect apparent risks, and is a particular problem if different regional cancer registries identify the site or histology of a cancer with different degrees of precision. For instance, if one registry records the specific histology of leukaemia cases, while another more often records simply 'leukaemia unspecified', then risks of specified cell types of leukaemia (e.g. monocytic) will tend to appear greater in the better-specified registry area. It is to counteract this tendency that in the analysis we combined groups such as 'all leukaemias' (see p. 9). Lack of specificity of diagnostic labelling may nevertheless have had an effect in certain of the maps where it could not be counteracted so easily. For instance, in an appreciable number of cases, melanomas of unspecified site (which are coded to the three-digit ICD code for cutaneous melanoma) on further enquiry transpire to be eye melanomas (Swerdlow 1989). Thus registries which ascertain diligently the site of melanomas will tend to have higher recorded risks of eye cancer than registries which do not gain this detail.

In order to give an indication of the extent of ill-specification of cancer site, Table 2 shows the proportion of all uterine cancers in each county for which corpus/cervix was not stated. This specificity was poorest in several counties in north-west England (Lancashire, Cumberland, and Westmorland), in Wales, and in the Isle of Wight. However, nowhere did it exceed 15 per cent. Swerdlow (1989) shows sites for which, judging from mortality data, ill-specification is likely to affect apparent risks of cancer at three-digit ICD level. We do not have information on other data quality indicators by county; sources of such information by registration region are referenced on p. 7.

Late registrations

Cancer registration may occur many years after the incidence of a cancer, for instance because a cancer notified to a registry from a death certificate may lead the registry to information about an ante-mortem diagnosis of which they were previously unaware. The extent of 'late' registration of cancer varies considerably by cancer site and also by region of registration (Swerdlow 1986). Almost all registrations are received by five years after the incidence date, however, and late registrations should therefore be a negligible problem for the present Atlas, in which registrations beyond 1985 were not included (deliberately, in order to avoid this problem — see p. 5).

Site coding

After cancers have been registered, the site of malignancy must be coded. Differences in coding practice could affect apparent geographical distribution of specific cancers. Coding of cancer site in the England and Wales registration system was at one time undertaken centrally by the Office of Population Censuses and Surveys from paper registration records submitted by the regional registries, and therefore should not have led to geographical artefacts. Over the years it has been devolved to the regional cancer registries, as they have started to submit data on magnetic media. Table 3 shows the year at which each registry took over its own

Table 2 Percentage of all incident uterine cancers (ICD9: 179, 180, 182) coded as 'part unspecified' (ICD9: 179), by county of residence, England and Wales, 1968–85

County	% uterine cancers unspecified	County	% uterine cancers unspecified
Bedfordshire	2·70	Shropshire	4·14
Berkshire	1·38	Somerset	1·77
Buckinghamshire	0·73	Staffordshire	4·03
Cambridgeshire	3·51	Suffolk (East)	1·17
Cheshire	6·74	Suffolk (West)	3·82
Cornwall	3·64	Surrey	0·70
Cumberland	15·04	Sussex (East)	0·29
Derbyshire	3·27	Sussex (West)	0·71
Devon	4·55	Warwickshire	4·94
Dorset	6·22	Westmorland	8·10
Durham	4·17	Wight (Isle of)	8·51
Essex	4·62	Wiltshire	4·38
Gloucestershire	0·98	Worcestershire	5·26
Hampshire	4·46	Yorks. (East)	6·37
Herefordshire	3·45	Yorks. (North)	6·64
Hertfordshire	2·33	Yorks. (West)	6·14
Huntingdonshire	2·65	Anglesey	5·13
Kent	0·50	Breconshire	13·77
Lancashire	9·22	Caernarvonshire	9·76
Leicestershire	3·65	Cardiganshire	11·47
Lincolnshire (Holland)	5·48	Carmarthenshire	12·53
Lincolnshire (Kesteven)	2·85	Denbighshire	9·35
Lincolnshire (Lindsey)	6·11	Flintshire	8·15
London (Greater)	2·22	Glamorgan	11·30
Norfolk	1·91	Merionethshire	12·26
Northamptonshire	0·93	Monmouthshire	10·03
Northumberland	4·32	Montgomeryshire	11·03
Nottinghamshire	1·54	Pembrokeshire	13·43
Oxfordshire	1·14	Radnorshire	10·26
Rutland	3·28		

coding. For data coded regionally, differences in risk between regions might be due to differences in usage of specific codes, and in miscoding. One would expect such artefacts to affect all counties in a registry region,[1] and to affect similarly males and females.

Coding of second cancers

Particular potential for coding artefacts occurs from differences between registries in coding of multiple cancers occurring in the same person. The England and Wales registry files do not differentiate between first and subsequent cancers in an individual, and all cancers are included in the maps in this Atlas. It is not easy to discriminate between multiple primary cancers, recurrences of the same cancer, and duplicate registrations, and registries may differ in their policies, definitions, and methods for so doing, with consequences for apparent cancer risks. Artefacts may occur particularly for registration of multiple tumours at the same site, and of

1 Or bureau area in regions where, for parts of the study period, sub-regional bureaux coded the data — see Appendix 1.

Table 3 Year of first magnetic tape submission of data to OPCS by regional registries

Registry	First data year of tape submission
Newcastle/Northern	1969
Leeds/Yorkshire	1975
Sheffield/Trent	1979
East Anglia	1981
NW Metropolitan/Thames*	1985
NE Metropolitan/Thames*	1985
South Metropolitan/Thames*	1969‡
Wessex†	1983
Oxford	1985
South-western	1981‡
Wales	1980
Birmingham/West Midlands	1971
Manchester/North-western	1970¶
Liverpool/Mersey	1970

* Amalgamated to form the Thames registry, 1985
† The registry was started in 1973; the region was previously covered by the South Metropolitan registry
‡ Only part of data for the year submitted on tape
¶ Some data for registrations previous to this were submitted on punch cards
Table modified from Swerdlow (1986)

tumours occurring in opposite paired organs (breast, testis, etc.) which could potentially be recorded as one or as two tumours. A source of artefact specifically in registrations from the Mersey registry during the period covered by this Atlas, is that this registry coded cancers of mixed histology (i.e. two histologies present) as two registrations, whereas the other registries in England and Wales coded them as one. The only malignancy this is likely to have affected appreciably is testicular cancer (see p. 62).

Coding of place of residence

For most of the population, place of residence is not an ambiguous variable, but for certain groups, notably students, members of the armed forces, and prisoners, this is not the case. Thus in Oxfordshire and Cambridgeshire, an appreciable proportion of young people are students, for whom tumours might be treated and registered locally or in their home (parental) town. In a denominator-based analysis, this might bias rates seriously if cancer registration and the Census defined 'place of residence' differently, but it should not result in bias in analyses based on odds ratios (since the same definition of residence should apply to both the cases and controls), except to the extent that place of first treatment is greatly influenced by site of tumour.

Migration

The maps presented here are based on place of residence at 'incidence' of cancer (usually at first treatment, see p. 9). The geographical distribution would therefore be affected if there were selective migration, for instance to nursing homes or retirement areas, of persons already ill but not yet treated for cancer. This seems unlikely to be an appreciable effect in the present data. Later migration to be close to the place of treatment should not affect geographical registration rates, however, unless the new residence were mistaken by the cancer registry for the place of residence at incidence. It should be noted that migration *within* the geographical units used in this Atlas (i.e. counties) anyway will be irrelevant to the risks.

Migration unrelated to disease, for instance an influx of a particular ethnic group into a county, might explain geographical differences in risk, but for aetiological rather than artefactual reasons. That is, the immigrant group resident in the area may actually have high or low risk of a particular tumour. We have therefore shown in Tables A4.9–4.10 and Maps E6 and E7 the distribution of migrant groups by county. It will be noted that, even in the county with the highest proportion, immigrants constitute a small proportion of the population, and therefore they are only relevant to cancer risks where their relative risk of a tumour is very high.

Aetiology

Finally, to the extent that none of the above artefactual explanations hold, geographical variation in registration risks may be due to differences between areas in factors aetiological for, or preventive of, cancer: differences in environment, or in behaviour of the individuals who live there (for instance in occupation, or smoking, or diet), or screening programmes, or in genetic and ethnic composition. We have therefore published here various maps and tables of some factors which may be relevant to aetiology or prevention of cancer, and have given references to where the geographical distribution of others can be found. There are many more such factors — for which we could not present geographical data — which could explain differences in cancer risk and need to be considered. It should be noted, however, that the exposures found to cause cancer have largely been behavioural or environmental exposures which can be altered, not immutable features of geography to which the population is inevitably exposed. Therefore to the extent that the patterns of cancer are not due to chance or artefact, they are likely to be, in principle, preventable. For some (for instance, lung cancer and pleural cancer), the major preventive measures required are already clearly known (to decrease smoking and asbestos exposure respectively). For others, such as testicular and prostatic cancers, the measures are not known: it is the major aim and interest of cancer epidemiology to try to identify them.

7

Geographical distribution of 'exposures' which may cause or prevent cancer

The main way in which mapping of cancer distribution can rise above the purely descriptive is to consider how the distribution of a particular tumour relates to that of putative aetiological exposures, just as Snow in the nineteenth century (see p. 3) considered how the distribution of cholera related to the pattern of supply of polluted and of unpolluted drinking water. Such comparisons can prove useful in two different ways. On the one hand, close geographical similarity between the distribution of a cancer and that of an exposure may add to evidence for aetiology. On the other, particularly high or low values in the cancer distribution not 'explained' by the distribution of known major risk factor(s) may point to a risk worth more detailed investigation. Thus, for instance, the atlas of cancer mortality in the United States, published several years ago (Mason *et al.* 1975), led to several field studies in high risk areas (Blot and Fraumeni 1982), including studies in coastal Georgia and Tidewater, Virginia, which demonstrated the effect of wartime shipyard employment on lung cancer risk in these areas, and to a study of nasal cancer in North Carolina which was the first in the US to show a raised risk of these tumours from furniture-making.

It should be noted, however, that comparisons at a population level between the distribution of cancer and of 'exposures' must be interpreted with caution. Such correlations do not necessarily indicate an association at the level of individuals (since different individuals might have the exposure and the disease), and this weakens them as evidence about aetiology.

Anyway there are many reasons why the geographical patterns of particular exposures might not correlate with that of the cancers (for instance, because the attributable risk is low, or the years for which exposure data are available are not optimal). Nevertheless, when preparing the maps, we have often been curious about how the cancer patterns relate to those of known or suspected aetiological factors, and we think that readers may also be intrigued by this.

A large number of factors are known or suspected to be causative or preventive of cancer (Tomatis *et al.* 1990). This chapter lists, in alphabetical order of the exposures, sources of data on geographical distribution of some of them in England and Wales. Often the data are for proxies or indirect measures of exposure, since direct data on exposure are not available. Similarly, the calendar years of data presented reflect availability of data, and often are not as early as would be ideal for considering aetiology.

The range of exposures presented cannot be comprehensive. We are aware, however, that much of the interest in cancer maps is in their relation to exposure distributions, and that these are not easy to ascertain, particularly for non-British readers. On the principle that half a loaf is better than no bread, we therefore include some 'exposure' data here. We have provided maps for a few of the factors, as space permits, and tables for others.

ABO blood group

The distribution of ABO (and rhesus) blood groups in the United Kingdom, based on data from the National Blood Transfusion Service, is given in Kopeć (1970). Data are not available by conventional administrative geographical areas such as counties or standard regions, but by the areas covered by the transfusion service. There is a general trend for the proportion of the population with blood group O to decrease and the proportion with group A to increase from west to east and from north to south of England and Wales.

Abortions (Table A4.1)

The number of legally induced abortions performed in each county is available since April 1968 when abortion became legal. We used data for the years 1968–73 (OPCS 1970–74) to calculate crude abortion rates for women aged 10–49, and the results are shown in Table A4.1. There was a north–south gradient with high rates mainly in the south-east of England; London and Cambridgeshire showed the highest values.

Age at first birth (Map E3)

Using data specially tabulated from the 1971 Census, we calculated the mean age at first birth for married women aged 50–54 years in 1971. We had to restrict the age group analysed because of the large clerical effort required to calculate age at first birth. The data were solely for children born within marriage, because the Census only collected information relating to legitimate births. No data were available for Huntingdonshire, Hertfordshire, and Kent because of an OPCS computer fault. Age at first birth tended to be highest in the south-east and the north-west of England, although there were also a few counties elsewhere with high values.

Agricultural work

See occupation.

Air pollution (Table A4.2)

Data on air pollution are available by standard regions. They are based on daily measurements made at about 700–800 sites, mainly in urban areas, intended to give systematic data on air pollution throughout the country (Department of the Environment 1978). Smoke concentrations were high in the North-west, North, and Yorkshire and Humberside regions, whereas sulphur dioxide concentrations were greatest in Greater London, the North-west, and Yorkshire and Humberside regions (Central Statistical Office 1972).

Alcohol consumption (Tables A4.3, A4.4)

Alcohol consumption data by region are available, but only for recent years, from the General Household Survey (OPCS 1980). Table A4.3 shows data for the earliest year published, 1978, based on 19 500 persons. A detailed survey of drinking by adults in England and Wales was conducted in the same year by Wilson (1980), and data from that survey of almost 2000 adults are also shown in the table.

Data on alcohol consumption by region are also available from a 1982 survey of a national 1946 birth cohort (Braddon *et al.* 1988) (not shown in Table). The information was collected from 2000 individuals by the use of a seven-day dietary diary in the 36-year follow-up of this cohort. Alcohol intake was high in the north and south-east of England for men and in the south-east for women. Regional data on expenditure on alcohol, by household, at earlier dates can be found in the Household Expenditure Enquiry (Ministry of Labour and National Service 1957).

Data on alcohol intake are not available at county level. As an indirect indicator, we calculated the number of liquor-licensed premises ('on-' plus 'off'-licences) per 1000 inhabitants in 1968 (Table A4.4), which are provided by county (Home Office 1969). Values were high in the Isle of Wight and in most Welsh counties, in particular Radnorshire, Breconshire, and Pembrokeshire.

Another marker of alcohol consumption is the frequency of cirrhosis: 1968–78 mortality rates are mapped by county in England, but by only two subdivisions of Wales, in Gardner *et al.* (1984).

Asbestos (occupational exposure)

There are no direct measures available of the extent of asbestos exposure by county. However, we obtained unpublished data from the Health and Safety Executive's Asbestos Survey, on factories at which medical examinations have been made because of asbestos exposure. It is believed that no fixed locations involving substantial current exposure have been missed by the Survey. The data that we received, however, are for examinations since the Survey started in 1971, and therefore necessarily omit factories closed before then. The Survey does not record the date at which factories opened, but does record the earliest date of exposure for any current worker at the factory. To gain information as far as possible on the extent of past exposures, we therefore identified the factories in each county at which any workers had pre-1951 exposures. We then tabulated the number of such factories in each county, and also the numbers of examinations[1] made in such factories divided by the size of population of the county.

The counties with the largest numbers of asbestos factories are Lancashire (24/22)[2], London (15/13), Yorkshire West Riding (15/12), Cheshire (11/10), Durham (11/9), Glamorgan (10/7), Hertfordshire (10/2), Warwickshire (9/7), Essex (8/7), Staffordshire (8/6), Gloucestershire (8/6), and Nottinghamshire (8/5). Counties with no such factories are Lincolnshire Holland, Rutland, Westmorland, the Isle of Wight, Cardiganshire, Carmarthenshire, Montgomeryshire, and Radnorshire. In addition, in Herefordshire, Huntingdonshire, Shropshire, East Sussex, Anglesey, Breconshire, Denbighshire, and Pembrokeshire there are no factories with any pre-1951 exposed workers. Highest concentrations of asbestos-examined factory workers as a rate per general population, are in Caernarvonshire, Merionethshire, Breconshire, Cambridgeshire, Cheshire, Lancashire, Gloucestershire, Derbyshire, and Durham. Highest concentrations of workers in factories with any pre-1951 exposed workers were in Caernarvonshire, Gloucestershire, Cheshire, Merionethshire, Lancashire, Derbyshire, Cambridgeshire, Yorkshire East Riding, Durham, and Northumberland.

Diet (Tables A4.5, A4.6)

Representative information on diet across the country is available, but only at regional level, from the National Food Survey since 1955 (MAFF 1957). Table A4.5 shows data on the average consumption 1970–75 per person of different foods, from the 1975 annual report (MAFF 1977). An earlier survey (Rowett Research Institute 1955) collected detailed dietary information using a one-week dietary diary from a sample of families with children in six areas in England (Barrow-in-Furness,

1 For each factory, the largest number of examinations made in a single year since 1971.

2 Figures in brackets are the current number of factories, and the number of current factories with any pre-1951 exposed workers.

Liverpool, Yorkshire West Riding, Wisbech (in the Isle of Ely), Fulham, and Bethnal Green) and none in Wales, during 1937–9. A survey in 1949 presented regional data (MAFF 1956), but it was limited to urban working-class households.

More detailed information on regional differences in nutrient intakes, but based on smaller numbers, is available from follow-up of a cohort formed from a national sample of 1946 births (Braddon *et al.* 1988). A seven-day dietary diary (assisted by an interviewer) was used to collect dietary information in the 36-year follow-up of this group; some of the results are shown in Table A4.6. Men in the south-east of England had lowest mean intakes of energy, protein, fat, and carbohydrate, whereas women in this region had the highest intakes of fibre, calcium, and vitamin C. For a number of nutrients, intakes were particularly low in women who lived in the north of England.

Education (Table A4.11)

Various statistics on education by county have been published in Statistics of Education (Department of Education and Science 1969). Table A4.11 shows data for 1968 relating to pupils remaining at school beyond the compulsory minimum school-leaving age. At that time compulsory school attendance ended before age 16.[1]

Within England, continuation of education beyond the minimum was greatest in central southern England and the south-east, but not East Anglia or the south-west, and was generally low in the north of the country. The greatest levels of continuing education, however, were in Wales, particularly those counties furthest from the border with England.

Ethnic groups

See immigrants.

Fallout from nuclear explosions

Fallout radiation from atmospheric nuclear weapon tests was estimated in Great Britain in 1977 by measuring the deposits of caesium (^{137}Cs) and plutonium ($^{239+240}$Pu and ^{238}Pu) in soils from 58 grassland and woodland locations in the country (Cawse and Horrill 1986). There was a general trend for the radionuclide concentrations in the soil to increase from east to west and from south to north, being proportional to the average annual rainfall (see Rainfall, p. 31). These concentrations did not represent more than 1 per cent of the generalized derived limits proposed by the National Radiological Protection Board (NRPB) (Haywood and Simmonds 1983). The doses in 1977, however, were very low compared with those around 15 years earlier (greatest doses were in the late 1950s and early 1960s (Hughes *et al.* 1989)).

Gamma radiation

See indoor radiation.

Geochemistry

Description of the geochemistry of England and Wales, based on 50 000 stream sediment samples taken in 1969, can be found in great geographical detail in an atlas by

1 Attendance was compulsory to the following Easter if the child reached age 15 during 2 September to 1 February, and to the end of the summer term in the same year if he/she became 15 years old during 2 February to 1 September.

Webb *et al.* (1978). The maps, which are by 6·5 km^2 squares rather than counties or other administrative areas, show the distribution of 21 elements, including arsenic, chromium, cobalt, copper, nickel, strontium, and zinc, and four combinations of elements. Many of the maps show a broadly similar pattern, with greatest levels of, for instance, aluminium, arsenic, cobalt, gallium, iron, lithium, and vanadium in the westernmost counties of Wales, the Lake District, and Cornwall and Devon, and for some but not all of these elements high levels in an area around Northamptonshire and Huntingdonshire.

Height, weight, and obesity (Table A4.7, Maps E4, E5)

Data on adult height and Body Mass Index, but only at a regional level, are available from the first representative survey carried out among the adult (ages 16–64) population of Great Britain, by Knight (1984). Men in the South-west region, East Anglia, and the South-east except Greater London, and women in South-west, South-east, and East Midlands regions were taller than people in the rest of England and Wales (Table A4.7). Body Mass Index (weight/height^2), a measure of obesity adjusted for height, was greatest in Wales, East Anglia, and the East Midlands for men and in the South-west, East Midlands, and East Anglia for women (Table A4.7).

Some information on adult height at a county level was collected as part of studies of 1958 and 1970 national birth cohorts (Davie *et al.* 1972; Butler *et al.* 1982). These investigations collected information on height not only of the children in the cohorts but also of their parents. The British Perinatal Mortality Survey (Davie *et al.* 1972) studied a national birth cohort that included practically all children born during one week in 1958, and collected information on mother's height measured at antenatal examination and father's height when the child was aged eleven. The British Births Survey (Butler *et al.* 1982) followed up 97·5 per cent of all children born in Britain during one week in 1970. At examination of the (surviving) children at age 10, the parents' heights were reported. We combined the data on parents in both surveys to map average adult height by county of England and Wales (Maps E4, E5). Heights were generally greatest south of a line from the Severn to the Wash, but there were also some high values in the east Midlands, north and mid-Wales, and the Lake District.

Hepatitis B (Table A4.8)

Unpublished data on laboratory reports of acute hepatitis B were obtained from the Communicable Disease Surveillance Centre (CDSC). Table A4.8 shows the distribution by hospital region of reporting, for the years 1980–84 (data are not available for previous years). There were high crude rates in North-west Thames, South-western, East Anglia and Yorkshire regions, but it should be noted that these rates are influenced by completeness of reporting to CDSC by different centres, as well as underlying incidence and detection.

Immigrants/ethnic groups (Tables A4.9, A4.10/Maps E6, E7)

Using data on country of birth from the 1971 Census (OPCS, unpublished), we calculated the proportion of residents in each county who were born outside the United Kingdom and the Republic of Ireland. In Tables A4.9 and A4.10, results are shown for different countries of birth, grouped as explained in the footnote.

Census data are not available by ethnic group, but Haskey (1991) has estimated the size of populations of different ethnic groups by 'new county' (see Appendix 1) of England and Wales, using data from the 1981 Labour Force Survey in conjunction with 1981 Census data. The Labour Force Survey is an annual sample survey of approximately 150 000 residents in private households, which includes questions on both country of birth and ethnic group (asking for the group to which the respondent felt that he/she belongs). The method used by Haskey probably underestimated ethnic minority populations to some extent where they formed a high proportion of the overall population, and overestimated them where the proportion was low (J. Haskey, personal communication). Maps E6 and E7 show this estimated distribution in 1981 for the two largest groups, those from the Indian subcontinent and the West Indies. The other groups for which data were available were Africans, Chinese, and Arabs. Counties with the greatest proportions of Africans were London (0·65 per cent), Leicestershire (0·16 per cent), and Greater Manchester (0·16 per cent). Greatest proportions of Chinese were in London (0·36 per cent), the West Midlands (0·34 per cent), and Lincolnshire (0·28 per cent), and of Arabs in London (0·27 per cent), South Glamorgan (0·19 per cent), and Oxfordshire (0·13 per cent).

Income (Table A4.11)

Data from '*The Survey of Personal Incomes 1970–71*' (Board of Inland Revenue 1973) (one of the earliest tax years when the data were based on county of residence rather than county of business) were used to calculate the mean total net income per tax-paying unit (husbands and wives may pay tax together as a 'unit') in each county of England and Wales. It should be noted that the data available relate to income after allowable deductions, relate to tax-paying units rather than individuals, do not include income from non-taxable sources, and omit entirely those households whose income falls below the tax base. The results are shown in Table A4.11. Highest values were concentrated in the south-eastern counties, but Surrey had a surprisingly low value.

Indoor radiation (Map E8)

Data on natural radiation exposure in United Kingdom dwellings are available from national and regional sample surveys conducted during 1981–5 (Wrixon *et al.* 1988). The distribution of mean indoor radon concentration (Bq m^{-3}) by county (only available for the post-1974 reorganization county boundaries, see Appendix 1) is shown in Map E8. Data for gamma-ray dose rates (nGy h^{-1}) can be found in that publication. The highest concentrations of radon were in south-western counties (Somerset, Cornwall, and Devon). Gamma-ray dose rates showed a north–south and east–west gradient, with high concentrations in northern and Welsh counties. (While this Atlas was in press, more extensive radon data for England, based on measurements up to the end of 1991, were published from the same source as the above (Green *et al.* 1992). These data broadly confirm the pattern shown in Map E8, except that the value for Somerset based on this larger data set is somewhat lower — between those for Devon and Northamptonshire.)

Industry

See occupation.

Medical conditions (Tables A4.12, A4.13)

Data on hospital discharges for certain conditions of interest in relation to cancer risk were obtained from the Hospital In-Patient Enquiry, which collected information on a 10 per cent sample of discharges and deaths of National Health Service patients from NHS non-psychiatric hospitals in England and Wales (DHSS and

OPCS 1972). The diagnostic groups and degree of geographical detail for which data are available have varied over the years. Most of the data were published by hospital region, but in 1959 and 1960, for some medical conditions, tables by county were published (Ministry of Health and General Register Office 1963*a*,*b*). Tables A4.12 and A4.13 show the geographical variation in hospital discharges for selected conditions.

Maps of mortality from various non-malignant conditions which may affect risk of cancer can be found in Gardner *et al.* (1984) and OPCS (1981), for deaths 1968–78 and 1969–73 respectively. Earlier geographical mortality data can be found in the Registrar General's Decennial Supplements (e.g. GRO 1958, 1967).

Nuclear installations (Map E9)

Map E9, based on Cook-Mozaffari *et al.* (1987), shows the location of nuclear establishments in the United Kingdom. The years of first criticality/time of first waste release and of shut-down for each establishment are given in that publication. The first to release waste were Amersham (1946), Harwell (1947), Springfields (1948), Windscale (1950), Aldermaston (1952), Capenhurst (1953), and Calder Hall (1956). At all of the sites shown except Wylfa (1971), Hartlepool (1981), and Heysham 1 (1983), waste release began before the period of cancer incidence covered by this Atlas.

Obesity

See Height, weight, and obesity.

Occupation and industry (Tables A4.14–A4.16)

The numbers of people employed in certain occupations and industries whose activities might be associated with increases in cancer risk were extracted from the 1961 Census (GRO 1965*b*, 1966). The proportions of males and of females aged 15 and over in these occupations and industries were calculated by county, and the results are shown in Tables A4.14–A4.16. Data on the geographical distributions of occupations and industries at earlier dates can be found in previous censuses and in Langton and Morris (1986).

Operated conditions (Tables A4.17, A4.18)

Geographical differences in the rates of surgical interventions for particular conditions might be of interest as markers of the frequency of operated diseases which affect cancer risk, or because removal of an organ may itself affect risk of cancer. For example, circumcision affects risk of penile cancer, and orchidopexy relates to the frequency of undescended testis and also its correction, both of which, it has been postulated, may affect testicular cancer risk. An operation can also sometimes affect the risk of cancer in distant organs. For instance, breast cancer risk is decreased by oophorectomy, probably because of the hormonal changes brought about by this operation.

The Hospital In-patient Enquiry (HIPE) collected information on a 10 per cent sample of discharges and deaths from hospitals in England and Wales. The data collected related to spells in hospital rather than individuals (there was no linkage between successive admissions of an individual), and therefore are most useful for the present purpose for operations which it is rare or impossible to repeat on an individual. Table A4.17 shows from HIPE (Ministry of Health and General Register Office 1967; Department of Health and Social Security and OPCS 1970) estimated numbers of selected operations per 100 000 population by regional health authority for 1960–1 (circumcision) and 1967 (other operations). The data years for circumcision and orchidopexy are the earliest available.

Murphy *et al.* (1987) compiled data from HIPE to estimate age-standardized hysterectomy ratios 1967–83 by hospital region of England and Wales (Table A4.18). Hysterectomy ratios were highest in Oxford, Wessex, and Yorkshire and lowest in West Midlands and Mersey regions. These ratios do not include private operations, but Murphy *et al.* (1987) showed that, at least for 1981, the inclusion of private operations did not greatly change the overall pattern.

Overcrowded dwellings (Table A4.19)

The percentage of dwellings overcrowded in each county was determined in a national survey in 1936 (Ministry of Health 1936). The overcrowding standard applied was that defined in the Housing Act of 1935. It was somewhat complex, depending on the number and sex of inhabitants and number and size of rooms of the dwelling. Results are shown in Table A4.19. Overcrowding was greatest in northern counties (Durham and Northumberland) and north Wales (Anglesey, Caernarvonshire, and Denbighshire).

Data on household occupancy are also collected at the decennial national population Censuses of England and Wales. Persons per room in 1951 and 1961 (GRO 1954–5, 1965*c*) were greatest in Durham, Northumberland, and London, but not particularly high in north Wales (Table A4.19).

Parity (Map E10)

Data on children born within marriage were collected at the 1971 Census of England and Wales for women aged under 60, but parity data were not published by county. Using data specially tabulated from the 1971 Census, we mapped by county the average parity of women aged 35–59. Since Census information on parity was only collected for married women, we have assumed that single women were nulliparous. There was little variation across the country: highest values were in northern counties (Durham, North Yorkshire, and Lincolnshire Lindsey) and lowest in the south (London and East Sussex). Due to an OPCS computer fault, no data were available for Huntingdonshire, Hertfordshire, and Kent.

Population mobility (Map E11)

Data on the numbers of people by age in each county who had migrated from elsewhere in Great Britain[1] in the year preceding the 1971 Census (OPCS, unpublished) were used to calculate the proportion of each county population (both sexes combined) aged 1–14 who were immigrants (Map E11). There was a north–south gradient with high rates in the south of the country, but London had a low rate.

Post-neonatal mortality (Map E12)

Data on geographical variation in post-neonatal mortality (deaths between ages four weeks and one year) are given in the Registrar General's Annual Statistical Reviews of England and Wales. This mortality rate is widely regarded as a good marker of social conditions (Pharoah and Morris 1979). Map E12 shows the distribution for 1950 (General Register Office 1952), but the pattern has remained fairly constant over the years: there was a clear north–south and east–west gradient, with high rates in the northern and Welsh counties.

1 Data were not available by county and age for persons who had migrated from abroad in the previous year.

Rainfall (Table A4.20)

Data on rainfall are available from the Monthly Weather Reports (Meteorological Office 1956–65). We calculated the average annual total rainfall at meteorological stations in each county of England and Wales for the years 1955–64 and the results are shown in Table A4.20. (These years were selected because they represent the period when fallout radiation was highest in the country; see Fallout from nuclear explosions, p. 26.) Highest levels of rainfall in 1955–64 were in the western part of the country, particularly in Westmorland and mid-Wales.

Screening (Table A4.21)

There are only two cancers presented in this volume for which there was appreciable screening activity in England and Wales during the study period — breast and cervix (J. Chamberlain, personal communication).

For breast cancer, there was substantial screening during the study period only in Guildford (Surrey), where population-based screening was conducted from 1979 onwards.

Cervical screening programmes began in 1964, but data at a regional level are only available from 1967 onwards. The screening programmes were population-based before 1986 in West Sussex, Bristol (Gloucestershire), Cardiff (Glamorgan) and in the North-west region. Murphy *et al.* (1987) analysed data on cervical smears performed in 1967–84 in each region of England and Wales, and results are shown in Table A4.21. Cervical smear rates were highest in North-western, North-west Thames, and South-west Thames regions, and lowest in Mersey and Northern regions. It should be noted, however, that these rates are based on numbers of smears, not numbers of women with any examination in the period, and are for all ages, including those at which smears are likely to be relatively unproductive. They are for region of screening rather than region of residence (but related to residential region population denominators); this is likely to have had little effect on rates except between Manchester and Liverpool regions, and between the Metropolitan regions (Murphy *et al.* 1987).

Smoking (cigarettes) (Table A4.22)

Smoking data by region, but not by finer geographical divisions, are available for 1984 and 1986 (but not earlier) from the General Household Survey (OPCS 1986, 1989). We have pooled the data for 1984 and 1986 at ages 50 years and above in Table A4.22, to estimate the smoking behaviour most nearly relevant to the 1968–85 cancer maps (although data for much earlier years would of course be preferable). The highest cigarette consumptions were in the North, and Yorkshire and Humberside regions, and Wales for males, and in the North, Yorkshire and Humberside, and North-west regions for females. Regional data on expenditure on tobacco by household, but not individual expenditure or consumption, at earlier dates are given in the Household Expenditure Enquiry (Ministry of Labour and National Service 1957).

Social class (Table A4.11)

Data on the social class distribution of economically active males by county are available from the 1971 Census (OPCS 1975). Social class was determined from occupation by the Registrar General's classification (OPCS 1970). We calculated the percentage of men in social classes I, II, and III(N) (generally non-manual occupations) in each county (Table A4.11). There was a north–south gradient: men of the upper classes tended to concentrate in the south of the country. At first sight surprisingly, there were also some high percentages in Welsh counties (particularly Cardiganshire, Montgomeryshire, and Radnorshire). However, farmers and farm managers (but not agricultural labourers working as employees), are coded as social class II, and these counties have high proportions of farmers.

There are many other measures or proxies which might be used to map socio-economic conditions. Each of those examined has some disadvantages. Apart from social class, others for which data are presented here are education (p. 26), income (p. 28), post-neonatal mortality (p. 30), and overcrowding of dwellings (p. 30). Maps by county can be found in Coates and Rawstron (1971) for further measures; for instance, the percentage of children receiving free (means-tested) school lunches, and the extent of private schooling. Maps of several other measures at the 1971 Census — for instance, one-person households, and unemployment — can be found in Clarke *et al.* (1980), but with display of the data by kilometre squares, not counties or other administrative geographical units.

Sunshine (Map E13)

Data on bright sunshine were available from the Monthly Weather Reports (Meteorological Office 1954, 1959, 1964, 1969, 1974). The daily mean hours of bright sunshine by county in selected years during 1953–73 were calculated and are shown in Map E13. County values were calculated as the arithmetic average of the values registered throughout the year in all of the meteorological stations located in each county (no measurements were taken in Montgomeryshire during the period). There was a north–south gradient, with highest values in southern counties, East Anglia, Lincolnshire, and some coastal Welsh counties.

Venereal diseases (Table A4.23)

Geographical data on incidence of venereal diseases are not available, but Table A4.23 shows data on new attendances at venereal disease clinics by region of attendance. These statistics are for gonorrhoea and syphilis (primary and secondary) attendances in 1963, using information obtained from the Department of Health (unpublished). There was a strong correlation between the geographical distributions of the two diseases, and for each disease between the two sexes. In each sex, the four highest crude attendance rates (per 100 000 population) for gonorrhoea were in North-west Metropolitan, Liverpool, North-east Metropolitan, and Manchester regions. Crude syphilis rates were highest in North-west Metropolitan, South-west Metropolitan and Liverpool regions, in each sex.

Geographical mortality data for syphilis in 1959–63 (GRO 1967), which may reflect incidence considerably earlier, showed a fairly similar pattern, with greatest rates in certain Metropolitan regions, Newcastle, Manchester, and Liverpool regions (Table A4.23).

Welsh language speaking (Table A4.24)

Welsh-speaking may correlate with other cultural behaviours. The extent of Welsh-speaking has been ascertained in Wales at the decennial Censuses of population (OPCS 1973*a*), and data on the proportions by county in 1971 are given in Table A4.24.

8

Distribution of cancer incidence in England and Wales

The maps are presented and discussed here in the order in which the cancer sites appear in the International Classification of Diseases (ICD) (WHO 1978). The text gives a brief description of the major patterns of incidence in the published maps, and also of the patterns in the maps by urbanization and age, which could not be published because of space constraints. Also outlined are the main known risk factors for the tumours, and the extent to which these factors can be related to the cancer patterns observed. A detailed discussion of risk factors for each cancer is beyond the scope of this Atlas. Such information can be found in great detail in Schottenfeld and Fraumeni (1982, but a new edition is in press), and more briefly in Doll and Peto (1981) and Tomatis *et al.* (1990). Extensive references on cancer aetiology can be found in these volumes, and therefore we have not attempted full referencing of aetiological issues here. We have concentrated instead on references to raised risks found in specific geographical locations in England and Wales, certain recent publications on causation, and references on likely attributable risks in England and Wales.

Tables giving the numbers of cancer cases and odds ratios underlying the maps, and confidence intervals for the odds ratios, are presented in Appendix 5.

Lip cancer (Maps 1 and 2)

This ICD site comprises tumours of the vermilion border of the lip, but not of the internal surface of the lip, or of the (hair-bearing) external skin beyond the vermilion border (a potential source of misclassification error in registration). The great majority of the tumours are on the lower rather than the upper lip. Survival is good, so that a mortality map would be a relatively poor indicator of incidence patterns. Incidence rates of this tumour have been decreasing greatly for men in the country in recent years, but less for women.

The known causes of this cancer are sun exposure and tobacco use: characteristically it occurs in elderly male farmers and fishermen. Greatest risks in England and Wales are in these occupations and in building workers (Swerdlow *et al.*, unpublished). Correspondingly, relative risks of lip cancer in men in England and Wales (Map 1) were twice as great in rural as in urban and metropolitan areas. The geographical distribution of this cancer in men was as striking as for any site examined in this Atlas: risks in each county in East Anglia were two-and-a-half- to threefold those in the country overall, and there were also high risks in the westernmost counties of Wales. Highest risks (all significant) were in Anglesey (odds ratio 3·12), Huntingdonshire (3·09), Norfolk (3·08), and Pembrokeshire (3·03). There were particularly low risks in the Midlands and north of England, especially the north-west.

This distribution was not simply due to the greater proportion of rural residents in East Anglia and Wales than in many other areas. Within rural populations, there were still twofold raised risks in East Anglia, south Lincolnshire, and parts of Wales, and generally low risks in the Midlands and north-west and much of the north. Highest risks were in Pembrokeshire (2·38), West Suffolk (2·38), Huntingdonshire (2·32), Lincolnshire Holland (2·24), and Norfolk (2·24) (all significant). In males in urban areas, highest risks were in Rutland (3·38, NS), Anglesey (3·14, significant), East Suffolk (2·99, significant), and Pembrokeshire (2·87, significant). In metropolitan areas, which do not exist in most of Wales, greatest risks were in Norfolk (2·73), East Suffolk (2·62), and Berkshire (2·22) (all significant).

Lip cancer is far less common in women than men (Table 1). For women (Map 2) the urban–rural gradient in risk was less than that for men, but in the same direction. The county distribution was also similar to that for men but less consistent. Some parts of East Anglia, but not all, had high risks, and there were also high risks in some counties in central southern England, as well as in the westernmost parts of Wales, where risks were two- to threefold those in the country overall. Highest odds ratios were in Montgomeryshire (3·79), Norfolk (2·79), Cardiganshire (2·68), and Wiltshire (2·52) (all significant).

Rural females again had high risks in counties in East Anglia, and in south-west Wales, but also in several other areas. Greatest were in Lincolnshire Kesteven (3·61, significant), Wiltshire (2·98, significant), Cardiganshire (2·36, NS), and Kent (2·33, significant). In urban areas, greatest risks were in Norfolk (2·76, significant), Pembrokeshire (2·63, NS), Carmarthenshire (2·60, significant), and Cambridgeshire (2·50, significant). Greatest metropolitan risks were in Berkshire (3·39), Oxfordshire (3·11), Somerset (2·63), and Essex (2·55) (all significant).

The cluster of high-risk areas in East Anglia might suggest an artefact of coding by the regional cancer registry, but this seems unlikely since the registry adopts a particularly conservative and careful policy with regard to coding this site, and excluding tumours of the skin of lip from this heading (M. Page, personal communication).

The association of lip cancer with sun exposure might lead one to expect a north–south gradient in risk, but this was not clearly present. Compare, for instance, the distribution of hours of sun in Map E13, and also that of melanoma in Maps 39 and 40 . This fits with geographical data from elsewhere that lip cancer does not simply follow levels of solar UV radiation or proximity to the equator: internationally, the highest recorded rates of lip cancer are in parts of Canada and rural Romania, as well as in parts of Australia (Muir *et al.* 1987). In analyses within countries, there were not consistently higher rates closer to the equator in Scandinavia (Jensen *et al.* 1988), whites in the US (Mason *et al.* 1975), or in Scotland, where rates were greatest in the north (Kemp *et al.* 1985).

The reasons for the high risks of lip cancer in East Anglia and western Wales, particularly compared with other rural areas, are not clear. The highest-risk counties are among those with high proportions of farmers[1] in the population (see Tables A4.14, A4.15), but there are also some farming counties (for instance, Westmorland and Radnorshire) where lip cancer risk was low. Climatic differences between these counties may be relevant. The excess does not appear to have been noted previously, and would merit local investigation.

Cancer of the salivary glands (Maps 3 and 4)

These uncommon tumours occur mainly in the parotid glands. Their aetiology is largely unknown. Radiation is a risk factor, and there have been some indications that salivary stones are also.

1 Fishermen are less relevant, since they constitute less than three per cent of the population in each county (see Table A4.14).

In each sex, in England and Wales, there was a slight gradient of higher risk in rural than urban than metropolitan areas. The counties with the highest risk coincided, to an extraordinary extent, between the sexes — in males and in females the highest risk was in Radnorshire (males 2·88, females 2·73 (both significant)) and the next highest risk was in Oxfordshire (males 2·00, females 2·21 (both significant)). The next-ranking risks were again similar between males and females, although not in identical order. In males, the next-highest significant risks were in Northumberland (1·58), Norfolk (1·54), Worcestershire (1·52), Berkshire (1·50), Durham (1·45), and West Sussex (1·41), with non-significant high risks in Breconshire (1·86), Merionethshire (1·67), Montgomeryshire (1·49), and Flintshire (1·33). In females, the next-highest risks were in Norfolk (1·93), Northumberland (1·79), Durham (1·70), Worcestershire (1·57), West Suffolk (1·56), Berkshire (1·35), and West Sussex (1·34) (all significant).

In metropolitan areas, greatest risks in males were in Worcestershire (2·19), Oxfordshire (2·15), and Essex (1·91) (all significant), and in females in Oxfordshire (2·27), Norfolk (2·16), and Northumberland (2·11) (all significant). In urban areas, highest risks for males were in Radnorshire (3·18, significant), Breconshire (2·58, NS, based on four cases), and Northumberland (2·03, significant), and for females in Radnorshire (3·21), Oxfordshire (2·38), and Durham (2·07) (all significant). In rural areas greatest risks in males were in Oxfordshire (1·92), Worcestershire (1·81), and Norfolk (1·80) (all significant) and in females in Radnorshire (2·49, NS, based on two cases), Norfolk (2·08, significant), and Northumberland (2·03, significant).

The geographical similarity in high risks of this tumour between the sexes, in widely separated counties, is striking. If it does not indicate a diagnostic or registration artefact (which seem possible particularly for borderline malignant tumours (Muir 1987), and would be expected to affect both sexes similarly), it would appear to be worth further investigation. Weighing against a registration artefact explanation is the fact that the high-risk counties came from many different registry regions, and involved only a few of the counties within each region. Data on the geographical distribution of salivary gland stones in England and Wales are not available. Data are published on salivary gland operations (Table A4.17), which are mainly (80 per cent) for non-malignant conditions, with salivary gland calculi accounting for about a quarter (Ministry of Health and General Register Office 1967). These statistics are available only by region, at which level there is no obvious correspondence with salivary gland cancer distribution, but the pattern found for salivary gland cancer was very much a county pattern rather than regional.

Cancers of the tongue, mouth, and pharynx (Maps 5–8)

These tumours are often considered together in epidemiological studies.[1] They are not individually common, and therefore in many studies there are insufficient cases for separate investigation. Moreover, it is sometimes difficult to decide the exact site of origin of these cancers.

Incidence rates in England and Wales are greater in men than women. Risks of these tumours in men in England and Wales are low by European standards, but risks in women are fairly high (Jensen *et al.* 1990; Smans *et al.*, in press). The tumours have well-established associations with alcohol and smoking, with a particularly high risk in individuals who both smoke and drink heavily (Rothman and Keller 1972). Over half of the cancers of these sites in England and Wales may be attributed to these two habits (based on Tomatis *et al.* 1990). Chewing of tobacco

1 The analyses of these sites exclude cancers of the nasopharynx and salivary glands, which we have mapped separately since they have certain clear epidemiological features differentiating them from other oral and pharyngeal malignancies.

increases oral and perhaps pharyngeal cancer risks. There is also some indication of risk from nutritional deficiencies, for instance in the Plummer–Vinson syndrome. Consumption of raw vegetables and fresh fruits appears to be protective. In the Indian subcontinent, where some of the highest rates of these cancers have been recorded, chewing of betel quids, with or (probably) without tobacco, is a risk factor. Rates in Indian migrants to England and Wales are raised (Swerdlow *et al.*, unpublished), and the locations of Indian communities within the country may therefore influence the geography of risk.

We initially mapped tongue, mouth, and pharyngeal cancers separately, then mapped the sites combined. For males, the sites separately showed different patterns of risk, and we therefore show the individual sites in Maps 5–7. For females, patterns of risk were similar between the three sites, and therefore only the distribution for the tongue, mouth, and pharynx overall is shown (Map 8).

Tongue cancer in males (Map 5) showed high incidence in south and mid-Wales, and in the north-east of England, with no clear pattern elsewhere. Highest risks were in Carmarthenshire (1·75, significant), Pembrokeshire (1·41, NS), Cardiganshire (1·39, NS), and Breconshire (1·37, NS). Malignancies of the mouth (Map 6) showed uniformly low risks in southern and eastern Britain as far as Lincolnshire and south Wales, but no cluster of high risks in any particular area north of this. Greatest risks were in Radnorshire (2·23, significant), Durham (1·69, significant), Montgomeryshire (1·67, NS), and Northumberland (1·65, significant). Pharyngeal cancer (Map 7) showed a well-demarcated area of high incidence in mid-Wales, the west Midlands, and north-west of England. Highest risks for this site were in Radnorshire (2·04, significant), Breconshire (1·68, significant), and Herefordshire (1·66, significant). Risks for oral and pharyngeal cancers overall in men (not shown in the maps) were greatest in the north-east of England and mid- and west Wales, with the highest county risks in Radnorshire (1·88, significant), Montgomeryshire (1·54, significant), Herefordshire (1·43, significant), and Durham (1·35, significant). For tongue, oral, and pharyngeal cancers, both separately and overall, there was a gradient of increasing risk with increasing degree of urbanization.

Examining risks of tongue, oral, and pharyngeal cancers overall in males by urbanization stratum: in metropolitan areas greatest risks were in Northumberland (1·40), Durham (1·34), and Lancashire (1·24) (all significant); in urban areas in Radnorshire (1·75, NS), Herefordshire (1·75, significant), and Pembrokeshire (1·63, significant); and in rural areas in Radnorshire (2·67, significant), Montgomeryshire (2·14, significant), and Breconshire (1·63, significant).

In females (Map 8), highest risk of cancers of the tongue, mouth, and pharynx were in Montgomeryshire (1·53, significant), Pembrokeshire (1·28, NS), Radnorshire (1·21, NS), and Glamorgan (1·21, significant). Several of the highest risks were in Wales, but otherwise there was no pattern. Risk was slightly greater in metropolitan and urban than in rural areas. There was no clear pattern in metropolitan, urban and rural areas separately: in metropolitan areas highest risks were in Berkshire (1·30, NS) and Glamorgan (1·24, significant); in urban areas in Montgomeryshire (1·64, NS) and Radnorshire (1·51, NS), and in rural areas in Monmouthshire (1·83, significant), and Merionethshire (1·61, NS).

The areas with high risk of these tumours correspond with the general pattern found in mortality data (OPCS 1981; Gardner *et al.* 1983), although these were not published in quite the present degree of detail. Recent survey data show high levels of smoking and drinking in the northern regions of England and generally fairly high levels in Wales (see pp. 31 and 24). Data for subdivisions of Wales are not available, however, and neither are data for earlier, more appropriate, years. Most of Wales is well supplied with licensed premises (see Table A4.4), and risks of other alcohol- (and poor nutrition-)related tumours were high there (see Maps 11, 12, 17,

18, 25, 26), suggesting that alcohol and diet may be important to the oral and pharyngeal risks. Lung cancer risks, as an indicator of past smoking, were generally low in Wales (see Maps 27–30). Risks of cancers of the tongue, mouth, and pharynx were not especially high in counties where persons of Indian subcontinent-origin congregate (see Tables A4.9, A4.10 and Map E6), but it should be noted that in no county do they form more than a small proportion of the overall population.

Nasopharyngeal cancer (Maps 9 and 10)

This tumour is notable for extreme variations in incidence internationally, with exceptionally high rates in southern China and South-east Asia compared with other countries, and very high risks also in individuals of south Chinese origin who have migrated to other countries. The highest recorded incidence is in Hong Kong (Ho *et al.* 1987), from which there has been appreciable migration to England and Wales. The high risks of nasopharyngeal cancer in certain populations appear to be at least in part environmental — diet and viral infection (Epstein–Barr virus) have been the principal aetiological hypotheses (*Lancet* 1989), but also there appears to be a degree of genetic susceptibility. An association of risk has been shown with a particular HLA antigen, and the existence of a susceptibility gene at the HLA locus has been demonstrated by a linkage study (Easton and Peto 1990). Recent evidence has suggested that eating of salted fish and other fermented foods at a young age may be a causal factor (Yu *et al.* 1988). There may be some relation of risk to smoke and fume exposure.

There has been no previous examination of the geography of this tumour within England and Wales. Maps 9–10 show no consistent pattern. Significant raised risks of nasopharyngeal cancer were present in London in each sex (males 1·72, females 1·31), Lancashire in females (1·32) and Cambridgeshire in males (1·77). Non-significant highest risks in males were in Radnorshire (1·89) and Rutland (1·84) and in females in Rutland (1·88) and the Isle of Wight (1·82), but based on small numbers.

There was a gradient of higher risks in more urbanized areas, stronger in males than in females. The male gradient was, with the exception of scrotal cancer, the largest excess related to urbanization in the tumours analysed in males. Examining risk in urban, rural, and metropolitan areas separately, there was no coherent pattern. In males, greatest risks in metropolitan areas were in Oxfordshire (2·01, significant) and London (1·59, significant), in urban areas in Cambridgeshire (2·53, significant) and West Suffolk (2·05, NS), and in rural areas in Radnorshire (6·27, significant, based on two cases) and Rutland (5·31, significant, two cases). In females, highest risks in metropolitan areas were in Kent (2·20, NS) and Essex (1·90, NS) and highest significant risks in Lancashire (1·31) and London (1·23); in urban areas greatest risks were in Merionethshire (2·25, NS) and East Yorkshire (2·15, NS) and greatest significant risk in Lancashire (1·42); and in rural areas highest risks were in Rutland (4·23, NS) and Huntingdonshire (2·90, NS) and greatest significant risks in Durham (2·51) and Wiltshire (2·21).

The high risks of nasopharyngeal cancer in London and (based on small numbers) Rutland, correspond with counties with high concentrations of Chinese-born inhabitants (see Tables A4.9, A4.10), and London also had the highest proportion of ethnic Chinese in the country[1] (see p. 28). Otherwise the distribution of the cancer does not correspond with that of Chinese-origin inhabitants, but the Chinese-origin population of England and Wales is small.

1 No data were available on ethnic Chinese in Rutland.

Oesophageal cancer (Maps 11 and 12)

The main known aetiological factors for this tumour in Western populations are alcohol and smoking, which when combined increase risk synergistically (Tuyns *et al.* 1977). There is some evidence that spirits are greater risk factors than wine and beer. There appears also to be a relationship to poor diet — perhaps micronutrient deficiencies. Risk is increased in patients with coeliac disease. A notable descriptive feature of oesophageal cancer epidemiology has been the sharp changes in incidence over relatively short distances in certain parts of the world — there are very high rates in central Asia in populations of Turkic origin in China, Iran, and the USSR, and high rates also in the Transkei, and in Brittany and Normandy (Day 1984). National risks in England and Wales are among the highest in Europe for this tumour, particularly in females (Jensen *et al.* 1990; Smans *et al.*, in press).

Within England and Wales risk in males tended to be high in Wales and the north-west of England (Map 11) (although not as strikingly as in females; see below). Greatest risks in men were in Rutland (1·51, significant), Merionethshire (1·42, significant), Westmorland (1·23, NS), and Cheshire (1·21, significant). Risk was particularly low in the Oxford region: the lowest risks in the country were in Northamptonshire (0·66, significant) and Oxfordshire (0·68, significant).

In metropolitan areas, risk in men was greatest in coastal counties of the north of England (greatest in North Yorkshire (1·37, significant)). In urban areas, risks were high in north Wales and the north-west of England, with some high risks also in other areas; greatest risks were in Rutland (1·80, NS), Merionethshire (1·73, significant), and Westmorland (1·55, significant). In rural areas, greatest risks were in Wales and parts of the north of England (highest in Pembrokeshire (1·46, significant), Rutland (1·46, NS), and Herefordshire (1·39, significant).

In females (Map 12), the distribution of oesophageal cancer was very different from that of any other cancer in women in this Atlas: high risks were present almost exclusively in the most western counties of the country, with no north–south gradient. Greatest risks (all significant) were in Merionethshire (1·59), Caernarvonshire (1·59), Montgomeryshire (1·49), and Denbighshire (1·40). Low risks were present in most of the south of England, notably in the Oxford region (lowest risks nationally were in Oxfordshire (0·72, significant) and Northamptonshire (0·74, significant)), but also in Yorkshire and the north-east of England. Greatest risk in metropolitan areas was in Cumberland (1·69, significant); there are no metropolitan areas in most of Wales (see Table A1.1). Urban areas showed a similar pattern to that overall, with greatest risks in Carmarthenshire (1·64, significant), Rutland (1·64, NS), and Caernarvonshire (1·45, significant), while in rural areas high risks were almost restricted to Wales (greatest in Caernarvonshire (2·21, significant) and Westmorland (2·12, significant)). There was no gradient of risks between metropolitan, urban, and rural areas in males or in females.

The distribution of oesophageal cancer in England and Wales in 1968–85 is almost the opposite of that found by Stocks (1936) 50 years ago. At that time risks in males[1] (see Map S1) were high in the south-east of England, and indeed the greatest risk was recorded in Berkshire which now has the third-lowest risk nationally. Our data concur, however, with recent mortality maps, although these have not been published by county (OPCS 1981; Gardner *et al.* 1983). It is of interest that oesophageal cancer risks in Welsh migrants to Australia have been found to be much higher than in English migrants, especially in females (Armstrong *et al.* 1983).

Whether the high risks of oesophageal cancer in west Wales and the north-west of England and the low risks in the Oxford region are explicable by tobacco,

1 Stocks did not publish data for females.

alcohol consumption, and diet is not clear. Geographical data on these variables unfortunately are available only for relatively recent years, and by region (see Chapter 7): tobacco and alcohol consumption have been fairly high in the north-west of England and in Wales. Risks of upper aerodigestive tract tumours also believed to be associated with alcohol, tobacco, and poor diet were high in parts of Wales and north-western England (Maps 5–8), as were laryngeal cancer risks (maps 25–26). Liver (Maps 17–18) and lung (Maps 27–30) cancer distributions were less like the oesophageal cancer pattern. The distribution of high risk of oesophageal cancer in women showed considerable similarity to the distribution of high levels of several elements in geochemical maps of the country (see p. 26). Individual-based studies of oesophageal cancer in the west of Wales may be worthwhile.

Stomach cancer (Maps 13 and 14)

Stomach cancer in England and Wales, as in most Western countries, is one of the main causes of cancer death in each sex, although a diminishing one. Mortality rates at younger ages now are a quarter of those 35 years ago (Doll 1990). Risk is about twice as great in men as in women. The incidence of the tumour internationally and within countries is related to poor socio-economic conditions. Stomach cancer is probably mainly of dietary aetiology, although the causal agents or deficiencies responsible have yet to be ascertained. Suggested factors have included deficiencies of fresh fruit and vegetables, and use of methods of food preservation prevalent before the era of refrigeration (salting, pickling, and smoking). In several studies, raised risk of stomach cancer has been found in persons who have been smokers, but whether this is causal is not clear. An association has also been shown with infection with *Helicobacter pylori* (Forman *et al.* 1991), but again the aetiological importance of this is uncertain. Raised risk is also found in persons with blood group A, and persons exposed to ionizing radiation.

The pattern of risks of stomach cancer was very similar between the sexes in the present data, with greatest risks in north Wales (Maps 13–14). There were also high risks in several other counties of Wales, in Staffordshire, and northern England, and low risks south of a line from the Severn estuary to the Wash. In males, greatest risks were in Caernarvonshire (1·37), Staffordshire (1·37), Merionethshire (1·25), and Anglesey (1·24) (all significant), and in females in Merionethshire (1·49), Caernarvonshire (1·47), Durham (1·44), and Staffordshire (1·36) (all significant). The distribution of stomach cancer was similar at young and at older ages (Swerdlow and dos Santos Silva 1991). Risks increased a little with increasing urbanization. The geographical distribution was very similar in urban, rural, and metropolitan areas considered separately. In males, greatest risk in metropolitan areas was in Staffordshire (1·36), in urban areas in Anglesey (1·42) and Caernarvonshire (1·38), and in rural areas in Denbighshire (1·65) (all significant). In females, greatest metropolitan risks were in Staffordshire (1·41) and Durham (1·35), greatest urban in Merionethshire (1·52) and Caernarvonshire (1·50), and greatest rural in Caernarvonshire (1·82) and Durham (1·77) (all significant). The distribution is little changed from that in 1921–30 described by Stocks (1936) (Map S2), although the relative difference between counties has diminished. Stocks also described the high risk in north Wales in incidence data for 1953–54 and mortality data for 1947–54, and at a smaller area level showed high mortality particularly in the east of Caernarvonshire (Stocks 1957). It is notable that the greatest relative risks in north Wales and the north of England in each sex now are in rural areas, where it might be expected that traditional dietary habits and food preservation methods might have persisted longest. It is also of interest that risks of stomach cancer incidence (McCredie and Coates 1989) and mortality (Armstrong *et al.* 1983) in Welsh migrants to Australia are increased compared with risks in English migrants.

The distribution of high risk of stomach cancer by county in England and Wales in general parallels that of poor social conditions (see p. 31), and, from available data, low consumption of fresh fruit and green vegetables (see p. 25), but these do not specifically explain the high incidence in north Wales. Stocks and Davies (1964) took soil samples in north Wales, Cheshire, and two localities in Devon from houses of stomach cancer cases and of controls, and found high zinc and zinc/copper ratios at houses of cases. The atlas of geochemistry of England and Wales (Webb *et al.* 1978) shows the distributions of zinc and copper in the country to be fairly similar to each other, with some high values in north Wales and Devon, but also in many other areas of the country where stomach cancer risk is not particularly high. Recent papers have suggested that housing overcrowding (Barker *et al.* 1990) or bracken infestation (Galpin *et al.* 1990) might be aetiologically associated with stomach cancer and explain the particularly high risks in north Wales, but these correlate no better with the county distribution of stomach cancer than do socio-economic conditions (Swerdlow and dos Santos Silva 1991). Blood group A is associated with increased risk of stomach cancer in individual-based studies, but the national distribution of blood group A (see p. 24) does not parallel the stomach cancer risks.

Cancers of the colon and rectum (Maps 15 and 16)

These sites represent collectively one of the major causes of cancer death in each sex in England and Wales (Table 1). Recorded incidence rates are rising a little at older ages but declining in younger adults. In contrast to stomach cancer, colorectal cancer is most common in 'developed' populations. Rates in England and Wales are fairly high by European standards (Jensen *et al.* 1990; Smans *et al.*, in press). The aetiology of these tumours is probably dietary — current evidence points to lack of vegetables or fibre and excess of fat (particularly saturated fat) as likely causal factors. There is evidence of increased risk of colon cancer, and less consistently of rectal cancer, in relation to a sedentary life-style (Nomura 1990; Whittemore *et al.* 1990). Ionizing radiation exposure is a minor risk factor. A few cases are due to inflammatory bowel disease, and familial polyposis of the colon. There may be a raised risk from infection with *Schistosoma japonicum*, a parasite endemic in South-east Asia which can cause chronic colitis. There is inconsistent evidence for a relation of cancer of the rectum with high beer consumption, and of cancer of the colon with prior cholecystectomy and (in women) with low parity.

The aetiology of colorectal cancers may vary somewhat by subsite, but they are often considered together in epidemiological studies: the distinction between them is sometimes difficult anatomically (Muir 1987), their aetiological features are probably fairly similar, and there is potential for registration artefact in the separate data (cancers of the large intestine not further specified are coded with rectal cancers in the ICD[1]). The separate maps for colon and rectum prepared from the present data were similar, so we have shown maps for colorectal cancers combined.

The range of risks across England and Wales was particularly low for this tumour in each sex. In males (Map 15) and females (Map 16), high risks were present in an area centering on the west Midlands, and there were also high risks, but not consistent between the sexes, in some other counties. Greatest risks in males were in Montgomeryshire (1·26), Shropshire (1·24), and Worcestershire (1·20) (all significant), and in females in Staffordshire (1·14) and Caernarvonshire (1·14) (both significant). For males there were low risks of colorectal cancer in the area south of a line from the Severn estuary to the Wash, and for females this was often so but with some exceptions, for instance in East Sussex (1·11) and Bedfordshire (1·11) (both significant). There was no urban–rural gradient of risk, and in urban, rural,

1 International Classification of Diseases.

and metropolitan areas examined separately there was no clear deviation from the overall geographical pattern. For males, greatest risks in metropolitan areas were in Worcestershire (1·22) and North Yorkshire (1·20), in urban areas in Merionethshire (1·32) and Shropshire (1·28), and in rural areas in Worcestershire (1·31) (all significant). In females, the greatest metropolitan risk was in Staffordshire (1·17), greatest urban risk in West Suffolk (1·22), and rural in Cumberland (1·20) (again all significant).

Examining rectal and colon cancer geography separately (maps not published), risks south of the Severn–Wash line were more uniformly low for the rectum than for the colon, but otherwise their distributions were similar. Greatest risks of rectal cancer in males were in Shropshire (1·31, significant), Montgomeryshire (1·29, significant) and Staffordshire (1·26, significant) and in females were in Pembrokeshire (1·29, significant), Bedfordshire (1·15, significant) and Herefordshire (1·14, significant). For colon cancer in males, greatest risks were in Merionethshire (1·22), Cumberland (1·18), and Lincolnshire Kesteven (1·17) (all significant) and in females were in Caernarvonshire (1·18), West Suffolk (1·14), and Staffordshire (1·12) (all significant).

The maps produced by Stocks (1936) 50 years ago for England and Wales did not show high risk of intestinal cancer in the west Midlands in females, but for rectal cancer in males[1] there was some indication of high risk in the same counties as in the present maps. Mortality maps by region for recent years show highest risk of rectal but not colon cancers in the west Midlands (OPCS 1981).

There is no obvious reason for the greater risk of colorectal cancer found in the west Midlands than elsewhere, but the geographical differentials in risk of the tumour within England and Wales are modest.

Cancer of the liver (Maps 17 and 18)

This is a tumour with great international variation in incidence, with risks being particularly high in China, south-east Asia, sub-Saharan African, and some other developing countries. In England and Wales, tumours at this site are mainly hepatocellular carcinomas. They occur more often in men than women. The main known aetiological factors for liver cancer are chronic hepatitis B virus infection, and alcohol intake. Also, probably aflatoxin ingestion in developing countries. (Aflatoxins are contaminants of food produced by fungi in warm climates.) More rarely liver cancers may occur in relation to various hereditary metabolic diseases, use of combined oral contraceptives, and probably with the use of anabolic steroids. Hepatic angiosarcomas result from vinyl chloride monomer exposure. Liver cancers have also been caused by thorotrast, a radioactive substance which was at one time injected for diagnostic purposes, but is no longer used. For cholangiocarcinoma, an uncommon histological type in Britain, liver fluke infection in Japan and eastern Asia appears to be aetiological.

British risks of this tumour are low by European standards (Jensen *et al.* 1990). In England and Wales, liver cancer risk is particularly high in immigrants from developing countries (Grulich *et al.*, unpublished).

In the present analyses, liver cancer risks were greatest in Wales in each sex. In males the greatest odds ratios were in Pembrokeshire (1·88), Flintshire (1·66), Denbighshire (1·63), and Caernarvonshire (1·44) (all significant), and in females in Merionethshire (3·08), Pembrokeshire (2·73), Breconshire (1·86), and Flintshire (1·79) (all significant). For females, there were almost no high risks outside Wales, whereas in males there were some elsewhere, notably in London (1·33, significant) where female risks were not particularly high. It was notable that the range of relative risks for females was extremely wide.

1 He did not publish a map for colon cancer or for colorectal cancer in this sex.

Risks were greatest in the most urban areas for males, but did not vary appreciably by urbanization in females. Considering metropolitan, urban, and rural areas separately, highest risks in males in metropolitan areas were in Kent (1·62, NS) and Northumberland (1·47, significant). There are no metropolitan areas in north and mid-Wales (see Table A1.1). In urban males, highest risks were in Denbighshire (1·75, significant), Breconshire (1·73, NS), and Flintshire (1·69, significant), and in rural males in Flintshire (2·43), Caernarvonshire (2·36), and Breconshire (2·06) (all significant). In females in metropolitan areas, greatest risks were in Kent (3·43, significant) and Monmouthshire (1·91, significant); in urban areas in Merionethshire (3·88), Pembrokeshire (3·26), and Carmarthenshire (2·35) (all significant); and in rural areas in Pembrokeshire (3·56, significant), Merionethshire (2·61, significant), and Breconshire (2·05, NS).

The liver is a frequent site of secondary malignancy, and there is therefore a risk that poor-quality data might lead to inflation of apparent liver cancer rates by erroneous inclusion of metastatic tumours. A possible artefactual explanation for the high risks of liver cancer recorded in Wales might be a particular tendency in the Welsh registry for secondary metastases to the liver to be misclassified as primary liver cancers. We cannot be certain whether this occurred, but as an approach to the problem we reanalysed Maps 17 and 18 excluding cases occurring at ages 70 years and above, for whom such misclassification might be expected to occur more often than at younger ages. These analyses showed the same pattern, and about the same magnitude of the highest relative risks, as those in the all-age maps presented. Greatest overall risks for men under age 70 were in the counties of Pembrokeshire (1·98), Flintshire (1·65), and Denbighshire (1·61) (all significant), and in women were in Merionethshire (2·93), Pembrokeshire (2·89), and Breconshire (2·66) (all significant).

Another potential source of artefact in Welsh cancer incidence data is duplication of registrations, which is known to have been a particular problem in Wales compared to the English registries. Such duplication would only be of concern in the present odds ratio calculations, however, if it were greater for liver cancer than for other sites. Although this remains a possibility, there is no obvious reason why it should be so. Finally, it is possible that misclassification of gallbladder cancers as liver cancers might have occurred to a greater extent in Wales than in other areas. This would be consistent with the low risks of gallbladder cancers in Wales in Maps 19 and 20, but we do not know whether it indeed occurred.

The reasons for the apparently high risks of liver cancer in Wales are unclear, and merit further investigation. The only data available on alcohol consumption (see Table A4.3) are more recent than is desirable to assess aetiology, but show Welsh alcohol consumption to be high but not exceptional (and availability of licensed premises in Welsh counties is high; Table A4.4). Acute hepatitis is not reported at high rates in Wales (Table A4.8). It is notable that cirrhosis death rates are greater in metropolitan than urban than rural areas of England and Wales, and have generally been found to be greater in Wales and the North region of England than elsewhere in the country[1] (OPCS 1981; Gardner *et al.* 1984). Also the data for other alcohol-related cancer sites in this Atlas (mouth and pharynx, oesophagus, and larynx) would suggest high alcohol consumption in much of Wales. This offers some support for alcohol consumption being responsible for the liver cancer pattern. On the other hand, favouring registration artefact as an explanation, available mortality data for liver cancer (Gardner *et al.* 1983), which only divide Wales into two areas, do not indicate high risk of mortality in Wales, whereas for other

1 North- plus mid-Wales, and south Wales, in men; only south Wales in women; greater detail of Welsh data was not published. Risks in the north of England have been high, but not entirely consistently, and there were also some raised risks in the Midlands.

sites in this Atlas registration data have generally accorded well with mortality distributions, as far as available.

Cancer of the gallbladder (Maps 19 and 20)

Cancer of the gallbladder (including extrahepatic bile ducts) accounts for under one per cent of cancers in England and Wales (see Table 1). It is more common in women than men. The most important known risk factor is gallstones, but ulcerative colitis and liver flukes (in tropical countries) are also risk factors. The geographical distribution of gallbladder cancer will also be affected by the frequency of cholecystectomy (usually for gallstones) in different areas, since this operation removes the organ at risk.

In the maps for England and Wales there was an excess of gallbladder cancer in each sex in the centre of England, which occurred across three cancer registry regions and was therefore unlikely to be a registration artefact. There was also a smaller excess in the north of England. Both mirror closely the distribution in mortality data (Gardner *et al.* 1983). Greatest risks in males were in Bedfordshire (1·43), Oxfordshire (1·37), and Durham (1·24) (all significant), and in females were in Warwickshire (1·37, significant), Anglesey (1·36, NS), and Staffordshire (1·33, significant).

Risks were similar in metropolitan, urban and rural areas. Examining risks in strata by urbanization, in each sex in urban areas there was some tendency for high risk to occur in counties in the centre of England: greatest risks in males were in Northamptonshire (1·84, significant), Anglesey (1·64, NS) and Buckinghamshire (1·50, significant), and in females in Northamptonshire (1·48), Durham (1·46), and Worcestershire (1·44) (all significant). For rural and metropolitan areas the pattern of distribution was less marked or there was no clear pattern. Highest rural risks for males were in Bedfordshire (1·87, significant), Westmorland (1·63, NS), and Durham (1·49, significant), and for females in Herefordshire (1·84, significant), Staffordshire (1·84, significant), and Anglesey (1·62, NS). In metropolitan areas, greatest male risks were in Kent (1·69, NS) and Oxfordshire (1·43, NS), and greatest female risks in Northamptonshire (1·52), Warwickshire (1·36), and North Yorkshire (1·28) (all significant).

Barker *et al.* (1979) have published data on the prevalence of gallstones at necropsy in nine towns in England and Wales, but these show no obvious relation to the gallbladder cancer risks in the present material. Admissions to hospital for non-malignant gallbladder disease in 1959 (Table A4.12) (the only year for which county data were published), were greatest in counties with generally low gallbladder cancer rates. Data specifically for cholelithiasis and cholecystitis (Table A4.13) and for gallbladder operations (Table A4.17) are available only by region: they show greatest rates in Wales, where gallbladder cancer is uncommon, and low rates in the west Midlands, where gallbladder cancer is most common, but for other regions they show less of an inverse relationship. Mortality data for non-malignant gallbladder disease 1968–78 (ICD8: 574–6) (Gardner *et al.* 1984), showed high risks in several counties in the centre of England and most of the north of England, with a particularly high risk in both sexes in Northamptonshire and the North Riding of Yorkshire. Since gallstones are a risk factor for gallbladder cancer, while cholecystectomy (often for gallstones) reduces the number of persons at risk of the tumour, the relation of the geography of these to gallbladder cancer cannot be understood without more detailed analysis.

Cancer of the pancreas (Maps 21 and 22)

This is one of the major causes of cancer death in England and Wales (see Table 1); it is a tumour which is usually rapidly fatal. Diagnosis of pancreatic cancer is not simple and there is therefore potential for diagnostic artefact, particularly at older ages. Its aetiology is not well understood. Smoking is a cause, but with much lower relative risks than apply to lung cancer; up to 40 per cent of pancreatic cancers in males and 20 per cent in females might be attributed to this cause (Tomatis *et al.* 1990). Ionizing radiation exposure is aetiological, and possibly also diabetes mellitus.

There were several counties with high risk of pancreatic cancer in each sex in the south-east of England but also some in the north, and to a lesser extent elsewhere. Highest risks in males were in East Sussex (1·16, significant), Kent (1·14, significant), and Cardiganshire (1·11, NS) and in females in Rutland (1·27, NS), Berkshire (1·21, significant), and Westmorland (1·14, NS). The small range of risks within the country is notable, particularly given the high potential for diagnostic artefact in this deep-seated abdominal tumour. Risks were very similar in different urbanization strata. There was no obviously different pattern from that overall in the metropolitan, urban, and rural maps considered separately. Metropolitan highest risks in males were in East Sussex (1·24, significant) and Kent (1·19, NS) and in females in Berkshire (1·41, significant) and Monmouthshire (1·20, NS); urban highest risks in males were in Kent (1·23, significant) and Merionethshire (1·21, NS) and in females in Oxfordshire (1·33, significant) and Buckinghamshire (1·23, significant); and rural greatest risks in males were in Cardiganshire (1·43, significant) and Lincolnshire Lindsey (1·28, significant) and in females in Monmouthshire (1·53, significant) and the Isle of Wight (1·51, significant). In mortality maps by region (OPCS 1981), variation in risk was also small, and greatest risks were in the south-east of England for women, but were similarly high in several regions for men. (Pancreatitis mortality rates (Gardner *et al.* 1984) in contrast were generally low in the south-east of England, with high-risk counties mainly in the north of England and the Midlands.)

Cancers of the nose, ear, and nasal sinuses (Maps 23 and 24)

The main malignancies under this heading are cancers of the nose and nasal sinuses. There are very high risks of these in certain well-defined occupational groups, some of which have given rise to risks in specific geographical areas of England and Wales. Risk is much raised in furniture- and cabinet-makers, boot and shoe manufacturers and repairers, possibly workers exposed to other organic dusts such as textiles, nickel refinery workers (with several hundred-fold risks found for workers employed before 1920 at a nickel refinery in south Wales (Kaldor *et al.* 1986)), chromate workers, workers manufacturing isopropyl alcohol by the strong acid process, workers making mustard gas, radium dial painters, and possibly workers in gas manufacture. There may also be a raised risk from smoking and from snuff inhalation. Highest risk of these tumours in males in England and Wales was in Buckinghamshire (1·87, significant), where a very high risk in High Wycombe furniture makers was shown over 30 years ago (Macbeth 1965; Acheson *et al.* 1967). There were also significant raised risks in men in Herefordshire (1·55), Northamptonshire (1·50) (where Acheson *et al.* (1970) showed raised risk in leather workers) and Derbyshire (1·23). Non-significant high risks occurred in Merionethshire (1·47, based on six cases) (which has a particularly high percentage of woodworkers, although not cabinet-makers, in the population (see Table A4.14)) and Breconshire (1·44, seven cases). In females, the only significant risks were in Buckinghamshire (1·39) and Essex (1·33), with greater but not significant risks in Rutland (2·10, three cases) and Lincolnshire Holland (1·55, 12 cases). Apart from these risks, there was no obvious pattern of distribution. There was also no urban/rural gradient in risk for males, and a slight gradient of higher risks in more urban areas for females.

Metropolitan, urban, and rural areas considered separately showed some similarities to the pattern seen for the data overall. For males in metropolitan areas, no risks were significant, and highest risks were in Lincolnshire Lindsey (1·67, NS) and Northamptonshire (1·63, NS). In urban areas, highest male risks were in Lincolnshire Kesteven (2·22, significant), Cardiganshire (2·21, NS), Buckinghamshire (1·91, significant), and Northamptonshire (1·66, significant); and in rural areas in Merionethshire (2·67, significant), Rutland (2·52, NS), and Herefordshire (2·19, significant). For females, there was no obvious pattern of risk in metropolitan or in rural areas; highest risks in metropolitan areas were in Lincolnshire Lindsey (2·36, significant), Leicestershire (1·62, significant), and Essex (1·60, significant). In rural areas, the only significant risk was in Buckinghamshire (1·87), with other substantial risks in Rutland (2·80, NS), Lincolnshire Holland (2·00, NS), and the Isle of Wight (1·96, NS). In urban areas there were no significant raised risks, but there was a cluster of the highest risks in three neighbouring counties in south Wales — Cardiganshire (2·02, NS), Carmarthenshire (1·72, NS), and Breconshire (1·66, NS).

The areas of high risk of nasal cancer shown here seem particularly worth further investigation where their origin is not already known. The very high relative risks which have typified occupational risks of nasal cancer, and the substantial proportion of nasal cancers that appear to be of occupational origin, suggest that additional occupational risk factors for this tumour might be found by geographical analyses (as indeed they have been found in the past). Risk in Herefordshire males was notably high, with few wood- or leather-workers in the county (see Table A4·14). Risk in males in Derbyshire was significantly high, with few wood- or leather-workers, but a large textile industry which might be relevant. The coincidence of highest metropolitan risk in each sex in Lincolnshire Lindsey (i.e. the town of Grimsby — see Table A1.1) is striking, and seems to be worth further investigation. The high-risk counties for females are not obviously explicable by wood- or leather-work. Less than 0·3 per cent of female workers in each county in England and Wales were engaged in woodworking, and leather-work accounted for over 2·0 per cent of the female work-force only in Northamptonshire (8·2 per cent) and Leicestershire (3·0 per cent), where risks of nasal cancer were 0·92 (NS) and 1·25 (NS) respectively.

Laryngeal cancer (Maps 25 and 26)

Cancer of the larynx is far more common in men than women (Table 1). Risks in men in England and Wales are low by European standards, but this is less so for women, particularly in north-west Wales (Jensen *et al.* 1990; Smans *et al.*, in press). The tumour is known to be caused by alcohol and by smoking of tobacco. Several studies have suggested that the joint effect of these two factors is approximately multiplicative. In North American studies it has been found that 80 to 90 per cent of cases may be attributable to these habits (Tomatis *et al.* 1990). More uncommon and less-certain causes may be work in mustard gas manufacture, nickel manufacture, and ethanol production by the strong acid process, and perhaps asbestos exposure.

Risks in males were consistently high in the north of England, and there were also some high risks around London and in Wales. For females, highest risks were in the north of England and much of Wales. Greatest risks in males were in East Yorkshire (1·27, significant), Breconshire (1·25, NS), Pembrokeshire (1·19, NS), and Lancashire (1·19, significant), and in females in Carmarthenshire (1·36, NS), Montgomeryshire (1·32, NS), Lancashire (1·31, significant), and Glamorgan (1·28, significant). In each sex risks were low in the south-west of England.

In each sex there was a gradient of higher risks in more urban areas. In males, risks in metropolitan, urban, and rural areas separately showed a less clear pattern than for the data overall. Highest metropolitan risks were in Lincolnshire Lindsey (1·36, significant) and East Yorkshire (1·30, significant); in urban areas greatest risks were in Pembrokeshire (1·80, significant) and Westmorland (1·54, significant); and in rural areas in Rutland (1·63, NS) and Warwickshire (1·35, significant). In women, the excess risk in the north of England was strongly present for urban and for metropolitan areas, but not for rural areas, for which no clear pattern was seen. Highest risks in metropolitan areas were in Cheshire (1·49, significant) and Lancashire (1·30, significant); in urban areas in Carmarthenshire (1·95, significant), Breconshire (1·79, NS), and Cumberland (1·73, significant); and in rural areas in Radnorshire (2·50, NS) and Denbighshire (2·22, significant).

The distribution in males has changed greatly from that found by Stocks (1937) for 1921–30 (Map S3).[1] At that time, risks in the north of England were low, and risks almost uniformly highest in the south-east. The change in high-risk areas is similar to that seen for lung cancer, which must have been influenced strongly by smoking behaviour (see p. 47).

Since most laryngeal cancers are attributable to smoking and drinking of alcohol, one would expect the distribution in England and Wales to reflect these factors, and also to parallel the distribution of other smoking- and drinking-related tumours. The high risks of laryngeal cancer in the north of England accord with high levels of smoking and drinking (in the available, too recent, data — Tables A4.3, A4.22), and with high risks of lung (Maps 27–30), oropharyngeal (Maps 5–8) and oesophageal (Maps 11–12) cancers, although not generally liver cancer (Maps 17–18). The high laryngeal cancer risks in Wales fit well with the alcohol-related cancer sites, but not with lung cancer as a marker of past smoking. Current smoking and drinking there were high but not exceptional.

Lung cancer (Maps 27–30)

Cancers of the trachea, bronchus, and lung (largely bronchial cancers, but conventionally abbreviated as 'lung cancer') are the most common cause of cancer death in men in England and Wales. In women they are the second most common, after breast cancer (see Table 1).

Lung cancer is probably the most common cancer in the world (Tomatis *et al.* 1990). British rates have been exceptionally high in international terms, but for males have been decreasing in recent years. These rates and trends reflect past cigarette-smoking, which is the major risk factor for lung cancer in England and Wales. Other forms of tobacco-smoking also cause the tumour. It has been estimated that 94 per cent of lung cancer deaths in men and 83 per cent in women in England and Wales are attributable to smoking (Tomatis *et al.* 1990). Several occupational exposures have been shown to raise risk of lung cancer[2] (in several instances with the earliest studies conducted in England and Wales) — inorganic arsenic, asbestos, talc containing asbestiform fibres, chloromethylmethyl ether and bischloromethyl ether, hexavalent and possibly other chromium compounds, mustard gas production, nickel refining, several occupations which involve heavy exposure to polycyclic hydrocarbons — coal-gas and coke production, and work with coal-tar pitch — and exposure to radon and its decay products in mining. In England and Wales raised

1 Stocks did not publish a map of laryngeal cancer in females.

2 The history of these discoveries is recounted by Doll (1975). Some specific geographical associations in England and Wales are: nickel-refining in Clydach, Glamorgan (Kaldor *et al.* 1986); chromate production in Bolton, Lancashire, and Eaglescliffe, Durham (Davies *et al.* 1991); mustard gas manufacture in Cheshire (Easton *et al.* 1988); and inorganic arsenic exposure in sheep dip manufacture at Berkhamstead, Hertfordshire (Doll 1967; Hill and Faning 1948). Also the mining exposures detailed below, and the asbestos exposures described on p. 49. Several of the above also gave rise to other respiratory cancers, as noted when discussing those cancers.

risk has been demonstrated in tin miners in Cornwall (Fox *et al.* 1981) and haematite miners in Cumberland (Boyd *et al.* 1970). Raised risks of lung cancer also occur in iron and steel foundry-workers and in painters. There are many other occupational exposures which are probable causes of lung cancer — for instance, crystalline silica inhalation and work with diesel engines. Around 15 per cent of lung cancers in men and five per cent in women may be attributable[1] to occupational factors (Doll and Peto 1981). Risk is also increased by ionizing radiation exposure. Indoor residential exposures to smoke (Gao *et al.* 1987) and radon (Darby and Doll 1990) in air are suspected aetiological factors. The latter may account for around 6 per cent of lung cancers[1] in England and Wales (Darby and Doll 1990). It is not clear whether urban (outdoor) air pollution contributes to lung cancer aetiology.

The geography of lung cancer risk in England and Wales (Maps 27–30) differs by age, particularly in men, with greatest risk in the north of England at younger ages, and in the south-east of England and the north at older ages. At ages 0–44, greatest significant risks in males (Map 27) were in Lancashire (1·63), Durham (1·52), and North Yorkshire (1·30), with non-significant high risks in Radnorshire (1·76), Caernarvonshire (1·47), and Anglesey (1·44). The risk in London was significantly low (0·88). In females aged 0–44 (Map 28) greatest risks were in Northumberland (1·74), Durham (1·58), Cumberland (1·57), and Lancashire (1·51) (all significant), and risk in London was 1·17 (significant). Lowest risks in males were in Montgomeryshire (0·14, one case), East Suffolk (0·44), and Pembrokeshire (0·47) (all significant) and in females in Breconshire (0·25, NS, one case), Herefordshire (0·31, significant), and Somerset (0·33, significant).

At age 45 years and over (Maps 29–30), however, greatest risks in men were in London (1·18), Lancashire (1·17), Northumberland (1·16), and Staffordshire (1·14) (all significant) and in females were in London (1·33), Northumberland (1·21), Rutland (1·17), and North Yorkshire (1·17) (all significant except Rutland). Lowest risks in men were in Radnorshire (0·53), Cornwall (0·68), and Carmarthenshire (0·69) (all significant) and in women in Carmarthenshire (0·46), Cardiganshire (0·51), and Breconshire (0·57) (all significant).

The all-age risks (not shown) inevitably reflect mainly the risks at older ages, at which the great majority of cases occur: in males greatest all-age risks were in Lancashire (1·18), London (1·17), and Northumberland (1·16) (all significant), and in females risks were highest in London (1·33), Northumberland (1·22), and North Yorkshire (1·17) (all significant). Lowest risks in males were in Radnorshire (0·55) and Cornwall (0·68) (both significant), and in females in Carmarthenshire (0·47) and Cardiganshire (0·51) (both significant).

The differences in geography of lung cancer by age appear to be part of a long-term change, probably reflecting mainly geographical differences in adoption and cessation of smoking habits in different generations (Swerdlow and dos Santos Silva 1991). In 1921–30 the pattern found by Stocks (1936, 1939) was of high risks concentrated around London, and relatively low risks in the north of England (Maps S4, S5). He concluded that these probably reflected real differences in incidence, although there might also be an element of diagnostic artefact. In the present data at older ages, high risks persisted around London particularly for women, whereas for men and women under 45 years of age, and to a lesser extent for older men, the pattern has changed greatly: the epidemic has moved north, and highest risk is in Northumberland and Durham. This movement appears to have occurred earlier for men than for women, and for the most urban than for less-urban areas,

1 The percentages of lung cancers thought to be attributable to different agents (smoking, occupation, etc.) cannot be added to give the percentage attributable to these agents in combination, because there can be interaction between their effects.

Table 4 Lung cancer incidence risks by degree of urbanization: counties with significant odds ratios greater than 1·10 in each sex, age-group, and urbanization stratum

Sex	Age	Metropolitan	Urban	Rural
Males	0–44 years	Lancashire (1·62) Durham (1·56) North Yorks. (1·45) Staffordshire (1·26) West Yorks. (1·26)	Lancashire (1·61) Durham (1·55) West Yorks. (1·37) Cheshire (1·22)	West Yorks. (1·47) Glamorgan (1·45)
	45+ years	North Yorks. (1·18) Northumberland (1·16) Staffordshire (1·13) East Yorks. (1·13)	Northumberland (1·24) Lancashire (1·16) Durham (1·14) Shropshire (1·11) Kent (1·11)	Kent (1·27) Hertfordshire (1·22) West Sussex (1·16) Bedfordshire (1·15) Durham (1·13) Buckinghamshire (1·13)
Females	0–44 years	Northumberland (1·73) East Yorks. (1·65) Durham (1·45) Lancashire (1·45)	Durham (1·94) Northumberland (1·87) West Yorks. (1·40) Lancashire (1·36)	Lincoln. Kesteven (1·98) Bedfordshire (1·97) Cheshire (1·87) Durham (1·67) Kent (1·61) West Yorks. (1·56)
	45+ years	London (1·24) Northumberland (1·21) North Yorks. (1·21)	Hertfordshire (1·27) Surrey (1·27) Kent (1·27) West Sussex (1·26) Buckinghamshire (1·25) Northumberland (1·21) Norfolk (1·19) Berkshire (1·14) Essex (1·14)	Hertfordshire (1·49) Rutland (1·47) Surrey (1·45) Buckinghamshire (1·40) West Sussex (1·39) Oxfordshire (1·33) Berkshire (1·31) Kent (1·31) Essex (1·23) Hampshire (1·19) East Sussex (1·12)

occurring latest of all for women in rural areas (Table 4). Regional disparity has also increased, especially in males: risks in the northern regions are now over twice those in much of Wales and the south.

Lung cancer risk showed a strong gradient of greater risks in more urban areas in each sex and age group. The gradient was greater at younger ages than older.

The major cause of lung cancer in England and Wales is smoking, but geographical data on smoking are not available for past periods relevant to the aetiology of the lung cancers in the present maps. The smoking data available (Table A4.22) are too recent, and do not fit well with the distribution of lung cancer shown here. Certain industrial exposures, notably to asbestos and in foundry work, are responsible for a small proportion of lung cancers in England and Wales, and thus high risks in ship-building areas and areas where steel foundries are situated (Tables A4.14, A4.16) might in part be explicable by industrial exposures. However, comparison with the maps for pleural cancer (Maps 31–32), which is almost entirely caused by asbestos (see below), does not show close similarities.

Cancer of the pleura (Maps 31 and 32)

These tumours are mainly mesotheliomas caused by asbestos exposure, usually occupational, although cases have been reported in non-occupationally exposed wives of asbestos workers who brought dusty clothes home, and there may be cases due to neighbourhood exposures around factories, and other asbestos exposures. Incidence rates in England and Wales are over three times as great in men as women, and are rising in men but probably not now in women. Risks in England and Wales were higher in metropolitan than urban than rural areas, particularly in males, presumably reflecting industrial uses of asbestos in cities and towns. Highest risks in males were in Northumberland (2·42), Hampshire (1·89), the Isle of Wight (1·82), and Devon (1·76) (each significant): all counties where shipbuilding[1] has been an important industry (see Table A4.16). There were also appreciably raised risks in Cheshire (1·57), Kent (1·52), Durham (1·47), and Lancashire (1·37) (all significant), each of which had shipyards (and in some instances also other major asbestos-using facilities), and in Buckinghamshire (1·42, significant), which did not. It is not obvious why risk should have been raised in Buckinghamshire: its work-force does not include a particularly large number of asbestos workers now (see p. 25), although there are, as in most counties, several factories in the county registered under the Asbestos Survey.

In females, significant raised risks were in Durham (1·80), Nottinghamshire (1·72), Lancashire (1·50), and London (1·41). Risks were also high but not significant for women in Merionethshire (2·14, based on three cases), Cardiganshire (1·51, three cases), Northumberland (1·39, 34 cases), and Leicestershire (1·32, 26 cases). The Nottinghamshire risk is likely to relate to work by women in gas-mask manufacture, using filter pads containing asbestos, during World War II (Wignall and Fox 1982). In Lancashire there was also gas-mask manufacture (Gardner *et al.* 1982), as well as an asbestos textile factory in Rochdale (Peto *et al.* 1985). In London, Newhouse showed very high risks in women workers at an asbestos factory in the east of the city (Newhouse and Berry 1979), and there were other asbestos factories in the same area (Gardner *et al.* 1982). The significant risk in Durham is more surprising. In other counties where raised risk in men appears to relate to shipyard employment (apart from, to a lesser extent, Northumberland), there was not such an unexplained raised risk in women. It is of interest that apart from the Isle of Wight, where numbers were small, Durham and Northumberland had the highest proportion of the female work-force employed in shipbuilding in 1961, although percentages were low (0·20 per cent and 0·39 per cent for the two counties respectively (GRO 1966)), but also at earlier dates when more women were employed in shipyards (0·75 per cent and 0·98 per cent in 1951 (GRO 1957), and 0·41 per cent and 0·70 per cent in 1931 (GRO 1934)). In Merionethshire there were raised risks, although not significant, in each sex (males 1·21, based on five cases; females 2·14, three cases); the county appears to have had one of the highest rates of asbestos factory employment in England and Wales according to the crude data available to us (see p. 25).

Table 5 shows the significant risks in metropolitan, urban, and rural districts separately; in general the high risks in these analyses were in the counties where significant risks occurred overall, but there were also raised risks for males in urban East Suffolk and rural Anglesey and Berkshire, and for females in urban Leicestershire and rural Hertfordshire.

A reason for caution in interpreting mesothelioma data is that there is an appreciable error in attributing cause of death on death certificates for this tumour (McDonald 1979), which may be influenced by knowledge of asbestos exposure or prospects of compensation payments.

In summary, most of the raised risks of mesothelioma in the maps appear to be explicable by asbestos use at known locations, although there may have been some

1 Which can involve heavy exposure to asbestos.

Table 5 Pleural cancer incidence risks by degree of urbanization: counties with odds ratios significantly raised in each sex and urbanization stratum

Sex	Metropolitan	Urban	Rural
Males	Devon (2·95) Northumberland (2·57) Hampshire (2·16) Cheshire (1·94) Durham (1·48) Lancashire (1·27)	Northumberland (2·32) Isle of Wight (2·26) East Suffolk (2·00) Kent (1·70) Essex (1·61) Durham (1·52) Hampshire (1·41) Hertfordshire (1·39) Cheshire (1·31) Lancashire (1·21)	Anglesey (3·89) Buckinghamshire (1·83) Berkshire (1·67) Lancashire (1·56)
Females	Nottinghamshire (2·54) London (1·43)	Durham (2·60) Leicestershire (2·00) Nottinghamshire (1·82) Lancashire (1·38)	Lancashire (2·72) Hertfordshire (2·32)

artefactual effect from doctors' knowledge of these locations. Risks based on appreciable numbers of cases but not clearly explicable, and which may merit further investigation, are that for men in Buckinghamshire, and the risks for women in Durham and Northumberland.

Bone cancer (Maps 33–36)

Bone cancer is not common (Table 1). The epidemiology of this tumour differs by age. At older ages, a major aetiological factor is Paget's disease of the bone (Price 1962), for which the UK has exceptionally high rates. A peak of bone cancer incidence occurs in young people in their teens, which is thought to relate to growth during adolescence; the tumours are incident mainly in the bones which grow most rapidly, the femur and tibia. Aetiological factors for bone cancer include ionizing radiation (both deposited radio-isotopes and external radiation) and certain rare genetic conditions.

Because of their different epidemiological characteristics, we mapped separately bone cancers occurring at ages 0–24, and those at ages beyond this. Bone tumours below the age of 25 (Map 33–34) showed no particular pattern of distribution across England and Wales. In males, the only significant raised risk was in Flintshire (2·24), with high non-significant risks in Pembrokeshire (2·34, based on seven cases) and Rutland (2·21, two cases), while in females there were significant risks in Herefordshire (3·01), Huntingdonshire (2·80), Bedfordshire (1·82), and Essex (1·54), and high non-significant risk in Rutland (2·41, one case). In each sex, risks were slightly higher in metropolitan and urban than in rural areas. (We have not analysed geography within urbanization strata for bone cancer at these ages because of small numbers.) Since deposited radionuclides concentrate particularly in the bone, there might be concern that rates of the tumours would be increased in those areas where fallout from atomic weapons testing has been greatest. There was no indication, however, that areas where high fallout occurred, in the west and north of the country (see p. 26), were at increased risk. There was also no relation to available data on the distribution of adult height in the country (see p. 27).

Above age 25 (Maps 35–36), by contrast, bone cancer risks showed a clear geographical pattern, with greatest risks in Wales. In males, risks were highest in Montgomeryshire (3·15), Caernarvonshire (2·36), Denbighshire (2·04) (all significant), and other Welsh counties. Greatest risks in England were much lower — in Shropshire (1·32, NS), Surrey (1·29, significant), and Lancashire (1·29, significant). In females, risks were again greatest in Welsh counties: Pembrokeshire (2·77), Denbighshire (2·40), and Glamorgan (1·91) (all significant). Risks were much lower in England, being greatest in Hampshire (1·24, significant). In each sex, risks were slightly higher in metropolitan and urban than in rural areas. High-risk areas for bone cancer were seen in north Wales in both rural and urban strata. In rural areas, greatest risks for males were in Anglesey (4·15), Carmarthenshire (2·65), and Caernarvonshire (2·60) (all significant) and for females in East Yorkshire (2·22, significant), Hampshire (2·01, significant), Cardiganshire (1·95, NS), and Cheshire (1·95, significant). For urban areas, significant high risks in males were in Montgomeryshire (4·79), Flintshire (1·92), Lancashire (1·34), and Cheshire (1·33), with non-significant high risks in Breconshire (1·82) and West Suffolk (1·77); in females significant high risks were in Denbighshire (2·77), Pembrokeshire (2·27), Flintshire (1·98), and Cheshire (1·37), with non-significant high risks in Anglesey (2·19) and West Suffolk (1·75). In metropolitan areas, significantly raised risks in males were in Northumberland (1·49) and Lancashire (1·49), with a non-significant risk of 1·82 in Lincolnshire Kesteven, while in females there were significant risks in Hampshire (1·47) and Devon (1·46), and non-significant but high risk in Kent (2·30).

In New South Wales, Australia, a significant excess of bone cancer has been noted in Welsh migrants but not English migrants, but based on small numbers and only in males (McCredie and Coates 1989).

Barker *et al.* (1980) have published data on the distribution of radiological prevalence of Paget's disease in 31 towns in England and Wales. This showed high prevalence in each sex in towns in Lancashire, but gave no data for Wales other than for Cardiff, where prevalence was around the average for the towns investigated. In the present data, urban and metropolitan risks of bone cancer at older ages in Lancashire in men were significantly raised and among the highest in England, and in women were non-significantly raised and fairly high.

A map of bone cancer mortality by county at ages under 65 was published for 1951–3 by Court Brown *et al.* (1961), but based on few deaths in many of the counties. It shows no clear resemblance to the present maps.

In older people the bone is a site for which there is particular potential for secondary malignancies from elsewhere in the body to be misclassified at cancer registration, or misdiagnosed, as primary tumours (of the bone). The distribution therefore needs further investigation — initially to determine whether there is indeed a high-risk area for primary bone cancers in Wales, and, if so, to try to find its cause.

Cancer of soft tissues (Maps 37 and 38)

These constitute a diverse range of tumours of different tissue origins — fibrous tissue, muscle, blood vessels, and other tissues of mesenchymal origin, excluding bone and cartilage. A few such malignancies occur in persons at high risk because of genetic conditions, and there is also high risk in immunologically depressed subjects, for instance after renal transplantation. There is inconclusive evidence of a raised risk from herbicide exposure. Kaposi's sarcoma, which comes within the soft tissue tumours, has recently been strongly related to human immunodeficiency virus (HIV) infection, and may be sexually transmitted (Beral *et al.* 1990). However, it was very rare in England and Wales during the study period.

In England and Wales, greatest risks of soft tissue tumours in males were in Radnorshire (2·36), the Isle of Wight (1·61), and East Suffolk (1·39) (all significant). In females the greatest risks were in Merionethshire (1·50, NS), Northamptonshire (1·44, significant), and the Isle of Wight (1·44, NS).

There was no appreciable difference in risk by degree of urbanization, and no clear pattern of risks in metropolitan, urban, and rural areas considered separately. In males, greatest risks in metropolitan areas were in Kent (2·18, significant) and Northamptonshire (1·46, NS); in urban areas in East Yorkshire (2·06, significant), Radnorshire (1·89, NS), and Devon (1·48, significant); and in rural areas in the Isle of Wight (2·73, significant) and Radnorshire (2·57, NS). In females, highest metropolitan risks were in Northamptonshire (1·78, significant), Kent (1·43, NS), and Lincolnshire Lindsey (1·42, NS); urban in Herefordshire (1·70, significant), Northamptonshire (1·60, significant), and Cambridgeshire (1·57, significant); and rural in Merionethshire (1·76, NS) and Westmorland (1·53, NS), with significant risks in Northamptonshire (1·51) and Essex (1·44). It is notable that in Northamptonshire there was a significant raised risk in each of the urbanization strata for females, and overall (although not within urbanization strata separately) for males.

Malignant melanoma of the skin (Maps 39 and 40)

Although not at present one of the most common cancers in England and Wales, the incidence of melanoma is increasing rapidly in these countries, as in all white populations around the world for which data are available. Incidence in England and Wales in females is about twice that in males, but survival is worse in men, so that the sex ratio is more nearly equal for deaths (see Table 1).

Intermittent recreational sun exposure of usually-covered skin is probably the main aetiological agent for melanoma, with particularly high risk in individuals with fair complexion and those with large numbers of benign naevi (moles) or with atypical naevi. A minority of melanomas, of the histological subtype lentigo maligna melanoma, have an aetiology which appears to relate mainly to cumulative sun exposure, and occur particularly in older outdoor workers. Raised risk of melanoma also occurs in some immunosuppressed groups, in certain rare genetic conditions, and in individuals with giant congenital naevi. The distribution of this tumour in whites internationally is generally closely correlated with solar ultraviolet levels, with highest rates in the world in whites in Queensland, Australia, and in other tropical areas. Despite the far smaller gradient in ultraviolet levels within England and Wales than internationally, it is interesting to note in Maps 39 and 40 that there is a north–south gradient of risk, and a clear correlation between melanoma incidence, especially in males, and hours of sunshine (see Map E13). Highest risks of melanoma in males were in the southernmost counties of England (highest in Cornwall (2·01), Dorset (1·58), Hampshire (1·55), and Surrey (1·55) (all significant)), with fairly high risks in much of East Anglia and Wales. In females, again highest risks of melanoma were in the south and particularly the south-west of England (highest in Cornwall (1·82), Dorset (1·80), the Isle of Wight (1·76), and Devon (1·72) (all significant)), with some high risks in East Anglia and in the Lake District (Cumberland and Westmorland). In each sex, risks were higher in rural than urban than metropolitan areas; geographical distribution of risks in each of these categories was similar to that for the analyses overall. In males in metropolitan areas, highest risks were in Essex (1·97), Kent (1·95), and Berkshire (1·73) (all significant); in urban areas in Rutland (4·28, significant), Breconshire (1·82, NS), and Cornwall (1·77, significant); and in rural areas in Huntingdonshire (1·76), Cornwall (1·75), and Dorset (1·46) (all significant). In females the greatest risks in metropolitan areas were in Devon (2·00), East Sussex (1·75), and Somerset (1·58) (all significant); in urban areas in Dorset (1·91), Cornwall (1·83), and East Sussex (1·71) (all significant); and in rural areas in Somerset (1·67), Hampshire (1·66), and Dorset (1·56) (all significant).

Melanoma risk is greater in higher social classes, so a possible reason apart from local UV levels for the greater risk in the south of England than further north could be social class-related behaviours of southerners, who tend to be of higher average social class than persons in areas to the north (see p. 31); for instance, more holidays in sunny countries abroad, or more time spent resident abroad. Another potential influence on the geographical distribution is skin type. Across Europe, for instance, this appears to be a greater influence than UV levels on geographical rates, with rates greater in the north of the continent (e.g. among fair-skinned Scandinavians) than the south (darker-skinned Mediterranean populations). While skin type does not seem a likely explanation of north–south differences in England and Wales, the high risks in Wales may partly reflect the presence of 'Celtic' skin types which are known to have high risk of the tumour (Swerdlow 1984). The proportion of non-whites (who have very low risk) in certain of the county populations (see p. 27) must also have had a small effect on the distribution.

Non-melanoma skin cancer

These tumours are common, but do not often metastasize and are rarely fatal. The majority are basal cell cancers, and most of the remainder are squamous cell. It is notoriously difficult to achieve complete registration of non-melanoma skin cancers since cases are usually not treated as in-patients, histological confirmation is sometimes not undertaken, and probably an appreciable number of cases are never diagnosed. Therefore there is a particular potential for the 'incidence' of these tumours from routine data to reflect artefacts of registration, and we have not shown the maps produced; they can be obtained on application to the authors. In brief, the data showed a slight gradient of higher risks in rural than urban than metropolitan areas in males but not clearly in females. In both sexes, risks of registered non-melanoma skin cancers were high in East Anglia, Kent, Surrey, Devon, Cornwall, and Herefordshire, but beyond this there was no clear pattern of risks.

Breast cancer in women (Maps 41 and 42)

Breast cancer is the most common cancer in women in England and Wales (Table 1), and indeed in women world-wide (Tomatis *et al.* 1990). Some 20 000 new cases occur in women in England and Wales each year, and more than 11 000 women per year die of it. Risks in England and Wales, especially in the south and east of England, are among the highest in Europe (Jensen *et al.* 1990; Smans *et al.*, in press). Incidence and mortality appear to be decreasing a little at pre-menopausal ages, but are increasing at post-menopausal ages.

The main known risk factors for breast cancer in women are related to reproduction, probably via the effect of reproductive factors on endocrine status. It has been hypothesized that increased exposure to oestrogen and/or progesterone is the underlying risk factor (Preston-Martin *et al.* 1990). Risk is increased for women with early menarche, nulliparity, and late first full-term pregnancy, and decreased with early natural menopause or oophorectomy before the menopause. There may also be a long-term protective effect of high parity (for post-menopausal tumours at least) and an adverse effect of late age at last birth, independent of age at first birth. Abortions may increase risk. Lactation has been shown to be protective in some studies, but its effect is not well established. Risk may be increased after post-menopausal hormone replacement therapy, diethylstilboestrol treatment during pregnancy, and prolonged use of oral contraceptives from a young age, but evidence on these remains unclear. Adipose tissue is the main source of oestrogens in post-menopausal women, and obesity is a risk factor for breast cancer at post-menopausal ages.

Some cases of breast cancer are related to ionizing radiation exposure, with greater relative risks for exposures at a young age. Certain benign breast diseases, mainly proliferative lesions, increase risk. Associations of breast cancer risk have been shown, mainly in population-based correlations, with high-fat diets. Several studies have found associations of breast cancer risk with alcohol consumption, but whether this is causal is not clear.

Breast cancer risk is particularly influenced by family history: raised risks occur for women whose mother or sister have had the disease. Genetic factors are strongest at young ages and for bilateral cancers. A recent study suggests that a few per cent of breast cancers may be attributable to heterozygote carriage of the gene for ataxia telangiectasia (Swift *et al.* 1987).

Screening programmes could affect apparent geographical risks of breast cancer, but there was not sufficient screening activity in England and Wales during the study period to affect appreciably the data presented (see p. 31).

There are indications of differences in aetiology of breast cancer before and after the menopause, and we have therefore mapped separately the distribution of the tumour for women aged 0–44 years and women aged 45 years and over.

For women under age 45 (Map 41), risks of breast cancer were low in the north of England, south Wales, the south-west and parts of the south of England. Risk was similar in metropolitan, urban, and rural strata. Highest risks, although not consistently, were in a band across the middle of England, with the greatest odds ratios in Lincolnshire Holland (1·39, significant), Leicestershire (1·13, significant), and Merionethshire (1·12, NS). This pattern was particularly clear in rural areas, for which there was a slight cluster of high-risk counties in the east Midlands. Highest risks were in Radnorshire (1·61, NS), Lincolnshire Lindsey (1·51, significant), and Westmorland (1·38, NS). There was no clear pattern in metropolitan or urban areas. In metropolitan areas, highest risks were in Essex (1·30, NS) and Lincolnshire Kesteven (1·20, NS) with no risks significantly raised. In urban areas, the greatest risks were in Merionethshire (2·71, significant) and Cardiganshire (1·47, NS).

In women aged 45 years and over (Map 42), by contrast, there was a clear north–south gradient of risk. Greatest risks were in Merionethshire (1·20), Bedfordshire (1·18), Leicestershire (1·15), and Surrey (1·13) (all significant), and lowest risks in Cumberland (0·79) and Northumberland (0·84) (both significant). There was a slight gradient of higher risks in rural than urban than metropolitan areas. In general the north–south pattern of risks was present in rural, urban, and metropolitan areas separately, except that in Wales the risks were uneven. Greatest risks in rural areas were in Merionethshire (1·23, NS), Leicestershire (1·17, significant), and Northamptonshire (1·16, significant); in urban areas in Merionethshire (1·20, NS), Leicestershire (1·20, significant), and Bedfordshire (1·18, significant); and in metropolitan areas in Essex (1·31, significant), Oxfordshire (1·18, significant), and Leicestershire (1·18, significant). There are no metropolitan areas in north and mid-Wales (Table A1.1). The consistency of high risks in Merionethshire and Leicestershire is notable.

The all-ages map for breast cancer closely resembled that for ages 45 years and over, at which most breast cancers occur, and has not therefore been shown. Greatest risks were in Merionethshire (1·20), Bedfordshire (1·17), Leicestershire (1·15), and Surrey (1·12) (all significant). Risks were slightly greater in rural than urban than metropolitan areas. Greatest rural risks were in Leicestershire (1·19, significant), Merionethshire (1·18, NS), and Northamptonshire (1·17, significant); greatest urban risks in Merionethshire (1·26), Leicestershire (1·19), and Denbighshire (1·17) (all significant); and greatest metropolitan risks in Essex (1·31), Leicestershire (1·17), and Oxfordshire (1·15) (all significant).

Greenwood (1925) and Stocks (1936), over half a century ago, analysed breast cancer mortality risks across England and Wales by county for 1911–20 and 1921–

30 (Map S6) respectively. Their maps, for all ages and ages 25–65 (*sic*) respectively, reflected mainly post-menopausal tumour risks, and resemble quite closely the present pattern at post-menopausal ages, except in north Wales (and for 1921–30 mid-Wales).

The distribution of pre-menopausal breast cancer in Map 41 does not parallel any of the relevant risk factors for which we had geographical data (see Chapter 7). The north–south gradient for post-menopausal breast cancer (Map 42) accords with the high social class characteristic of breast cancer patients (see p. 31). It also corresponds generally with the distribution of height of women in England and Wales (Map E5). The map of parity by county (Map E10) shows a general similarity to the breast cancer distribution in that parity is highest in the north of England and lowest in the south, but there is no more precise resemblance between the two maps. Age at first birth (Map E3) was high for women in the south-east of England, but also in certain other counties, with no close correspondence to breast cancer risks. Fat intakes recorded in the National Food Survey are higher in the north of England and in Wales than in the south (see Table A4.5), although another survey (see Table A4.6) shows the opposite, albeit with wide standard deviations. Regional variation in obesity is slight and not north–south (Table A4.7). More investigation would be needed to determine whether the breast cancer distributions correspond well with further reproductive and dietary variables.

Breast cancer in men (Map 43)

Breast cancer in men is far more rare than in women, and there has been relatively little study of its aetiology. A raised risk occurs in men with Klinefelter's disease — a chromosomal abnormality in men in which there are hormonal abnormalities and breast enlargement. There is evidence for a genetic element in risk. Several other factors — for instance, mumps infection at a relatively late age, testicular injury, and oestrogen treatment — have been found associated in particular studies but not yet established as risk factors.

Risk of male breast cancer in England and Wales was greatest in central southern England and the south-east. The area of high risk crossed registry boundaries and is therefore unlikely to be simply a function of registration. Highest risks were in West Suffolk (1·64), East Sussex (1·61), and Surrey (1·51) (all significant). Risks were fairly similar in urban, rural, and metropolitan areas. No clear pattern differing from that shown in Map 43 was present for urban, rural, and metropolitan areas separately. In urban areas, several counties in southern England showed significantly raised risks (greatest in East Sussex (1·84) and Surrey (1·71)), as did Derbyshire (1·48); in rural areas, only Hampshire (2·03) showed significant risk, with non-significant high risks in Merionethshire (1·87) and Pembrokeshire (1·72); and in metropolitan areas greatest risks were in Glamorgan (1·81) and East Sussex (1·75) (both significant).

The geographical distribution of breast cancer in men shows some resemblance to that for post-menopausal women, but there was not as clear a north–south difference as for women, and the range of risks was larger than for women, although of course based on far smaller numbers.

An unusual potential artefact in male breast cancer rates is that if a small proportion of females have their sex misclassified in registry records, this will appreciably affect apparent male risks because the tumour is over a hundred times more common in women than men.[1] Such an error was unlikely to occur in registrations coded to the Ninth Revision of the ICD[2], because there were

1 This sex ratio is far greater than for any other tumour in this Atlas (apart of course from sex-specific tumours), and therefore there is no other cancer presented for which sex miscoding is likely to be an appreciable problem.

2 International Classification of Diseases.

(deliberately) separate three-digit codes reserved for breast cancer in males and in females in this coding system.[1] The error may have occurred appreciably in ICD8, however, since breast cancer was coded there to the same ICD code regardless of sex. The present data consisted of 11 years coded to ICD8 and seven years to ICD9. We estimate that miscoding of female breast cancers as male gave 3 per cent error in sex in the recorded male tumours during the ICD8 years. The effect should therefore have been small compared to the spread of risks in the map.

Cervical cancer (Map 44)

Cervical cancer rates show great geographical variation internationally, with highest rates generally in less-'developed' countries, and some exceptionally high rates in South America. Mortality risks in England and Wales are among the highest in Europe (Jensen *et al.* 1990; Smans *et al.*, in press). Incidence and mortality rates in England and Wales have increased markedly in younger women in recent years.

The major risk factors relate to past sexual experience, notably early age at first intercourse and large numbers of sexual partners, strongly suggesting that the cancer is the result of a sexually transmitted infection. Several viruses have been shown to be associated (Singer and Jenkins 1991), but whether they are causal is not certain. There may also be an increasing risk with greater numbers of pregnancies, separate from the effect of sexual experience itself. Recent data suggest that smoking may also be associated, but whether it makes an independent contribution to risk is not yet clear. Risk is increased in users of oral contraceptives, but it is not known whether this is aetiological or reflects their sexual exposures. The great majority of cervical cancers are squamous, but about 5–10 per cent are adenocarcinomas, which appear to share with the squamous tumours the above risk factors, but also to share some risk factors with endometrial cancers (see p. 58). Prenatal exposure to diethylstilboestrol is a rare cause of cervical adenocarcinoma in young women.

Interpretation of geographical differences in cervical cancer registration rates is complicated by possible geographical variation in the extent to which cancer *in situ* and dysplasia of the cervix[2] have been counted mistakenly as invasive malignancies, variation in the extent to which registrations of cancer of the uterus have failed to identify the exact subsite[3], and variations in hysterectomy rates, since the operation will have removed women from risk. Highest hysterectomy rates during the study period overall were in the Oxford, Wessex, and Yorkshire regions (see Table A4.18), with high rates early in the period in South-west Metropolitan, South-western, and Oxford regions (see Table A4.17). Cervical screening might also affect registration rates: this could occur in two ways, one artefactual, the other not. Firstly, it might identify borderline malignant tumours which otherwise might not have been diagnosed, and, secondly but with opposite effect on the statistics, it might lead to a real decrease in rates of cancer by successfully preventing the development of malignant tumours. It is estimated that about 25–35 per cent of invasive cervical cancers in England and Wales during 1978 may have been prevented by the screening programme (Parkin *et al.* 1985). The programme was particularly active during the study period in the North-western region and in the Thames regions (i.e. in and around London) see p. 31).

In England and Wales, the risk of cervical cancer was highest in parts of Wales and in much of the north of England, although not the most northern counties

1 Hence accidental miscoding of sex should have been detected by validation checks made of the sex code against the site code in ICD9 years, but such checks were not possible under ICD8.

2 Which should be coded to non-malignant ICD codes and therefore *excluded* from the malignancies mapped here.

3 Although in England and Wales, these 'unspecified' tumours (ICD9: 179) appear mainly to be cancers of the body of uterus (Swerdlow 1989).

(Map 44). Risks were low south of a line from the Severn to the Wash. The counties with the greatest risks were Anglesey (1·48), Pembrokeshire (1·38), Carmarthenshire (1·32), and Lancashire (1·31) (all significant). The range of relative risks for this cancer was appreciably greater than for the hormonally-related reproductive cancers (i.e. breast, corpus uteri, and ovarian cancers), with extreme values of 0·70 in Oxfordshire and 1·48 in Anglesey (both significant).

Risk was slightly greater in metropolitan than urban than rural areas. Examining the data separately in metropolitan areas, there was a clear raised risk in all northern counties (greatest risks in North Yorkshire (1·38) and Lancashire (1·36) (both significant)), and generally lower risks were in the south (lowest risks in Oxfordshire (0·58, significant) and Kent (0·70, NS)). In urban areas there was a less-clear increase in northern regions, and highest risks were in Wales. Greatest risks were in Pembrokeshire (1·82) and Anglesey (1·69) (both significant) and least in West Sussex (0·63), Surrey (0·75), and Somerset (0·75) (all significant). In rural areas the high risk in the north was yet less evident — only West Yorkshire had a risk appreciably above unity (1·35, significant), and several Welsh counties had high risks (the highest were Anglesey (1·72), Denbighshire (1·56), and Carmarthenshire (1·53) (all significant). Lowest risks were in Lincolnshire Kesteven (0·76) and Oxfordshire (0·76) (both significant). Examination of the geographical distribution of percentages of cancer of uterus unspecified (Table 2) suggests that cervical cancer relative risks were not an artefact of the degree of uterine cancer specification — indeed, in general, high cervical cancer risks were in areas of comparatively[1] poor specification and low risks were in counties where specification was particularly good.

Perhaps surprisingly, the geographical distribution of cervical cancer was very similar at young and at older ages (maps not shown). For women under age 45, greatest risks were in Wales and much of northern England, but not the most northerly counties, where risks were well below unity: highest risks were in Pembrokeshire (2·12), Flintshire (2·11), Denbighshire (1·51), and North Yorkshire (1·41) (all significant). For older women, risks were again greatest in parts of Wales and northern England, although risks in the most northerly counties were nearer to unity. Greatest risks were in Anglesey (1·50), Carmarthenshire (1·30), Lancashire (1·29), and West Yorkshire (1·17) (all significant). At both age groups, risks were low south of a line from the Severn Estuary to the Wash, with lowest risks under age 45 in Surrey (0·54, significant) and West Sussex (0·57, significant) and at older ages in Oxfordshire (0·72) and West Sussex (0·75) (both significant).

Mortality mapped by region (OPCS 1981) similarly showed greatest risk in the north of England and in Wales for this tumour. Clinic attendance and mortality data for venereal diseases (Table A4.23) show some resemblances to the cervical cancer pattern — notably the high risks in Manchester and Liverpool regions — but also some striking differences: particularly the high venereal disease attendance and mortality rates in some Metropolitan regions and the high mortality rate in the Newcastle region.

The geographical distribution of cervical cancer was unusual in the degree to which it varied between urbanization strata. The reasons may well relate to variations in sexual behaviour (and perhaps screening). Particular scope for further aetiological investigation may relate to the highest risk, in Anglesey. If epidemics of cases relating to particular focuses of infection were to occur for this tumour, they might most easily be detected in rural island communities such as Anglesey. Furthermore, the highest risk of penile cancer, which probably has a similar aetiology to cervical cancer, was also in Anglesey (see p. 63).

1 In no county were more than 15 per cent of uterine cancers unspecified with regard to corpus/cervix.

Cancer of the placenta (Map 45)

These are choriocarcinomas, and are rare. Choriocarcinomas originate from trophoblastic tissue in the placenta, and there is very greatly increased risk (around 2000-fold) in women with a molar pregnancy (a benign cystic condition of the placenta). Risk increases greatly with increasing maternal age and possibly with parity, and appears to be high in southern and eastern Asia, and in Africa.

The map for England and Wales (Map 45) was based on far smaller numbers than any other tumour in this Atlas, and there were no cases in several counties. The risks presented are for women rather than for individual pregnancies (the latter would have some advantages for aetiological purposes, since the cancer can only occur in relation to a pregnancy, but is not a practical measure to calculate from the routine data). Highest risks were in Montgomeryshire (6·43, significant, based on two cases), Shropshire (3·02, significant, based on seven cases), and East Yorkshire (2·98, significant, based on 10 cases). The only other significant risk was in Staffordshire (1·89; 22 cases). Risk was 40 per cent (significantly) greater in urban than rural areas, with metropolitan risks intermediate (Table A5.45).

Cancer of the corpus uteri (Map 46)

Cancers of the body of the uterus arise mainly in its surface lining (endometrium). In the data for this map we have included uterine cancers not further specified, since the frequency of failure to specify varies considerably by county (see Table 2), and in England and Wales most such tumours are from the corpus uteri (Swerdlow 1989). Internationally the distribution of uterine corpus cancer resembles that of breast cancer, with high risk in 'developed' populations. Also like breast cancer, it is more common in women of high social class. Individuals who have uterine corpus cancer are at increased risk of breast cancer.

Risk factors for cancer of the uterine corpus are nulliparity, obesity, early menarche, late age of menopause, and, dramatically in recent years in the United States, post-menopausal treatment with oestrogens (oestrogen replacement therapy). It will be noted that many of these factors overlap with the risk factors for breast cancer. Use of combined oral contraceptives is protective against endometrial cancer, but sequential oral contraceptives increase risk. Increasing parity is protective. All of these risk factors may be explicable as a risk from exposure to unopposed oestrogen (i.e. oestrogen in the absence of progesterone (Preston-Martin *et al.* 1990)). Risks in the registration data will also have been affected by hysterectomy rates (see Tables A4.17, A4.18), since this operation removes the organ at risk.

The geographical distribution within England and Wales (Map 46) showed some similarity to that of breast cancer at older ages (Map 42), with lower risks in the north of England than elsewhere. Unlike breast cancer, however, there were also fairly low rates in much of the south-east of England, and highest risks in a band across the middle of England and Wales, and in the south-west of England. Greatest risks were in Radnorshire (1·36, NS), Lincolnshire Holland (1·34, significant), and Herefordshire (1·33, significant).

Risks were greatest for rural areas and least for metropolitan. The patterns of risk within metropolitan, urban, and rural strata separately were similar to those for the analyses overall. In metropolitan areas, highest risks were in Norfolk (1·36), Worcestershire (1·27), and Northamptonshire (1·24) (all significant); in urban areas in Radnorshire (1·46, NS), Breconshire (1·39, NS), and Devon (1·31, significant); and in rural areas in Carmarthenshire (1·38, significant), Lincolnshire Holland (1·32, significant), and Merionethshire (1·28, NS).

The overall distribution fits well with the regional distribution of non-cervix uterine cancer mortality in maps by OPCS (1981), which showed greatest risks in Wales, the east Midlands, and the south-west of England.

It is unlikely that use of post-menopausal oestrogen treatment appreciably affected the distribution of the tumour in England and Wales in the period covered by Map 46. There is no obvious relation of the corpus uteri cancer risks to the distribution of hysterectomy rates (Tables A4.17, A4.18). Geographical variation in obesity, in the data available (by region), was very slight (Table A4.7). Parity (Map E10) tended to be greater in the north than the south of England, but the north–south difference was not as consistent as that for uterine corpus cancer.

Ovarian cancer (Map 47)

Ovarian cancer accounts for five per cent of incident cancers and six per cent of cancer deaths in women in England and Wales (Table 1), but its causes have been less investigated than those of the other major reproductive neoplasms in women. The three-digit ICD category mapped includes cancers of the Fallopian tube and other uterine adnexa as well as of the ovary, but the non-ovarian cancers constitute only around one per cent of the total. The great majority of ovarian cancers are epithelial, and the major known risk factor for these is low fertility: risk is greatest in nulliparous women and decreases with increasing parity. Use of oral contraceptives leads to decreased risk, and it has been postulated that the underlying risk factor for the tumour may directly relate to the number of ovulatory menstrual cycles a woman has during her life, greater risk occurring with more cycles. An alternative explanation is that aetiology might result from hormonal factors which affect ovulation. More minor risk factors for ovarian cancer are ionizing radiation, Peutz–Jeghers syndrome (a rare hereditary condition), and possibly asbestos exposure. There is also a genetic element in risk. Risks in registration data may also be affected by oophorectomy rates (Table A4.17), and by hysterectomy rates (Tables A4.17, A4.18) since the ovaries are often removed at this operation.

A small proportion of ovarian cancers are of germ-cell origin, and possibly have an aetiology related to prenatal hormone exposure, similar to that postulated for testicular cancer (Walker *et al.* 1988). Dysgenetic gonads are a risk factor accounting for a few germ-cell ovarian cancers.

Internationally, risk of ovarian cancer is greatest in 'developed' populations in Europe and North America. By European standards the risks in England and Wales are high (Jensen *et al.* 1990; Smans *et al.*, in press).

The overall distribution of ovarian cancer in England and Wales (Map 47), like that for post-menopausal breast cancer (Map 42), showed lowest risks in the north and greater risks in the south — a pattern consistent with regional ovarian cancer mortality (OPCS 1981). Unlike breast cancer, however, there were also low risks in most of Wales, and the risks in the south of England were less uniformly high than for breast cancer, especially in central southern England. The range of relative risks across the country was small — from 0·78 to 1·28. Greatest risks were in Rutland (1·28, NS), Dorset (1·27, significant), Radnorshire (1·24, NS), Norfolk (1·20, significant), and West Sussex (1·20, significant), with significant raised risks also in several other southern and Midlands counties. There was a slight gradient of greater risks in rural than urban than metropolitan areas. The geographical pattern of risks within urban and metropolitan strata was similar to that for ovarian cancer overall, and this was generally true also for rural areas, although there was a particularly low risk in the rural areas of west Wales compared with the rest of the country. Highest risks in metropolitan areas were in Kent (1·31) and Norfolk (1·22) (both significant);

in urban areas in Radnorshire (1·41, NS) and East Sussex (1·26, significant); and in rural areas in Breconshire (1·32, NS) and Dorset (1·27, significant).

Comparing ovarian cancer geography with that of parity (Map E10) there was a general resemblance, in that high risks were in the south and lower risks in the north, but there was not a close similarity. Hysterectomy rates have tended to be high in the south of England (Tables A4.17, A4.18) and oophorectomy rates high around London and in Wales (Table A4.17). The distribution of ovarian cancer now is remarkably similar to that 50 years ago (Stocks 1939) (see Map S7). It will be difficult to understand the reasons for the geographical distribution of ovarian cancer in England and Wales further, until more is known about ovarian cancer aetiology generally.

Cancers of the vagina and vulva (Map 48)

These tumours are not uncommon (around 1000 cases per year in England and Wales), but they have received little epidemiological study. The three-digit ICD code which has been mapped includes, as well as cancers of the vulva and vagina, other and unspecified female genital cancers, but these constitute only two per cent of the total. A viral aetiology has been postulated, but without clear evidence as yet. Immunological suppression probably increases risks, since high risks have been seen in renal transplant patients. Exposure to diethylstilboestrol *in utero* (the drug was given to pregnant women, usually to treat threatened abortion) has been found to cause clear-cell vaginal adenocarcinoma in girls and young women, but this is a rare cause in Britain — only three cases have been reported (L. J. Kinlen, personal communication), and it is thought that about 7500 women in Britain received stilboestrol during pregnancy, mainly in the 1950s (Kinlen *et al.* 1974). Risks of these tumours were low south of a line from the Seven estuary to the Wash, except in East Anglia, where there was a group of high-risk counties, and in the Isle of Wight and Wiltshire. North of the line there was no clear pattern, but two of the highest-risk counties were adjacent to each other in south Wales. Greatest risks were in Rutland (1·93), Breconshire (1·57), and Carmarthenshire (1·42) (all significant). Risk was slightly greater in rural than in urban and metropolitan areas. Within urbanization strata there was no clear pattern: in rural areas greatest risks were in Rutland (2·21, significant), Breconshire (1·73, significant), and Radnorshire (1·64, NS); in urban areas in Rutland (1·53, NS), Derbyshire (1·45, significant), and Breconshire (1·40, NS); and in metropolitan areas in Norfolk (1·79, significant), Durham (1·38, significant), and Kent (1·25, NS).

In the map of vulval and vaginal cancers in England and Wales produced by Stocks 50 years ago (1939), there was a striking area of high risk in counties south and west of the Wash (Map S8): there is no sign of this in the present data.

Cancer of the prostate (Map 49)

Cancer of the prostate is one of the most common cancers in men in England and Wales. It occurs chiefly at older ages; more than four-fifths of cases are incident over the age of 65, and almost half over 75. The great majority of the tumours are adenocarcinomas. Registered incidence and mortality rates in England and Wales are increasing, but this may reflect increased diagnostic investigation. The large proportion of cases occurring at older ages, and the high frequency of latent prostatic cancers undetected clinically (Breslow *et al.* 1977), give particular potential for extra cases to be detected if the prostate is resected or removed during life for benign prostatic disease, or if post-mortem examination is undertaken. This makes geographical differences in apparent incidence of the tumour difficult to interpret.

The aetiology of prostatic cancer is obscure. Some studies have suggested relationships to endocrine levels and sexual activity, to occupational exposure to cadmium, and occupational exposure to external radiation and radionuclides (Beral *et al.* 1985; Beral *et al.* 1988). At the population level and in some individual-based studies there has been an association with high fat intake.

Two areas of high risk of registered cancer of the prostate can be seen in Map 49 — in East Anglia and in the south-west of England. There was also an area of fairly high risk in Surrey and Sussex. Particularly low risks were seen in the north of England and in north and south Wales. Highest risks were in Cambridgeshire (1·31), Somerset (1·29), and Norfolk (1·28) (all significant). The high-risk areas did not coincide with cancer registry boundaries, arguing against artefacts of registration completeness or coding as an explanation. Diagnostic artefacts might particularly occur at older ages. We therefore reanalysed the data for ages under 65 years, but with fairly similar results to those shown in the published map. Highest risks were in Cornwall (1·53), Cambridgeshire (1·34), Norfolk (1·31), Bedfordshire (1·30), and Somerset (1·22) (all significant). Also arguing against registration artefact as the explanation of the geographical pattern is the similar distribution seen in available mortality data (by region) (OPCS 1981) — greatest risks were in the south-west of England, East Anglia, and the south-east of England, and lowest risks in Wales and the north of England. There is some resemblance to the regional pattern of prostatectomies in England and Wales (which are mainly for benign hyperplasia) (see Table A4.17), but little resemblance to the limited data available on admissions for prostatic hyperplasia (Table A4.12).

There was a slight increase in risk of prostatic cancer with decreasing urbanization. There was a similar geographic pattern to that for prostatic cancer overall, when metropolitan, urban, and rural risks were examined separately. Highest metropolitan risks were in Norfolk (1·32) and Bedfordshire (1·31) (both significant); greatest urban risks were in Somerset (1·35) and Devon (1·27) (both significant); and greatest rural risks in Somerset (1·30) and Cambridgeshire (1·29) (both significant).

There is at present insufficient knowledge of the aetiology of prostatic cancer for the geographical distribution of the tumour in England and Wales to be linked to causative variables.

Cancer of the testis (Maps 50 and 51)

Cancer of the testis is mainly a tumour of young men, with a peak of incidence around age 30. A second increase in incidence occurs beyond the age of about 50. Although testicular cancers account for only one per cent of cancers in men overall in England and Wales (Table 1), at younger adult age groups it is the most common cancer in men, and is increasing in incidence. Mortality is decreasing, however, because of great advances in treatment. The tumours are mainly of germ-cell histology.

Maldescent of the testis is the principal known risk factor for testicular cancer; a history of maldescent is present in about 10 per cent of cases. It has been hypothesized (Henderson *et al.* 1983) that the underlying risk factor for both testicular cancer and undescended testis may be prenatal exposure to high levels of circulating free oestrogen *in utero*. Other minor risk factors are probably mumps orchitis, possibly inguinal hernia, and in rare instances dysgenetic gonads. Risk has been found to be increased for first-born boys, and in some but not all studies for males of low birth weight.

Both in international comparisons and in comparisons between groups within countries, high risk of testicular cancer has been associated with high socioeconomic development/position. One might therefore expect that risk within

England and Wales would be higher in the south than the north (see p. 31). At younger ages (0–49) this was true to some extent (Map 50), but not consistently. Greatest risks were in Rutland (1·72, NS), Westmorland (1·38, NS), Surrey (1·38, significant), and Norfolk (1·37, significant). Risks were particularly low in Wales and the most northerly counties of England — least in Merionethshire (0·28, significant), Denbighshire (0·67, significant), and Breconshire (0·70, NS).

Risks were greater in rural and urban than metropolitan areas. In each of the urbanization strata separately, risks tended to be greater in the south than the north of the country, but this pattern was far from consistent. In metropolitan areas greatest risks were in Norfolk (2·12, significant), Cumberland (1·46, NS), and Northamptonshire (1·39, NS); in urban areas in Rutland (4·43, significant) and Radnorshire (2·27, NS); and in rural areas in Westmorland (2·40, NS), Montgomeryshire (1·77, NS), and Surrey (1·68, significant).

At older ages (Map 51), in contrast, greatest risks of testicular cancer were mainly in Wales, with some high risks in East Anglia and southern England, and low risks throughout the north of England. Greatest risks were in West Suffolk (2·23, significant), Montgomeryshire (2·21, NS), Breconshire (1·95, NS), and Caernarvonshire (1·79, significant). As at younger ages, risks were greater in rural and urban than in metropolitan areas. There were insufficient cases for satisfactory analyses of geography within urbanization strata.

A potential registration artefact in testicular cancer data at older ages is that lymphomas of the testis, which are a relatively common histology at these ages, although not in young men, are coded in the International Classification of Diseases to lymphoma if the histology is stated, but to testis if the histology is not stated (i.e. if the information available is 'malignant testicular neoplasm, histological type not specified'). This may account for some of the high Welsh odds ratios in Map 51 (see p. 18 concerning the degree of specification of data in different counties). Another potential source of artefact, specifically in the area covered by the Mersey registry, is that during the period covered by this Atlas, this registry coded testicular cancers which were a mixture of two histologies (usually mixed seminoma and teratoma) as two registrations, whereas the other registries in England and Wales counted them as one registration. This will have tended to inflate somewhat the apparent risks in the registry's area; for the counties involved see Appendix 1.

All-ages risks (not shown) mainly reflect testicular cancers occurring at younger ages: highest significant risks were in West Suffolk (1·52), Surrey (1·39), Norfolk (1·36), and Berkshire (1·26) (with high non-significant risk in Rutland (1·44)), and were generally high around London and in East Anglia. Lowest risks were in Merionethshire (0·22, significant), Northumberland (0·75, significant), Denbighshire (0·77, NS), and Flintshire (0·79, NS), with a surprisingly low value in London (0·81, significant). There were generally low risks in the north of England, and in north and south Wales.

Risks in rural and urban areas were slightly higher than in metropolitan areas. Examining geographical distribution within the metropolitan stratum, the only much raised or significant risk was in Norfolk (2·09), and there was no clear overall pattern. In urban areas, greatest risks were in Rutland (3·54, significant), Radnorshire (2·23, NS), and Cardiganshire (2·05, significant), and risks were generally highest in the south of England and in mid-Wales. In rural areas, highest risks were in Westmorland (2·00, NS), Montgomeryshire (1·93, NS), and Surrey (1·50, significant), and there was no overall pattern.

The main known risk factor for testicular cancer is undescended testis, for which we have no direct evidence on geographical variation within England and Wales. Greatest orchidopexy rates in 1967 (although earlier data would be desirable) were in the South-west Metropolitan and East Anglia regions (Table A4.17), and undescended testis admissions, which will largely have been for orchidopexy, were also high in these regions (Table A4.13). The distribution of testicular cancer at younger ages showed some resemblance to the geography of other reproductive hormone-related cancers, in that there was a general north–south gradient.

Cancer of the penis (Map 52)

This is a rare tumour in England and Wales, as in other 'developed' countries, but far more common in some developing countries. It is probably of sexual aetiology, possibly a sexually transmitted infection, and is much more common in uncircumcised than circumcised men. Internationally, the geography of penile cancer strongly parallels that of cancer of the cervix (Tomatis *et al.* 1990), and geographical similarities between these tumours have been shown within China (Li *et al.* 1982) and Brazil (Franco *et al.* 1988). Raised risk of cervical cancer has been found in wives of men with cancer of the penis (Smith *et al.* 1980), suggesting that these tumours may have in common a sexually transmitted infectious aetiology.

Highest risks in England and Wales were in Anglesey (1·80, significant), Lincolnshire Holland (1·50, NS), Flintshire (1·43, NS), and Montgomeryshire (1·37, NS). It is notable that Anglesey was also the highest-risk county for cancer of the cervix (Map 44). Otherwise, however, there was little similarity between the highest-risk areas for the two tumours. Low risks of penile cancer were in the south-east of England and in south-west Wales and mid-west Wales, but apart from this the pattern of risk was uneven. The low risks in the south-east of England parallel low risks there for cancer of the cervix (Map 44), and indeed all of the lowest-risk counties for cancer of the cervix showed low risk also for penile cancer.

Greatest circumcision rates in 1960–61 (Table A4.17), the earliest years of published data, were in the Metropolitan regions (i.e. south-east of England), but the relevant circumcisions for the present cancer map would be those conducted early in this century.

Risk of penile cancer was a little greater in rural and metropolitan than in urban areas. There was no clear pattern of risk within urbanization strata. Within rural areas greatest risks were in Merionethshire (1·93, NS) and Anglesey (1·82, NS); in urban areas in Anglesey (3·14, significant) and Montgomeryshire (2·16, NS); and in metropolitan areas in Norfolk (1·68, significant) and Lincolnshire Kesteven (1·61, NS).

Cancer of the scrotum (Map 53)

Cancer of the scrotum was the first cancer to be recognized to have an occupational cause, when Percivall Pott in 1775 noted a large excess of the tumour among chimney sweeps in England (Pott 1775). The risk in this occupation appears to have been much greater in England than in other countries, and it continued well into the twentieth century (Doll 1975). Several other occupational groups have subsequently been found to be at high risk: men exposed to shale oils and to mineral oils (including mule-spinners in the cotton industry (Southam and Wilson 1922), tool-setters and tool-fitters, and machine operators exposed to lubricating oils (Cruickshank and Squire 1950)), workers in coal-gas and coke production, and workers exposed to pitch and tar.

The current distribution of scrotal cancer in England and Wales (Map 53) strongly reflects the influence of these occupational factors, with high risks in Lancashire and the west Midlands. Highest risk were in Warwickshire (2·43, significant), Lancashire (2·30, significant), Herefordshire (1·84, NS, six cases), the Isle of Wight (1·77, NS, five cases), and Worcestershire (1·70, significant)[1]. Lowest

1 There was also a risk of 1·96 (NS) in Rutland, but based on only one case.

risks were in Norfolk (0·13, significant) and Shropshire (0·16, significant). The Lancashire excess seems likely to be explained by mule-spinning in the cotton mills[1] (Lee *et al.* 1972), and the west Midlands excess by various mineral oil exposures (Waldron *et al.* 1984). The gradient of risk with urbanization for scrotal cancer was much the greatest for any tumour in this atlas, with risks almost four times as great in metropolitan as in rural areas. Relative risks over twofold within the metropolitan stratum were in Kent (3·21, significant, based on three cases), Lincolnshire Lindsey (2·96, significant, six cases), Somerset (2·46, significant, six cases), Warwickshire (2·40, significant, 65 cases), Bedfordshire (2·05, NS, seven cases), and Worcestershire (2·04, significant, 13 cases); in urban areas in Lancashire (3·07, significant, 61 cases), Cheshire (2·90, significant, 28 cases), and Derbyshire (2·83, significant, 14 cases); and in rural areas in Northamptonshire (5·23, significant, five cases), Lincolnshire Holland (4·55, significant, two cases), Flintshire (4·00, significant, two cases), Carmarthenshire (3·63, NS, two cases), and Lincolnshire Kesteven (3·43, NS, two cases). Further investigation for possible occupational causes would particularly be merited for the high-risk areas not previously identified.

Cancer of the bladder (Maps 54 and 55)

Cancer of the bladder is far more frequent in males than females in England and Wales, as in most other countries. Risks in females in England and Wales are high by European standards, while risks in males are around average (Jensen *et al.* 1990; Smans *et al.*, in press). The great majority of the tumours are transitional cell. This tumour is aetiologically associated with several occupational exposures. A raised risk in dye-stuffs workers was first suggested by Rehn in the nineteenth century, but it was not clearly demonstrated until the 1950s when Case *et al.* (1954) in England showed a large relative risk associated with work with aromatic amines, most clearly for benzidine and 2-naphthylamine. Risk was also raised in the rubber industry, where the same compounds were used (Case and Hosker 1954). Manufacture of auramine and magenta lead to increased bladder cancer risks, but the agent(s) responsible are not clear. Use of these substances ceased around 1950, and there was never appreciable use of another carcinogenic dye-stuff, xenylamine, in England and Wales. Since the induction period for bladder cancers appears to be long, dye-related cases could still have been occurring during the study period. There is also an occupational aetiology in coal-gas and coke production (Doll *et al.* 1972). The proportion of bladder cancers in men attributable to occupation in two studies in Yorkshire has been estimated at between 3 and 19 per cent (Vineis and Simonato 1986).

Cancer of the bladder is aetiologically associated with smoking, although with a far lower relative risk than for lung cancer. The attributable risk for smoking in Manchester, England, has been estimated as 46 per cent in men and 14 per cent in women (Morrison *et al.* 1984). Two agents which have been used in treatment of cancer, cyclophosphamide and chlornaphazine, the latter chemically related to 2-naphthylamine, have led to increased risk of bladder cancer. There is also a raised risk after pelvic irradiation and probably after infection with *Schistosoma haematobium* (a bladder parasite endemic in parts of Africa and the Middle East). An uncommon association which might result in small-scale geographical clustering of cases in England and Wales is with paraplegia and tetraplegia (El-Masri and Fellows 1981). Finally, there were much publicized concerns a few years ago that risk of bladder cancer might relate to coffee-drinking and to use of artificial sweeteners, but the evidence has not been supportive of this (there is considerable confounding by smoking).

1 Even though mule-spinning ceased soon after World War II (Waterhouse 1972).

The pattern of risks of bladder cancer in England and Wales was distinctive. The range of risks in England beyond the counties bordering Wales was, with few exceptions, narrow. Risks in north and mid-Wales and bordering English counties were generally far lower. The pattern was similar in each sex, with greater risks in the industrial and mining south Wales counties of Glamorgan and Monmouthshire than elsewhere in Wales. The extension of the low-risk areas into the border counties of England suggests that the low risk was not simply a registration effect. In males, highest risk was in Wiltshire (1·15, significant), but with similar levels of risk in many other counties. In females, the highest risk was in West Yorkshire (1·17, significant), with again similar risks in many other counties. Lowest risks in males were in Merionethshire (0·53, significant) and Montgomeryshire (0·58, significant), and in females in Merionethshire (0·45, significant) and Radnorshire (0·49, significant).

In each sex there was a slight gradient of greater risks in more urban areas. Within urban and rural strata there was a similar pattern to that seen overall, but in metropolitan areas this could not be examined fully since the only metropolitan Welsh areas are in Glamorgan and Monmouthshire. Highest risk in males in metropolitan areas was in Oxfordshire (1·19, significant); in urban areas in West Sussex (1·25, significant); and in rural areas in the Isle of Wight (1·62, significant) and Monmouthshire (1·34, significant). In females in metropolitan areas, greatest risk was in Northumberland (1·23, significant); in urban areas in Rutland (1·83, NS) and Gloucestershire (1·36, significant); and in rural areas in Westmorland (1·35, NS) and Buckinghamshire (1·33, significant). Lowest risks in males in rural areas were in Merionethshire (0·39, significant) and Montgomeryshire (0·48, significant); in urban areas in Rutland (0·28, significant) and Merionethshire (0·38, significant); and in metropolitan areas in Lincolnshire Lindsey (0·72, significant). In females, lowest rural risks were in Breconshire (0·43, significant) and Merionethshire (0·49, significant); in urban areas in Radnorshire (0·36, NS) and Cardiganshire (0·55, NS); and in metropolitan areas in Worcestershire (0·71, significant).

Comparability of bladder cancer data between registry regions could be affected by differences in classification and in recording of papillomas of the bladder. These comprise up to a third of bladder tumours (Tomatis *et al.* 1990), but are not coded in the ICD[1] as malignant and their ICD categories were not included in the present maps. Mortality maps by region of England and Wales for 1969–73 (OPCS 1981) (recent county maps are not available), however, also show clearly lowest bladder cancer mortality in north and mid-Wales for men, and in Wales and the south-west of England for women.

Fifty years ago, bladder cancer death rates in men were low in much of Wales but also in the south-west of England and northern England (Stocks 1937) (see Map S9). In Australia, lower risk of bladder cancer has been found in Welsh than English migrants of each sex in incidence data (McCredie and Coates 1989) but not mortality data (Armstrong *et al.* 1983).

Risk of bladder cancer was not clearly greater in the most industrial areas of England and Wales than in other areas. There was no relationship at county level to the extent of dye- and rubber-working (Tables A4.14–A4.16), but the proportion of dye-workers in each county was low (the greatest in 1961 was 4·27 per cent of males in Cheshire), and in no county was more than one per cent of the work-force involved in the rubber industry. It seems possible that the apparently low Welsh risks may be an artefact of registration. The areas of Wales concerned do, however, show low lung cancer risks[2] (Maps 29–30), as the best marker available of smoking habits,

1 International Classification of Diseases.

2 Indeed for females the maps for these two tumours are generally very similar.

and smoking is the main known risk factor for bladder cancer in the general population.

Cancer of the kidney (Maps 56 and 57)

Cancer of the kidney is substantially less common than bladder cancer, although they have several epidemiological similarities. Correspondingly there were resemblances between the geographical patterns of these tumours within England and Wales.

About three-quarters of kidney cancers are renal cell carcinomas (hypernephromas). The ICD[1] category mapped comprises cancers of the kidney including the renal pelvis, but also cancers of the ureter, urethra, and other urinary-tract cancers except bladder; the non-renal tumours constitute only around 10 per cent of the total.

Cancer of the kidney is related to smoking, with attributable risks probably of similar magnitude to those for bladder cancer (Tomatis *et al.* 1990), and also to use of analgesic mixtures containing phenacetin. Ionising radiation is a cause of renal cancer, although the sensitivity of the kidney to carcinogenesis by this factor is relatively low. High risks have been reported in areas of Yugoslavia and Bulgaria where 'Balkan nephropathy' is endemic. Balkan immigrants to England and Wales, however, are not numerous (there were 14 000 individuals born in Yugoslavia and Bulgaria in England and Wales at the 1981 Census). A small percentage of renal tumours occur in children, and are mainly nephroblastomas (Wilms' tumour), for which high risk occurs in relation to certain congenital malformations.

For males particularly, the geographical pattern of cancer of the kidney showed some resemblance to that of bladder cancer, although the low-risk area was smaller than that for bladder cancer, and did not spread across the border from Wales to England. Nevertheless, risks in each county in England (with the exception of Rutland) were greater than any in Wales except Monmouthshire, Montgomeryshire, and Anglesey. The greatest risk was in Westmorland (1·46, significant), and the lowest were in Merionethshire (0·59, significant), Rutland (0·61, NS), and Pembrokeshire (0·67, significant). In females generally the same pattern held, although there were some high risks in mid-Wales, and risks were high in the four northernmost counties of England. Highest risks were in Montgomeryshire (1·33, NS), and Westmorland (1·32, NS), and lowest in Anglesey (0·51, significant), Radnorshire (0·58, NS), and Carmarthenshire (0·66, significant).

In each sex, risks were approximately equal in rural, urban, and metropolitan areas. Risks within the separate urbanization strata showed a less clear pattern than the overall renal cancer maps. In males, some low risks occurred in Wales in rural and urban areas, but not consistently. In rural areas highest risks were in Anglesey (1·70, significant) and Monmouthshire (1·46, significant), and lowest were in Radnorshire (0·15, significant) and Rutland (0·54, NS). In urban areas, highest risks were in Radnorshire (1·63, NS) and Norfolk (1·35, significant), and lowest in Merionethshire (0·37, significant) and Pembrokeshire (0·41, significant). In metropolitan areas, highest risk was in East Suffolk (1·29, NS), and lowest were in Lincolnshire Lindsey (0·44, significant) and Lincolnshire Kesteven (0·75, NS). In females, risks in rural and urban strata were mainly lowest in the west of Wales but there were a few low risks also in England. In rural areas, highest risks were in Durham (1·45, significant) and Northumberland (1·40, NS), and lowest in Radnorshire (0·35, NS) and Pembrokeshire (0·42, significant). In urban areas, highest risks were in Breconshire (1·78, NS) and Rutland (1·71, NS), and lowest in Cardiganshire (0·40, NS) and Lincolnshire Holland (0·41, significant). In females

1 International Classification of Diseases.

in metropolitan areas, highest risks were in Durham (1·26, significant) and Monmouthshire (1·19, NS), and lowest in Bedfordshire (0·49, significant) and Norfolk (0·61, significant).

The distribution of renal cancer incidence did not follow closely the mortality data presented by Gardner *et al.* (1983), in which greatest risk was in the north-east of England, and risks in north and mid-Wales, although not presented by county, were around average (exact data were not presented). The low Welsh incidence of renal cancer, however, parallels low lung cancer risks (Maps 29–30), which imply low smoking in these counties.

Cancer of the eye (Maps 58 and 59)

There are two main histological types of eye cancer, which have different aetiologies and occur at very different ages. The major tumour in children is retinoblastoma, which is hereditary (a dominant gene which behaves like a recessive) in about 40 per cent of cases. Beyond childhood, most eye cancers are melanomas, for which there is some evidence that risk factors similar to those for skin melanoma may apply (Tucker *et al.* 1985). The two histological types can largely be distinguished by analysing data separately for 0–14 years of age and 15 and over (Swerdlow 1983); we therefore analysed in this way.

Analyses for ages 0–14 showed no consistent pattern of incidence (maps not shown), and there were no counties where risk was markedly raised in both sexes. Significant highest risks in males were in Kent (2·06) and Glamorgan (2·00), while there were higher but not significant risks in Breconshire (5·70, based on two cases), Westmorland (4·54, two cases), and Montgomeryshire (3·84, two cases). In females, the only significantly raised risk was in Somerset (2·80), and there were non-significant high risks in Pembrokeshire (3·30, two cases), Oxfordshire (2·60, six cases), and Herefordshire (2·53, three cases). There was no consistent pattern of risk by degree of urbanization (risk in males was greatest in urban areas, but risk in females was lowest in this category (Table A5.45)). The tumour was too uncommon to analyse geographical risk within urbanization strata.

Maps 58 and 59 show eye cancer incidence at ages 15 and above. (The results for all ages (not shown) are similar to these maps, since most eye tumours are in adults). For males (Map 58) there was no clear geographical pattern. Highest risks were in Rutland (2·26, NS), Montgomeryshire (1·85, NS), the Isle of Wight (1·85, significant), and Cornwall (1·71, significant). For females (Map 59) there was also no clear pattern of incidence, with highest significant risks in Derbyshire (1·32), and Hampshire (1·28), and high but not significant risks in several counties, greatest in Breconshire (1·73) and Anglesey (1·67). Only in the Isle of Wight was there high risk in both sexes (1·85, significant, in males; 1·50, NS based on 11 cases, in females). There was no gradient of risk with degree of urbanization in either sex (we have not analysed geography within urbanization strata for this uncommon tumour). There was also no clear north–south gradient of risk in either sex. This contrasts with the geography of cutaneous melanoma (Maps 39 and 40), and is not supportive of the view that skin and eye melanomas are of similar aetiology.

Cancer of the nervous system (Maps 60 and 61)

These are mainly tumours of the brain (89 per cent of the total), but some are of the cranial nerves, meninges, spinal cord, and other parts of the nervous system. There is considerable difficulty in separating malignant from benign lesions of this site on clinical grounds, since both can produce similar clinical effects, depending on their location. It is also a particular difficulty for study of neurological tumour epidemiology, that the brain is a frequent site of metastasis of tumours originating in other parts of the body, and diagnostic distinction from these can be difficult.

Apart from a small proportion of cases in rare genetic conditions, the aetiology of nervous system tumours is unknown. Registered mortality and incidence rates are increasing at older ages, but this may reflect diagnostic changes.

In England and Wales in males there was a slight gradient of greater risk of malignancies of the nervous system in less-urban areas, and virtually no gradient with urbanization in females. In males (Map 60), highest risk was around London and in parts of East Anglia, with significant highest risks in East Suffolk (1·39), Oxfordshire (1·37), and Surrey (1·28), and non-significant high risk in Westmorland (1·32). Rural, urban, and metropolitan areas each showed a pattern similar to that seen overall. Highest risks in rural areas were in Oxfordshire (1·32) and Cheshire (1·22) (both significant), in urban areas in East Suffolk (1·48) and West Sussex (1·43) (both significant), and in metropolitan areas in Oxfordshire (1·57) and East Suffolk (1·47) (both significant).

In females (Map 61) there was a marked area of raised risk in the south-east of England including East Anglia, with greatest risks in Surrey (1·35), Oxfordshire (1·31), West Sussex (1·28), and London (1·23) (all significant). The distribution within rural, urban, and metropolitan areas separately was similar to that seen overall. The highest risks in rural areas were in East Sussex (1·40) and Northamptonshire (1·37) (both significant), in urban areas in Surrey (1·47) and West Sussex (1·43) (both significant), and in metropolitan areas in Oxfordshire (1·45) and London (1·36) (both significant). In each sex there was particularly low risk in north Wales.

Surrey and Oxfordshire, notably, showed high risk of nervous system cancers in each sex and urbanization stratum. Diagnostic as well as registration artefacts need to be considered for this.

Reanalysis of nervous system tumour risks including benign and unspecified as well as malignant tumours for the years for which we had these data (1968–81) (maps not shown), did not appreciably alter the pattern for males, and made more consistent the north–south difference for females. Of counties south of a line from the Severn estuary to the Wash, only Cornwall (0·86, NS) had an odds ratio in women of less than 1·00.

Mortality data suggest that the present maps are not a reflection of registration biases or errors: lowest risks have generally been found north of the Severn–Wash line, and highest risks south of it (OPCS 1981; Gardner *et al.* 1983).

Cancer of the thyroid (Maps 62 and 63)

This tumour constitutes less than one per cent of cancers occurring at all-ages in England and Wales, but is of somewhat greater importance (one to two per cent) at young adult ages. It is over twice as frequent in women as men. Registered incidence rates are increasing. Occult thyroid cancers occur frequently (Weiss 1979), and the degree to which they are diagnosed is relevant to the interpretation of geographical patterns of incidence. Their potential extent has been shown in autopsy data (Ron and Modan 1982).

The thyroid is one of the sites most susceptible to radiation carcinogenesis, and there has been concern about the possible risks from fallout radiation. Relationships have been found with non-malignant thyroid disease, but it is not clear which specific thyroid conditions are involved. High parity has been found to be a risk factor in women (Kravdal *et al.* 1991). Medullary carcinoma of the thyroid, a rare histological type, is often of hereditary origin.

In each sex, thyroid cancers showed a large range of risk within England and Wales, with the greatest risks in counties in north Wales. In males (Map 62) highest risks were in Merionethshire (1·84, NS), Montgomeryshire (1·70, NS), Denbighshire (1·62, significant), and Cardiganshire (1·49, NS). Apart from the high risk in north

Wales there was no consistent pattern. Risks varied little by degree of urbanization. Within metropolitan, urban, and rural strata separately there was no geographical pattern except for inconsistent evidence of high risk in north Wales (based on small numbers): in metropolitan areas highest risks were in Essex (2·04, significant) and Derbyshire (1·58, NS); in urban areas in Cardiganshire (3·71), Westmorland (2·55), and Denbighshire (2·31) (all significant); and in rural areas in Merionethshire (4·47, significant), Montgomeryshire (3·36, significant), and the Isle of Wight (2·10, NS).

In females (Map 63), highest risks overall were in Flintshire (1·74, significant), Merionethshire (1·52, NS), the Isle of Wight (1·46, significant), and Huntingdonshire (1·34, significant). Risks tended to be low in the north of England, south Wales, and most of the south-east of England. There was a slight gradient of higher risks in more rural areas. The high risks in north Wales for females were present in rural and urban areas separately (there are no metropolitan areas in north Wales). In rural areas, highest risks were in the Isle of Wight (2·50, significant), Flintshire (2·25, significant), and Merionethshire (1·67, NS); in urban areas in Flintshire (2·10, significant), Merionethshire (1·80, NS), and Somerset (1·44, significant); and in metropolitan areas in Somerset (1·84, significant) and Norfolk (1·38, significant).

To investigate the above patterns further, we subdivided the data by age. At younger ages (under 55) there was limited evidence of highest risk in north Wales and mid-Wales, but only present for males, and otherwise with no coherent pattern of risks. In males, greatest risks were in Cardiganshire (2·50, NS) and Merionethshire (1·97, NS), but greatest significant risks were in Norfolk (1·56) and Derbyshire (1·49). In females greatest risks were in the Isle of Wight (2·23), Huntingdonshire (1·63), Somerset (1·56), and Norfolk (1·49) (all significant).

At ages 55 years and above, in males there was a clear area of high risk centering on mid-Wales: greatest risks were in Montgomeryshire (2·09, NS), Denbighshire (2·06, significant), and Merionethshire (1·78, NS), with significant risk also in Norfolk (1·37). In females, there was less of a cluster of high-risk counties in north Wales, but nevertheless the highest risks were in Merionethshire (2·19, significant) and Flintshire (2·08, significant); the only other significant risks were in Dorset (1·27) and Somerset (1·22).

Mortality data for thyroid cancer are not available by county within Wales. For north- and mid-Wales combined, mortality rates were high in males, but not particularly so in females (Gardner *et al.* 1983). Thyroid cancer risks in Australia have been found to be greater in Welsh than English migrants in each sex, but based on small numbers (McCredie and Coates 1989).

The distribution of thyroid cancer incidence in England and Wales parallels strongly the distribution of past thyrotoxicosis mortality.[1] Stocks (1925) mapped mortality rates for exophthalmic goitre by county in 1913–22, excluding metropolitan areas and combining the sexes. Greatest rates were in Cardiganshire, Montgomeryshire, Radnorshire, Flintshire, Anglesey, and Westmorland. This corresponds particularly with the pattern seen now for thyroid cancer in older men, and in women in rural areas, although less clearly for women overall. Death rates from all thyroid disease (including tumours) in 1913–22 (again excluding metropolitan areas) were greatest in Radnorshire, Flintshire, Lincolnshire Kesteven, Merionethshire, Oxfordshire, Carmarthenshire, and Cardiganshire (Stocks and Karn 1927). McEwan (1938) mapped thyrotoxicosis mortality in 1936, and found high risk in north Wales, mid-Wales, Westmorland, and Huntingdonshire. More recent data on thyrotoxicosis mortality[2] showed highest risk in Wales (OPCS 1981;

1 There is also some similarity of the distribution in males to the pattern of several elements in geochemical maps (see p. 26).

2 Published for both sexes combined by region 1970–72 by OPCS (1981), and for females by county in England and Wales 1968–78 by Phillips *et al.* (1983).

Phillips *et al.* 1983), and high risks also in south-western England, the Lake District, certain English counties close to Wales, Northamptonshire, and Derbyshire. The focus of high thyroid cancer risks in Wales was in an area where there has been high fallout radiation (see p. 26). This is discussed further in dos Santos Silva and Swerdlow (in press).

Hodgkin's disease (Maps 64–67)

Hodgkin's disease was first described in 1832 by Thomas Hodgkin, a British physician. It is distinguished from other lymphomas on histological criteria: the presence of Reed–Sternberg cells plus appropriate surrounding stroma. There are several histological subtypes, whose aetiological homogeneity is unclear. The prognosis of Hodgkin's disease has improved greatly, due to better treatment, over the last 25 years. Understanding of its aetiology has not progressed as greatly, however. There is some support for the hypothesis that Hodgkin's disease is a rare sequel of the late occurrence of a common infection: for instance there are raised risks in persons of high social class and from small sibships (Gutensohn and Cole 1981), which might accord with this. The evidence is not strong, however, and the aetiology remains unknown. Geographical and time–space clustering of the disease have repeatedly been sought, but not consistently found (Smith 1982). There is clear evidence for a genetic element in risk of Hodgkin's disease, with associations shown with various HLA antigens, and demonstration by linkage studies that these associations are due to a susceptibility gene (Easton and Peto 1990).

Hodgkin's disease shows different epidemiological characteristics in young adults and at older ages (MacMahon 1966). The age–incidence curve in England and Wales shows a peak in young adults, then a decline followed by an increasing incidence at older ages. We have therefore mapped the tumour separately for age groups 0–44, and 45 and over.

In males at younger ages (Map 64) risk generally showed an east-west gradient, with low risk in much of Wales and bordering English counties. Highest risks were in Westmorland (1·74, significant), Lincolnshire Kesteven (1·25, NS), West Suffolk (1·18, NS), and Cheshire (1·18, significant). Risks varied little by degree of urbanization. Within metropolitan, urban, and rural areas separately there was no consistent geographical pattern, with highest risks in metropolitan areas in Monmouthshire (2·18, significant) and Somerset (1·49, NS); in urban areas in Lincolnshire Kesteven (2·02, NS) and Westmorland (1·61, NS); and in rural areas in Westmorland (2·52, NS) and East Yorkshire (2·10, significant).

In females aged 0–44 (Map 65) there was a cluster of high risks around and to the north of London, but otherwise no pattern, and slightly higher risk in rural than in urban and metropolitan areas. Highest risks were in West Suffolk (1·66, significant), Cambridgeshire (1·48, significant), and Lincolnshire Holland (1·44, NS). In rural areas, highest risks were in West Suffolk (2·05, significant) and Rutland (1·82, NS); in urban areas in Lincolnshire Holland (2·17, NS) and Surrey (1·55, significant); and in metropolitan areas in Monmouthshire (1·72, significant) and Bedfordshire (1·51, NS).

At older ages in males (Map 66), risk of Hodgkin's disease showed a gradient of decreasing risk in more urban areas, and there was a clear pattern of high risks in the counties on the west coast of Wales and in the Lake District. Highest risks were in Merionethshire (2·73, significant), Westmorland (1·78, significant), Radnorshire (1·74, NS), and Anglesey (1·64, significant). The tendency for high risks to occur in counties near the coast of Wales was less clear in urban and rural strata separately (none of the counties in the west of Wales have metropolitan areas). Highest risks in rural areas were in Merionethshire (2·88, significant), Radnorshire (2·50, NS), and Westmorland (2·22, significant); in urban areas in Cardiganshire (2·60, significant) and Lincolnshire Holland (1·80, NS); and in metropolitan areas in Monmouthshire (1·99, significant), and Essex (1·84, significant).

In females aged 45 and over (Map 67), there was slightly greater risk in rural than in more urban areas, and, although risk was high in parts of Wales, there was no clear band of raised risks on its west coast. Highest risks were in Anglesey (1·96), Monmouthshire (1·74), Flintshire (1·67), and Denbighshire (1·59) (all significant). In rural areas, risk was highest in parts of Wales, but this was not as clearly true for urban and metropolitan areas: highest rural risks were in Westmorland (2·15, NS) and Monmouthshire (1·86, NS); urban in Anglesey (1·80, NS) and Montgomeryshire (1·78, NS); and metropolitan in Monmouthshire (2·77, significant) and Lincolnshire Lindsey (1·46, NS). It is notable that in each sex and age group the highest metropolitan risk of Hodgkin's disease was in Monmouthshire (i.e. in the town of Newport, the only metropolitan area in Monmouthshire — see Table A1.1).

We have not presented separately here maps of Hodgkin's disease overall, which reflect contributions from the maps already shown. Highest risks in males overall were in Wales and the Lake District: in Merionethshire (1·78, significant), Westmorland (1·76, significant), and Radnorshire (1·40, NS). In females, greatest risks were in West Suffolk (1·54, significant), Monmouthshire (1·42, significant), and Lincolnshire Holland (1·39, NS). In urban, rural, and metropolitan areas separately, highest risks again tended to be in Welsh counties.

Potential for artefact in registration of Hodgkin's disease comes from difficulties in distinguishing it from non-Hodgkin's lymphoma. The borderline between the two is a source of disagreement between pathologists, but also the tumours may be confused by registry clerks, and lymphomas not further specified are coded in the ICD[1] to the rubric for non-Hodgkin's lymphoma. Comparison of the Hodgkin's disease maps with those for non-Hodgkin's lymphoma (Maps 68 and 69), however, does not show the reciprocal differences which might be expected if such difficulties had caused major artefacts in the geographical pattern.

It is not obvious why, but the high-risk counties for Hodgkin's disease in older men were almost exclusively the Welsh-speaking counties (see Table A4.24), and the distribution also showed a similarity to the pattern in geochemical maps of high levels of several elements (see p. 26).

Non-Hodgkin's lymphoma (Maps 68 and 69)

This heading includes all lymphomas apart from Hodgkin's disease. Several different subclassifications have been proposed, on histological, immunological, and clinical grounds, and the aetiological homogeneity of non-Hodgkin's lymphomas (NHL) as a group remains unclear. They probably share aetiological factors, at least to some extent.

Known causes of NHL are immunological deficiencies and radiation exposure. Risk is greatly increased in individuals with various rare primary immunodeficiency disorders, for instance ataxia telangiectasia and Wiskott–Aldrich syndrome, and in persons given immunosuppressive therapy, for instance in renal and cardiac transplantation. In the latter, risk increases within a year of transplantation, which has been taken as suggesting that oncogenic viruses may be involved. Burkitt's lymphoma, a rare lymphoma in England and Wales (although far more common in children in parts of tropical Africa), has been linked to infection with Epstein–Barr virus, perhaps facilitated by the immunological effects of malaria. Raised risk of NHL has been noted in patients with certain immune-related diseases — Sjögren's syndrome, and coeliac disease. The risk of NHL is increased in AIDS patients, but

1 International Classification of Diseases.

this is too recent to have affected the data here appreciably. Various occupational exposures, including herbicides, have been claimed to be associated with NHL, but there is not yet firm evidence for this.

In England and Wales, NHL showed a striking excess in each sex south of a line from the Severn estuary to the Wash, but the range of risks was modest. This was similar to the pattern in mortality data (Gardner *et al.* 1983). In males, highest risks were in Rutland (1·53), the Isle of Wight (1·37), and Lincolnshire Holland (1·29) (all significant). Risk was slightly greater in rural than in more urban areas. There was a similar geographical distribution within metropolitan, urban, and rural areas separately to that seen overall, with highest risks in metropolitan areas in Essex (1·40) and Northamptonshire (1·36) (both significant), in urban areas in Rutland (1·72, NS), the Isle of Wight (1·70, significant), and Norfolk (1·63, significant), and in rural areas in Worcestershire (1·35, significant) and Montgomeryshire (1·32, NS).

In females, highest risks of NHL were in Berkshire (1·29), Northamptonshire (1·27), Somerset (1·27), and Buckinghamshire (1·25) (all significant), with a slightly greater risk in rural than urban and metropolitan areas. There was generally a similar pattern to that seen overall when risks within urbanization strata were examined separately — highest metropolitan risks were in Somerset (1·47, significant) and Kent (1·44, NS); urban risks in Cardiganshire (1·52, NS) and Bedfordshire (1·49, significant); and rural risks in Huntingdonshire (1·65, significant) and Northamptonshire (1·57, significant).

A potential artefact in the NHL data could arise from variation in the specificity of the histology data used by different regional registries, since lymphomas of sites such as the testis and brain are coded in the International Classification of Diseases (ICD) to lymphoma if this histology is specified, but to testis, brain, etc., if these sites are mentioned without specification of histology. It was not the case, however, that those counties where general specificity of registration data appeared to be worst (see p. 18) usually had raised odds ratios for NHL.

The three-digit ICD codes for NHL also include lymphomas not further specified, and hence the NHL maps could include ill-specified or ill-coded cases of Hodgkin's disease — a potential source of artefact. Comparing the maps for NHL and Hodgkin's disease, however, does not show evidence of compensating errors to suggest that this was a substantial problem.

The distribution of NHL in each sex showed a particularly clear difference between high risks south of a line from the Severn estuary to the Wash, and low risks north of it. Whether this was due to registration or diagnostic artefact, or was a real effect, would need further investigation.

Multiple myeloma (Maps 70 and 71)

Multiple myeloma is a malignancy of plasma cells; a lymphoproliferative tumour. The malignant plasma cells originate, although perhaps not solely, from the bone marrow, and they cause destruction of bone, especially of the skull. The tumour has undergone one of the greatest apparent increases in incidence and mortality in recent years of any cancer in England and Wales, particularly at older ages. There is reason to believe, however, that much or perhaps all of this increase has been an artefact of improved diagnosis. The tumour occurs mainly in the elderly, and its definitive diagnosis requires relatively sophisticated laboratory and bone marrow tests, so diagnostic artefact probably plays a large part in apparent differences in rates. We have therefore mapped myeloma at ages under 65, as well as for all ages, in the hope that diagnostic artefacts may have been of relatively minor importance for younger patients during the period examined.

There is evidence that radiation may be a cause of myeloma, and in England and Wales an excess has been noted in nuclear industry workers at Sellafield,

Cumberland (Smith and Douglas 1986). In general, however, the aetiology remains unknown.

In each sex in England and Wales, myeloma risk increased slightly with decreasing urbanization. There was an excess risk south of a line from the Severn to the Wash, particularly for males. This concurs with the pattern in mortality data (Gardner *et al.* 1983). In males, highest risks (all significant) were in Cardiganshire (1·52), Cambridgeshire (1·40), Dorset (1·28), and Wiltshire (1·27), and in females they were in Breconshire (1·64, significant), Anglesey (1·52, significant), Montgomeryshire (1·43, NS), and Wiltshire (1·36, significant). When the analyses were restricted to ages under 65 years, the results were similar. Greatest relative risks in males were in Cardiganshire (1·83, significant), Radnorshire (1·49, NS), and Wiltshire (1·33, significant), and in females in Radnorshire (1·95, NS), Breconshire (1·93, significant), and Huntingdonshire (1·59, significant).

Considering urban, rural, and metropolitan residents separately, in males there was a clear excess south of the Severn–Wash line for rural residents, and less clearly for urban and metropolitan residents. Highest risks in rural areas were in Cambridgeshire (1·43, significant) and Flintshire (1·33, NS); in urban areas in Wiltshire (1·33, significant) and West Sussex (1·33, significant); and in metropolitan areas in Kent (2·04, significant) and Oxfordshire (1·62, significant). For females there was a slight excess south of the Severn–Wash line in rural residents but no pattern for urban and metropolitan residents. In rural areas highest risks were in Montgomeryshire (2·06, significant) and Anglesey (2·03, significant); in urban areas in Breconshire (2·43, significant), Rutland (1·92, NS), and Westmorland (1·76, significant); and in metropolitan areas in Somerset (1·51, significant) and Berkshire (1·39, significant).

Leukaemia: all ages (Maps 72 and 73)

Leukaemias are malignant neoplasms arising from the precursor cells of white blood cells and tissue leucocytes. They are a little more common in males than females (Table 1). Leukaemias constitute about two-and-a-half per cent of malignancies in each sex in England and Wales (Table 1), and are notable for their low variation in incidence between countries with reasonably reliable data. Leukaemias can be subdivided by histological cell type, and by degree of acuteness/chronicity. Although there are differences in descriptive epidemiology between these categories (for instance, acute lymphocytic leukaemia occurs mainly in children, whereas chronic lymphoid leukaemia is largely a disease of old age), they do share aetiological factors to some extent (Tomatis *et al.* 1990). The proportion of leukaemias for which cell type and chronicity are specified varies greatly between regional registries in England and Wales, and we have therefore pooled all subtypes in the present analyses.

Ionizing radiation has long been known to be a cause of leukaemia, with excess risk shown in radiologists and in the survivors of the Hiroshima and Nagasaki atomic bombs, and also after therapeutic radiation. Risk is increased for acute leukaemia and chronic myeloid leukaemia, but appears not to be raised for chronic lymphoid leukaemia. *In utero* exposure to ionizing radiation is associated with increased risk of childhood leukaemia. Childhood leukaemia risk is also known to be greatly increased in persons with Down's syndrome as well as in certain other rarer congenital chromosome abnormalities. Therapeutic exposure to alkylating agents is a potent cause of leukaemia, and chloramphenicol treatment can probably also cause the disease. Benzene exposure is an occupational cause. Infection has long been seen as a likely cause, but only recently shown, in relation to human T-lymphotropic virus type 1 (HTLV 1), primarily in Japan and the West Indies. The known causes, however, account for only a small proportion of cases.

In England and Wales in each sex there was a tendency for raised risk of leukaemia to occur in the most southern counties of England, in north Wales, and in an area north-east of London (Maps 72 and 73). The range of risks across the country was not great, however, and the counties with the highest (and lowest) risks did not generally coincide between males and females. In males, greatest risks were in Lincolnshire Holland (1·46, significant), Flintshire (1·28, significant), and Anglesey (1·27, NS). In females, greatest risks were in Anglesey (1·18, NS), Huntingdonshire (1·16, NS), Cardiganshire (1·13, NS), and Somerset (1·12, significant).

In each sex there was a small gradient of higher risks in less-urban areas. Within the metropolitan stratum, there was some indication of greater risk in the south-east of England than elsewhere: in males greatest risks were in Cumberland (1·24, NS) and East Sussex (1·22, significant); in females greatest risks were in Lincolnshire Kesteven (1·35, significant) and Kent (1·31, NS). In urban areas, there was no pattern in either sex, but there was a similarity of distribution of high- and low-risk counties between the sexes in mid- and north Wales. In males, greatest risks were in Lincolnshire Holland (1·36, NS) and Devon (1·34, significant), and in females in Rutland (1·44, NS) and Merionethshire (1·40, NS), with greatest significant risk in East Suffolk (1·31). There was no pattern discernible in rural areas: greatest risks in males were in Lincolnshire Holland (1·48, significant) and Flintshire (1·34, significant), and in females in Huntingdonshire (1·32, NS) and Oxfordshire (1·23, NS) (with no significant raised risks).

Childhood leukaemia (Maps 74 and 75)

Leukaemias show a peak of incidence in childhood, and account for about one-third of malignancies incident in chidren in England and Wales. Eighty per cent are acute lymphocytic leukaemias. The known causes (see p. 73) may account for around a quarter of cases (Doll 1989; Doll and Darby 1990). Improvements in therapy have led to dramatic reductions in mortality rates in the last 20 years. The geographical distribution of childhood leukaemias in Britain has been the subject of intense epidemiological study since the finding of a much raised risk, but based on very few cases, in the vicinity of the Sellafield nuclear installation in Cumberland (Black 1984). Excesses have also been reported near other nuclear sites. Although this might be due to radiation exposures, it has been suggested that it might alternatively be part of a more general phenomenon — that childhood leukaemia may be a rare response to an unidentified infection whose transmission might be facilitated by increased population mixing, as occurred with influxes of workers and their families to certain areas, such as around nuclear installations, and with the creation of new towns (Kinlen *et al.* 1990).

The childhood leukaemia maps presented here are based on registrations by the Childhood Cancer Research Group, whose registry is virtually complete for this diagnostic group (see pp. 7 and 14). There was no obvious pattern of childhood leukaemia distribution in England and Wales, and no similarity between the sexes. Although in each sex there was a fivefold range of risks between counties, this resulted from statistically unreliable estimates of risks in small counties with few cases: in counties with larger numbers, the range was considerably smaller (Table A5.45). In males, highest rates of childhood leukaemia were in Radnorshire (2·11, NS), Montgomeryshire (1·97, NS), and Caernarvonshire (1·61, NS), and the only significant rates were in Wiltshire (1·50) and Surrey (1·28). In females, greatest rates were in Rutland (2·10, NS), Huntingdonshire (1·81, significant), and Westmorland (1·42, NS), and the only other significant result was a low rate in Nottinghamshire (0·72).

Comparison of the leukaemia maps with the extent of childhood population mobility (Map E11), which might indicate increased risks of a putative leukaemogenic infection (see above), shows no clear correspondence. The distribution of leukaemia also does not parallel indoor radon concentrations (Map E8).

We also analysed the risk of lymphocytic plus unspecified leukaemias in children, since this will effectively give analyses for the most common type of childhood leukaemia, acute lymphocytic, which constitutes about 80 per cent of childhood leukaemias.[1] The geographical pattern of this subgroup was very similar to that for leukaemias overall, and therefore has not been shown separately. Greatest rates in males were in Radnorshire (2·61, NS), Montgomeryshire (2·09, NS), Carmarthenshire (1·76, significant), and Wiltshire (1·59, significant). Greatest rates in females were in Rutland (2·68, NS), Huntingdonshire (1·91, significant), Westmorland (1·64, NS), and Lincolnshire Kesteven (1·45, NS). The only other significant raised or decreased rates in either sex were in Surrey (1·31) in males, and Berkshire (1·36), Nottinghamshire (0·70), and Caernarvonshire (0·18) in females. We did not have data by urbanization category available from the Childhood Cancer Research Group for childhood leukaemia.

1 All of the leukaemias categorized as lymphocytic are acute, and unspecified cases would also mainly be acute lymphocytic (if their diagnoses were known).

References

Acheson, E. D., Hadfield, E. H., and Macbeth, R. G. (1967). Carcinoma of the nasal cavity and accessory sinuses in woodworkers. *Lancet*, **i**, 311–12.

Acheson, E. D., Cowdell, R. H., and Jolles, B. (1970). Nasal cancer in the Northamptonshire boot and shoe industry. *British Medical Journal*, **i**, 385–93.

Armstrong, B. K., Woodings, T. L., Stenhouse, N. S., and McCall, M. G. (1983). *Mortality from cancer in migrants to Australia, 1962–1971*. National Health and Medical Research Council, Perth.

Barker, D. J. P., Gardner, M. J., Power, C., and Hutt, M. S. R. (1979). Prevalence of gall stones at necropsy in nine British towns: a collaborative study. *British Medical Journal*, **2**, 1389–92.

Barker, D. J. P., Chamberlain, A. T., Guyer, P. B., and Gardner, M. J. (1980). Paget's disease of bone: the Lancashire focus. *British Medical Journal*, **280**, 1105–7.

Barker, D. J. P., Coggon, D., Osmond, C., and Wickham, C. (1990). Poor housing in childhood and high rates of stomach cancer in England and Wales. *British Journal of Cancer*, **61**, 575–8.

Beral, V., Inskip, H., Fraser, P., Booth, M., Coleman, D., and Rose, G. (1985). Mortality of employees of the United Kingdom Atomic Energy Authority, 1946–1979. *British Medical Journal*, **291**, 440–7.

Beral, V., Fraser, P., Carpenter, L., Booth, M., Brown, A., and Rose, G. (1988). Mortality of employees of the Atomic Weapons Establishment, 1951–82. *British Medical Journal*, **297**, 757–70.

Beral, V., Peterman T. A., Berkelman R. L., and Jaffe, H. W. (1990). Kaposi's sarcoma among persons with AIDS: a sexually transmitted infection? *Lancet*, **335**, 123–8.

Black, D. (1984). *Investigation of the possible increased incidence of cancer in West Cumbria*. Report of the Independent Advisory Group (Chairman D. Black). HMSO, London.

Blot, W. J. and Fraumeni, J. F. Jr. (1982). Geographic epidemiology of cancer in the United States. In *Cancer epidemiology and prevention*, (ed. D. Schottenfeld and J. F. Fraumeni, Jr.), pp. 179–93. W. B. Saunders, Philadelphia.

Board of Inland Revenue (1973). *The Survey of Personal Incomes 1970–71*. London, HMSO.

Boyd, J. T., Doll, R., Faulds, J. S., and Leiper, J. (1970). Cancer of the lung in iron ore (haematite) miners. *British Journal of Industrial Medicine*, **27**, 97–105.

Braddon, F. E. M., Wadsworth, M. E. J., Davies, J. M. C., and Cripps, H. A. (1988). Social and regional differences in food and alcohol consumption and their measurement in a national birth cohort. *Journal of Epidemiology and Community Health*, **42**, 341–9.

Breslow, N. *et al.* (1977). Latent carcinoma of prostate at autopsy in seven areas. *International Journal of Cancer*, **20**, 680–8.

Breslow, N. E. and Day, N. E. (1987). *Statistical methods in cancer research*. Volume II: The design and analysis of cohort studies. International Agency for Research on Cancer, Scientific Publications, No. 82. IARC, Lyon.

Butler, N. R., Golding, J., Haslum, M., and Stewart-Brown, S. (1982). Recent findings from the 1970 child health and education study: preliminary communication. *Journal of the Royal Society of Medicine*, **75**, 781–4.

Campbell, W. J. and Nicholson, A. (1989). *PC Mapics*. Mapics Ltd, London.

Case, R. A. M. and Hosker, M. E. (1954). Tumour of the urinary bladder as an occupational disease in the rubber industry in England and Wales. *British Journal of Preventive and Social Medicine*, **8**, 39–50.

Case, R. A. M., Hosker, M. E., McDonald, D. B., and Pearson, J. T. (1954). Tumours of the urinary bladder in workmen engaged in the manufacture and use of certain dyestuff intermediates in the British chemical industry. Part I. The role of aniline, benzidine, alpha-naphthylamine, and beta-naphthylamine. *British Journal of Industrial Medicine*, **11**, 75–104.

Cawse, P. A. and Horrill, A. D. (1986). *A survey of caesium-137 and plutonium in British soils in 1977*. AERE Harwell Report, No. 10155. Harwell Laboratory, Oxfordshire.

Central Statistical Office (1958). *Standard industrial classification*, (2nd edn). HMSO, London.

Central Statistical Office (1972). *Social trends No. 3*. HMSO, London.

Clarke, J. I., Dewdney, J. C., Evans, I. S., Rhind, D. W., Visvalingam, M., and Denham, C. (1980). *People in Britain. A Census Atlas*. HMSO, London.

Coates, B. E. and Rawstron, E. M. (1971). *Regional variations in Britain. Studies in economic and social geography*. B.T. Batsford, London.

Cole, P. (1980). Introduction. In *Statistical methods in cancer research*. Volume 1: *The analysis of case-control studies*. (N. E. Breslow and N. E. Day), pp. 14–40. International Agency for Research on Cancer, Scientific Publications, No. 32. IARC, Lyon.

Cook-Mozaffari, P. J., Ashwood, F. L., Vincent, T., Forman, D., and Alderson, M. (1987). *Cancer incidence and mortality in the vicinity of nuclear installations, England and Wales, 1959–80*. SMPS No. 51. HMSO, London.

Court Brown, W. M., Doll, R., Heasman, M. A., and Sissons, H. A. (1961). Geographical distribution of primary tumours of bone in England and Wales. *British Journal of Preventive and Social Medicine*, **15**, 167–70.

Cruickshank, C. N. D. and Squire, J. R. (1950). Skin cancer in the engineering industry from the use of mineral oil. *British Journal of Industrial Medicine*, **7**, 1–11.

Darby, S. and Doll R. (1990). Radon in houses: how large is the risk? *Radiation Protection in Australia*, **8**, 83–8.

Davie, R., Butler, N., and Goldstein, H. (1972). *From birth to seven: the second report of the national child development study (1958 cohort)*. Longman, London.

Davies, J. M., Easton, D. F., and Bidstrup, P. L. (1991). Mortality from respiratory cancer and other causes in United Kingdom chromate production workers. *British Journal of Industrial Medicine*, **48**, 299–313.

Day, N. E. (1984). The geographic pathology of cancer of the oesophagus. *British Medical Bulletin*, **40**, 329–34.

Department of Education and Science (1969). *Statistics of education 1968*. Volume 1: *Schools*. HMSO, London.

Department of the Environment (1978). *Digest of environmental pollution statistics*. Pollution Report No. 4. HMSO, London.

Department of Health and Social Security and Office of Population Censuses and Surveys (1970). *Report on Hospital In-Patient Enquiry for the year 1967. Part I: Tables*. HMSO, London.

Department of Health and Social Security and Office of Population Censuses and Surveys (1972). *Report on Hospital In-Patient Enquiry for the year 1970. Part I: Tables*. HMSO, London.

Doll, R. (1967). *Prevention of cancer. Pointers from epidemiology. The Rock Carling Fellowship 1967*. The Nuffield Provincial Hospitals Trust, London.

Doll, R. (1975). Pott and the prospects for prevention (the 7th Walter Hubert Lecture). *British Journal of Cancer*, **32**, 263–72.

Doll, R. (1989). The epidemiology of childhood leukaemia. *Journal of the Royal Statistical Society*, Series A, **152**, 341–51.

Doll, R. (1990). Are we winning the fight against cancer? An epidemiological assessment. *European Journal of Cancer*, **26**, 500–8.

Doll, R. and Darby, S. (1990). Childhood leukaemia in the United Kingdom. *Radiation Protection in Australia*, **8**, 55–61.

Doll, R. and Peto, R. (1981). *The causes of cancer. Quantitative estimates of avoidable risks of cancer in the United States today*. Oxford University Press.

Doll, R. *et al.* (1972). Mortality of gasworkers — final report of a prospective study. *British Journal of Industrial Medicine*, **29**, 394–406.

dos Santos Silva, I. and Swerdlow, A. J. (in press). Thyroid cancer epidemiology in England and Wales: time trends and geographical distribution. *British Journal of Cancer*.

Easton, D. and Peto, J. (1990). The contribution of inherited predisposition to cancer incidence. *Cancer Surveys*, **9**, 395–416.

Easton, D. F., Peto, J., and Doll, R. (1988). Cancer of the respiratory tract in mustard gas workers. *British Journal of Industrial Medicine*, **45**, 652–9.

El-Masri, W. S. and Fellows, G. (1981). Bladder cancer after spinal cord injury. Incidence, presentation, histology and prognosis compared with bladder cancer in the non-paralysed population. *Paraplegia*, **19**, 265–70.

Farr, W. (1839). Letter to the Registrar General, from William Farr, Esq, respecting abstracts of the recorded causes of death registered during the half-year ending December 31, 1837, with numerous tables. London, 6 May, 1839. In *First Annual Report of the Registrar-General of births, deaths, and marriages in England*, pp. 86–166, Longman, Orme, Brown, Green, and Longmans for HMSO, London.

Forman, D. Newell, D. G., Fullerton, F., Yarnell, J. W. G., Stacey, A. R., Wald, N., and Sitas, F. (1991). Association between infection with *Helicobacter pylori* and risk of gastric cancer: evidence from a prospective investigation. *British Medical Journal*, **302**, 1302–5.

Fox, A. J., Goldblatt, P., and Kinlen, L. J. (1981). A study of the mortality of Cornish tin miners. *British Journal of Industrial Medicine*, **38**, 378–80.

Franco, E. L., Campos Filho, N., Villa, L. L., and Torloni, H. (1988). Correlation patterns of cancer relative frequencies with some socioeconomic and demographic indicators in Brazil: an ecologic study. *International Journal of Cancer*, **41**, 24–9.

Galpin, O. P., Whitaker, C. J., Whitaker, Rh., and Kassab, J. Y. (1990). Gastric cancer in Gwynedd. Possible links with bracken. *British Journal of Cancer*, **61**, 737–40.

Gao, Y.-T. *et al.* (1987). Lung cancer among Chinese women. *International Journal of Cancer*, **40**, 604–9.

Gardner, M. J., Acheson, E. D., and Winter, P. D. (1982). Mortality from mesothelioma of the pleura during 1968–78 in England and Wales. *British Journal of Cancer*, **46**, 81–8.

Gardner, M. J., Winter, P. D., Taylor, C. P., and Acheson, E. D. (1983). *Atlas of cancer mortality in England and Wales, 1968–1978*. Wiley, Chichester.

Gardner, M. J., Winter, P. D., and Barker, D. J. P. (1984). *Atlas of mortality from selected diseases in England and Wales, 1968–1978*. Wiley, Chichester.

General Register Office (1890). *Fifty-second Annual Report of the Registrar-General of births, deaths and marriages in England (1889)*. HMSO, London.

General Register Office (1933). *The Registrar-General's Decennial Supplement: England and Wales 1921. Part III: Estimates of population, statistics of marriages, births and deaths: 1911–1920 tables*. HMSO, London.

General Register Office (1934). *Census of England and Wales, 1931. Industry tables*. HMSO, London.

General Register Office (1952). *The Registrar General's Statistical Review of England and Wales for the year 1950. Tables: Part I: Medical.* HMSO, London.

General Register Office (1954–5). *Census 1951: England and Wales. County reports.* HMSO, London.

General Register Office (1957). *Census 1951, England and Wales. Industry tables.* HMSO, London.

General Register Office (1958). *The Registrar General's Decennial Supplement: England and Wales, 1951. Area mortality.* HMSO, London.

General Register Office (1960). *Classification of occupations, 1960.* HMSO, London.

General Register Office (1965*a*). *Census 1961: England and Wales. Index of place names* (2 volumes). HMSO, London.

General Register Office (1965*b*, 1966). *Census 1961: England and Wales. Occupation, industry, socio-economic groups.* County Volumes. HMSO, London.

General Register Office (1965*c*). *Census 1961: England and Wales. Housing tables. Part III: Local housing indices.* HMSO, London.

General Register Office (1967). *The Registrar General's Decennial Supplement: England and Wales, 1961. Area mortality tables.* HMSO, London.

Green, B. M. R.. Lomas, P. R., and O'Riordan, M. C. (1992). Radon in dwellings in England. NRPB-R254. National Radiological Protection Board, Chilton, Oxfordshire.

Greenwood, M. (1925). *Étude statistique sur le cancer du sein et de l'utérus.* In *Report on the Results of Demographic Investigations in Certain Selected Countries.* League of Nations Health Organization Cancer Commission, CH333, Vol. 1. 2nd Edition, pp. 36–104. League of Nations, Geneva.

Gutensohn, N. and Cole, P. (1981). Childhood social environment and Hodgkin's disease. *New England Journal of Medicine*, **304**, 135–40.

Haskey, J. (1991). The ethnic minority populations resident in private households — estimates by county and metropolitan district of England and Wales. *Population Trends*, **63**, 22–35.

Haviland, A. (1875). *The geographical distribution of heart disease and dropsy, cancer in females and phthisis in females, in England and Wales.* Smith, Elder & Co., London.

Haywood, S. M. and Simmonds, J. R. (1983). *Generalised derived limits for radioisotopes of caesium.* Report DL 7. National Radiological Protection Board, Chilton, Oxfordshire.

Henderson, B. E., Ross, R. K., Pike, M. C., and Depue, R. H. (1983). Epidemiology of testis cancer. In: *Urological Cancer* (ed. D. G. Skinner), pp. 237–50. Grune & Stratton, New York.

Hill, A. B. and Faning, E. L. (1948). Studies in the incidence of cancer in a factory handling inorganic compounds of arsenic. I. Mortality experience in the factory. *British Journal of Industrial Medicine*, 5, 1–6.

Ho, J. H. C., Man, K. K., Tsao, S. Y., and Chan, P. K. (1987). Hong Kong. In *Cancer incidence in five continents*, Vol. V. International Agency for Research on Cancer, Scientific Publication No. 88 (ed. C. Muir, J. Waterhouse, T. Mack, J. Powell, and S. Whelan), pp. 402–5. IARC, Lyon.

Home Office (1969). *Liquor licensing statistics for England and Wales, 1968.* HMSO, London.

Howe, G. M. (1970). *National atlas of disease mortality in the United Kingdom.* (Revised and enlarged edition). Nelson, London.

Hughes, J. S., Shaw, K. B., and O'Riordan, M. C. (1989). *Radiation exposure of the UK population — 1988 review*, NRPB-R227. National Radiological Protection Board, Chilton, Oxfordshire.

Jensen, O. M., Carstensen, B., Glattre, E., Malker, B., Pukkala, E., and Tulinius, H. (1988). *Atlas of cancer incidence in the Nordic countries.* Puna Musta, Helsinki.

Jensen, O. M., Estève, J., Møller, H., and Renard, H. (1990). Cancer in the European Community and its member states. *European Journal of Cancer*, **26**, 1167–1256.

Kaldor, J., Peto, J., Easton, D., Doll, R., Hermon, C., and Morgan, L. (1986). Models for respiratory cancer in nickel refinery workers. *Journal of the National Cancer Institute*, **77**, 841–8.

Kemp, I., Boyle, P., Smans, M., and Muir, C. (eds.) (1985). *Atlas of cancer incidence in Scotland 1975–1980. Incidence and epidemiological perspective.* International Agency for Research on Cancer, Scientific Publications, No. 72. IARC, Lyon.

Kinlen, L. J., Badaracco, M. A., Moffett, J., and Vessey, M.P. (1974). A survey of the use of oestrogens during pregnancy in the United Kingdom and of the genito-urinary cancer mortality and incidence rates in young people in England and Wales. *Journal of Obstetrics and Gynaecology of the British Commonwealth*, **81**, 849–55.

Kinlen, L. J., Clarke, K., and Hudson, C. (1990). Evidence from population mixing in British new towns 1946–85 of an infective basis for childhood leukaemia. *Lancet*, **336**, 577–82.

Knight, I. (1984). *The heights and weights of adults in Great Britain.* HMSO, London.

Kopeć, A.C. (1970). *The distribution of the blood groups in the United Kingdom.* Oxford University Press.

Kravdal, O., Glattre, E., and Haldorsen, T. (1991). Positive correlation between parity and incidence of thyroid cancer: new evidence based on complete Norwegian birth cohorts. *International Journal of Cancer*, **49**, 831–6.

Lancet (1989). Salted fish and nasopharyngeal carcinoma. *Lancet*, **ii**, 840–2.

Langton, J. and Morris, R. J. (1986). *Atlas of industrializing Britain 1780–1914.* Methuen, London.

Lee, W. R., Alderson, M. R., and Downes, J. E. (1972). Scrotal cancer in the north-west of England, 1962–68. *British Journal of Industrial Medicine*, **29**, 188–95.

Li, J.-Y., Li, F. P., Blot, W. J., Miller, R. W., and Fraumeni, J. F., Jr. (1982). Correlation between cancers of the uterine cervix and penis in China. *Journal of the National Cancer Institute*, **69**, 1063–5.

Macbeth, R. (1965). Malignant disease of the paranasal sinuses. *Journal of Laryngology*, **79**, 592–612.

McCredie, M. and Coates, M. S. (1989). *Cancer incidence in migrants to New South Wales: 1972 to 1984.* New South Wales Central Cancer Registry, New South Wales Cancer Council, Sydney.

McDonald, A. D. (1979). Mesothelioma registries in identifying asbestos hazards. *Annals of the New York Academy of Science*, **330**, 441–54.

McEwan, P. (1938). Clinical problems of thyrotoxicosis. *British Medical Journal*, **i**, 1037–42.

MacMahon, B. (1966). Epidemiology of Hodgkin's disease. *Cancer Research*, **26**, 1189–200.

Mantel, N. and Haenszel, W. (1959). Statistical aspects of the analysis of data from retrospective studies of disease. *Journal of the National Cancer Institute*, **22**, 719–48.

Mason, T. J., McKay, F. W., Hoover, R., Blot, W. J., and Fraumeni, J. F., Jr. (1975). *Atlas of cancer mortality for US counties: 1950–1969.* DHEW Publication No. (NIH) 75–780. US Department of Health, Education, and Welfare, Washington.

Meteorological Office (1954–65, 1969, 1974). *Monthly weather report. Summary for the years 1953–64, 1968, 1973.* Vols. 70–81, 85, 90. HMSO, London.

Miettinen, O. S. (1976). Estimability and estimation in case-referent studies. *American Journal of Epidemiology*, **103**, 226–35.

Miettinen, O. S. and Wang, J.-D. (1981). An alternative to the proportionate mortality ratio. *American Journal of Epidemiology*, **114**, 144–8.

Ministry of Agriculture, Fisheries and Food (1956). *Studies in urban household diets 1944–49. Second report of the National Food Survey Committee*. HMSO, London.
Ministry of Agriculture, Fisheries and Food (1957). *Domestic food consumption and expenditure: 1955. Annual Report of the National Food Survey Committee*. HMSO, London.
Ministry of Agriculture, Fisheries and Food (1977). *Household food consumption and expenditure: 1975, with a review of the six years 1970 to 1975. Annual Report of the National Food Survey Committee*. HMSO, London.
Ministry of Health (1936). *Housing Act, 1935. Report on The Overcrowding Survey in England and Wales, 1936*. HMSO, London.
Ministry of Health and General Register Office (1963*a*). *Report on Hospital In-Patient Enquiry for the year 1959. Part II: detailed tables and commentary*. HMSO, London.
Ministry of Health and General Register Office (1963*b*). *Report on Hospital In-Patient Enquiry for the year 1960. Part II: detailed tables*. HMSO, London.
Ministry of Health and General Register Office (1967). *Report on Hospital In-Patient Enquiry for the two years 1960 and 1961. Part III: commentary*. HMSO, London.
Ministry of Labour and National Service (1957). *Report on an Enquiry into Household Expenditure in 1953–54*. HMSO, London.
Morrison, A. S., Buring, J. E., Verhoek, W. G., Aoki, K., Leck, I., Ohno, Y., and Obata, K. (1984). An international study of smoking and bladder cancer. *Journal of Urology*, **131**, 650–4.
Muir, C. (1987). Classification. In *Cancer incidence in five continents*, Vol. V, International Agency for Research on Cancer, Scientific Publication, No. 88 (ed. C. Muir, J. Waterhouse, T. Mack, J. Powell, and S. Whelan), pp. 19–25. IARC, Lyon.
Muir, C., Waterhouse, J., Mack, T., Powell, J., and Whelan, S. (ed.) (1987). *Cancer incidence in five continents*, Vol. V. International Agency for Research on Cancer, Scientific Publication, No. 88. IARC, Lyon.
Murphy, M. F. G., Campbell, M. J., and Goldblatt, P. O. (1987). Twenty years' screening for cancer of the uterine cervix in Great Britain, 1964–84: further evidence for its ineffectiveness. *Journal of Epidemiology and Community Health*, **42**, 49–53.
Newhouse, M. L. and Berry, G. (1979). Patterns of mortality in asbestos factory workers in London. *Annals of the New York Academy of Science*, **330**, 53–60.
Nomura, A. (1990). An international search for causative factors of colorectal cancer. *Journal of the National Cancer Institute*, **82**, 894–5.
Office of Population Censuses and Surveys (1970). *Classification of Occupations, 1970*. HMSO, London.
Office of Population Censuses and Surveys (1972–1973). Census 1971, England and Wales. County Reports. HMSO, London.
Office of Population Censuses and Surveys (1973*a*). *Census 1971. Report on the Welsh language in Wales*. HMSO, Cardiff.
Office of Population Censuses and Surveys (1973*b*). *The Registrar General's Statistical Review of England and Wales for the year 1971. Part I(A)*: Tables, medical. HMSO, London.
Office of Population Censuses and Surveys (1970–1974). *The Registrar General's Statistical Reviews of England and Wales for the years 1968–1973. Supplements on abortion*. HMSO, London.
Office of Population Censuses and Surveys (1975). *Census 1971: England and Wales. Economic activity*. County leaflets. HMSO, London.
Office of Population Censuses and Surveys (1980). *General Household Survey 1978*. Series GHS No. 8. HMSO, London.
Office of Population Censuses and Surveys (1981). *Area mortality. The Registrar*

General's Decennial Supplement for England and Wales 1969–73. Series DS No. 4. HMSO, London.

Office of Population Censuses and Surveys (1986, 1989). *General Household Survey 1984, 1986*. Series GHS Nos. 14, 16. HMSO, London.

Office of Population Censuses and Surveys (1990). *Review of the national cancer registration system*. Report of the Working Group of the Registrar General's Medical Advisory Committee. Series MB1, No. 17. HMSO, London.

Owen, I. (1889). Reports of the collective investigation committee of the British Medical Association. Geographical distribution of rickets, acute and subacute rheumatism, chorea, cancer, and urinary calculus. *British Medical Journal*, **1**, 113–16.

Parkin, D. M., Nguyen-Dinh, X., and Day, N. E. (1985). The impact of screening on the incidence of cervical cancer in England and Wales. *British Journal of Obstetrics and Gynaecology*, **92**, 150–7.

Peto, J., Doll, R., Hermon, C., Binns, W., Clayton, R., and Goffe, T. (1985). Relationship of mortality to measures of environmental asbestos pollution in an asbestos textile factory. *Annals of Occupational Hygiene*, **29**, 305–55.

Pharoah, P. O. D. and Morris, J. N. (1979). Postneonatal mortality. *Epidemiologic Reviews*, **1**, 170–83.

Phillips, D. I. W., Barker, D. J. P., Winter, P. D., and Osmond, C. (1983). Mortality from thyrotoxicosis in England and Wales and its association with the previous prevalence of endemic goitre. *Journal of Epidemiology and Community Health*, **37**, 305–9.

Pott, P. (1775). *Chirurgical observations relative to the cataract, the polypus of the nose, the cancer of the scrotum, the different kinds of ruptures and the mortification of the toes and feet*. Hawes, Clarke, & Collins, London.

Preston-Martin, S., Pike, M. C., Ross, R. K., Jones, P. A., and Henderson, B. E. (1990). Increased cell division as a cause of human cancer. *Cancer Research*, **50**, 7415–21.

Price, C. H. G. (1962). The incidence of osteogenic sarcoma in South-west England and its relationship to Paget's disease of bone. *Journal of Bone and Joint Surgery*, **44B**, 366–76.

Ron, E. and Modan, B. (1982). Thyroid. In: *Cancer epidemiology and prevention* (ed. D. Schottenfeld and J. F. Fraumeni Jr.), pp. 837–54. W. B. Saunders, Philadelphia.

Rothman, K. and Keller, A. (1972). The effect of joint exposure to alcohol and tobacco on risk of cancer of the mouth and pharynx. *Journal of Chronic Diseases*, **25**, 711–16.

Rowett Research Institute (1955). *Family diet and health in pre-war Britain. A dietary and clinical survey*. Carnegie United Kindgom Trust, Dunfermline.

SAS Institute (1988). *SAS Release 6.03*. SAS Institute Inc., Cary, North Carolina.

Schottenfeld, D. and Fraumeni, J. F. Jr. (ed.) (1982). *Cancer epidemiology and prevention*. W. B. Saunders, Philadelphia.

Singer, A. and Jenkins, D. (1991). Viruses and cervical cancer. Genital virus infections warrant surveillance rather than radical treatment. *British Medical Journal*, **302**, 251–2.

Smans, M., Muir, C. S., and Boyle, P. (ed.) (in press). *The atlas of cancer mortality in the European Economic Community*. International Agency for Research on Cancer, Scientific Publication, No. 107. IARC, Lyon.

Smith, P. G. (1982). Spatial and temporal clustering. In: *Cancer epidemiology and prevention* (ed. D. Schottenfeld and J. F. Fraumeni Jr.), pp. 391–407. W. B. Saunders, Philadelphia.

Smith, P. G. and Douglas, A. J. (1986). Mortality of workers at the Sellafield plant of British Nuclear Fuels. *British Medical Journal*, **293**, 845–54.

Smith, P. G., Kinlen, L. J., White, G. C., Adelstein, A. M., and Fox, A. J. (1980). Mortality of wives of men dying with cancer of the penis. *British Journal of Cancer*, **41**, 422–8.

Snow, J. (1855). *On the mode of communication of cholera* (2nd edn, much enlarged). John Churchill, London.

Southam, A. H. and Wilson, S. R. (1922). Cancer of the scrotum: the etiology, clinical features, and treatment of the disease. *British Medical Journal*, **ii**, 971–3.

Stiller, C. A., O'Connor, C. M., Vincent, T. J., and Draper, G. J. (1991). The National Registry of Childhood Tumours and the leukaemia/lymphoma data for 1966–83. In: *The geographical epidemiology of childhood leukaemia and non-Hodgkin lymphomas in Great Britain, 1966–83*. (ed. G. J. Draper), pp. 7–16. SMPS No. 53. HMSO, London.

Stocks, P. (1925). Some further notes on cancer and goitre distributions. *Biometrika*, **17**, 159–65.

Stocks, P. (1928). On the evidence for a regional distribution of cancer prevalence in England and Wales. *Report of the International Conference on Cancer, London, 17th–20th July, 1928*. pp. 508–19, John Wright & Sons, Bristol.

Stocks, P. (1936). Distribution in England and Wales of cancer of various organs. In *13th Annual Report of the British Empire Cancer Campaign*, pp. 240–80. British Empire Cancer Campaign, London.

Stocks, P. (1937). Distribution in England and Wales of cancer of various organs. In *14th Annual Report of the British Empire Cancer Campaign*, pp. 198–223. British Empire Cancer Campaign, London.

Stocks, P. (1939). Distribution in England and Wales of cancer of various organs. In *16th Annual Report of the British Empire Cancer Campaign*, pp. 308–43. British Empire Cancer Campaign, London.

Stocks, P. (1950). *Cancer registration in England and Wales. An enquiry into treatment and its results*. SMPS, No. 3. HMSO, London.

Stocks, P. (1957). *Cancer incidence in North Wales and Liverpool region in relation to habits and environment. British Empire Cancer Campaign. Thirty-fifth Annual Report covering the year 1957*. Supplement to Part II, pp. 1–156. British Empire Cancer Campaign, London.

Stocks, P. and Davies, R. I. (1964). Zinc and copper content of soils associated with the incidence of cancer of the stomach and other organs. *British Journal of Cancer*, **18**, 14–24.

Stocks, P. and Karn, M. N. (1927). On the relation between the prevalence of thyroid enlargement in children and mortality from cancer and other diseases. *Annals of Eugenics*, **2**, 395–404.

Stocks, P. and Karn, M. N. (1930–1). The distribution of cancer and tuberculosis mortality in England and Wales. *Annals of Eugenics*, **4**, 341–61.

Swerdlow, A. J. (1983). Epidemiology of melanoma of the eye in the Oxford region, 1952–78. *British Journal of Cancer*, **47**, 311–13.

Swerdlow, A. J. (1984). Epidemiology of cutaneous melanoma. In: *Melanoma*. Clinics in Oncology, Vol. 3, No. 3. (ed. R. M. MacKie), pp. 407–37. W. B. Saunders, London.

Swerdlow, A. J. (1986). Cancer registration in England and Wales: some aspects relevant to interpretation of the data. *Journal of the Royal Statistical Society A*, **149**, 146–60.

Swerdlow, A. J. (1989). Interpretation of England and Wales cancer mortality data: the effect of enquiries to certifiers for further information. *British Journal of Cancer*, **59**, 787–91.

Swerdlow, A. J. and dos Santos Silva, I. (1991). Geographic distribution of lung and stomach cancers in England and Wales over 50 years: changing and unchanging patterns. *British Journal of Cancer*, **63**, 773–81.

Swift, M., Reitnauer, P. J., Morrell, D., and Chase, C. L. (1987). Breast and other cancers in families with ataxia-telangiectasia. *New England Journal of Medicine*, **316**, 1289–94.

Tomatis, L. *et al.* (ed.) (1990). *Cancer: causes, occurrence and control.* International Agency for Research on Cancer, Scientific Publications, No. 100. IARC, Lyon.

Tucker, M. A., Shields, J. A., Hartge, P., Augsburger, J., Hoover, R. N., and Fraumeni, J. F., Jr. (1985). Sunlight exposure as risk factor for intraocular malignant melanoma. *New England Journal of Medicine*, **313**, 789–92.

Tuyns, A. J., Pequignot, G., and Jensen, O. M. (1977). Le cancer de l'oesophage en Ille-et-Vilaine en fonction des niveaux de consommation d'alcool et de tabac. Des risques qui se multiplient. *Bulletin du Cancer*, **64**, 45–60.

Vineis, P. and Simonato, L. (1986). Estimates of the proportion of bladder cancers attributable to occupation. *Scandinavian Journal of Work and Environmental Health*, **12**, 55–60.

Waldron, H. A., Waterhouse, J. A. H., and Tessema, N. (1984). Scrotal cancer in the West Midlands 1936–76. *British Journal of Industrial Medicine*, **41**, 437–44.

Walker, A. H., Ross, R. K., Haile, R. W. C., and Henderson, B. E. (1988). Hormonal factors and risk of ovarian germ cell cancer in young women. *British Journal of Cancer*, **57**, 418–22.

Waterhouse, J. A. H. (1972). Lung cancer and gastro-intestinal cancer in mineral oil workers. *Annals of Occupational Hygiene*, **15**, 43–4.

Webb, J. S., Thornton, I., Thompson, M., Howarth, R. J., and Lowenstein, P. L. (1978). *The Wolfson geochemical atlas of England and Wales.* Clarendon Press, Oxford.

Weiss, W. (1979). Changing incidence of thyroid cancer. *Journal of the National Cancer Institute*, **62**, 1137–42.

Whittemore, A. S. *et al.* (1990). Diet, physical activity, and colorectal cancer among Chinese in North America and China. *Journal of the National Cancer Institute*, **82**, 915–26.

Wignall, B. K. and Fox, A. J. (1982). Mortality of female gas mask assemblers. *British Journal of Industrial Medicine*, **39**, 34–8.

Wilson, P. (1980). *Drinking in England and Wales*. HMSO, London.

World Health Organization (1967). *Manual of the International Statistical Classification of Diseases, Injuries, and Causes of Death.* Eighth Revision. WHO, Geneva.

World Health Organization (1978). *Manual of the International Statistical Classification of Diseases, Injuries, and Causes of Death.* Ninth Revision. WHO, Geneva.

Wrixon, A. D. *et al.* (1988). *Natural radiation exposure in UK dwellings.* Publication NRPB-R190. National Radiological Protection Board, Chilton, Oxfordshire.

Yu, M. C., Mo, C.-C., Chong, W.-X., Yeh, F.-S., and Henderson, B. E. (1988). Preserved foods and nasopharyngeal carcinoma: a case-control study in Guangxi, China. *Cancer Research*, **48**, 1954–9.

Maps of physical geography, population density, and geographical distribution of 'exposures'

MAP E1 PHYSICAL GEOGRAPHY OF ENGLAND AND WALES, AND COUNTY BOUNDARIES AT 31 MARCH 1974.

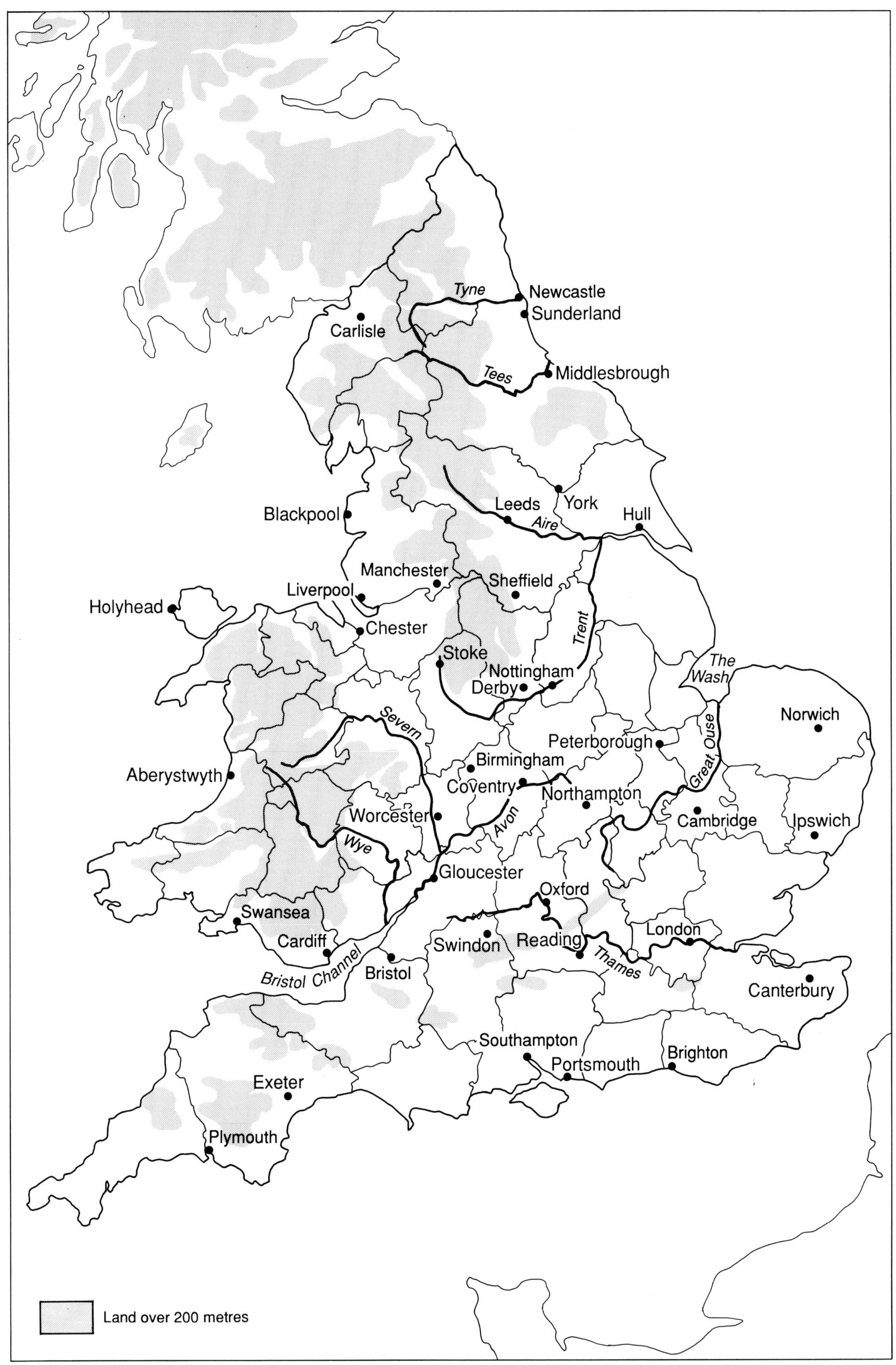

MAP E2 POPULATION DENSITY, ENGLAND AND WALES, 1971.

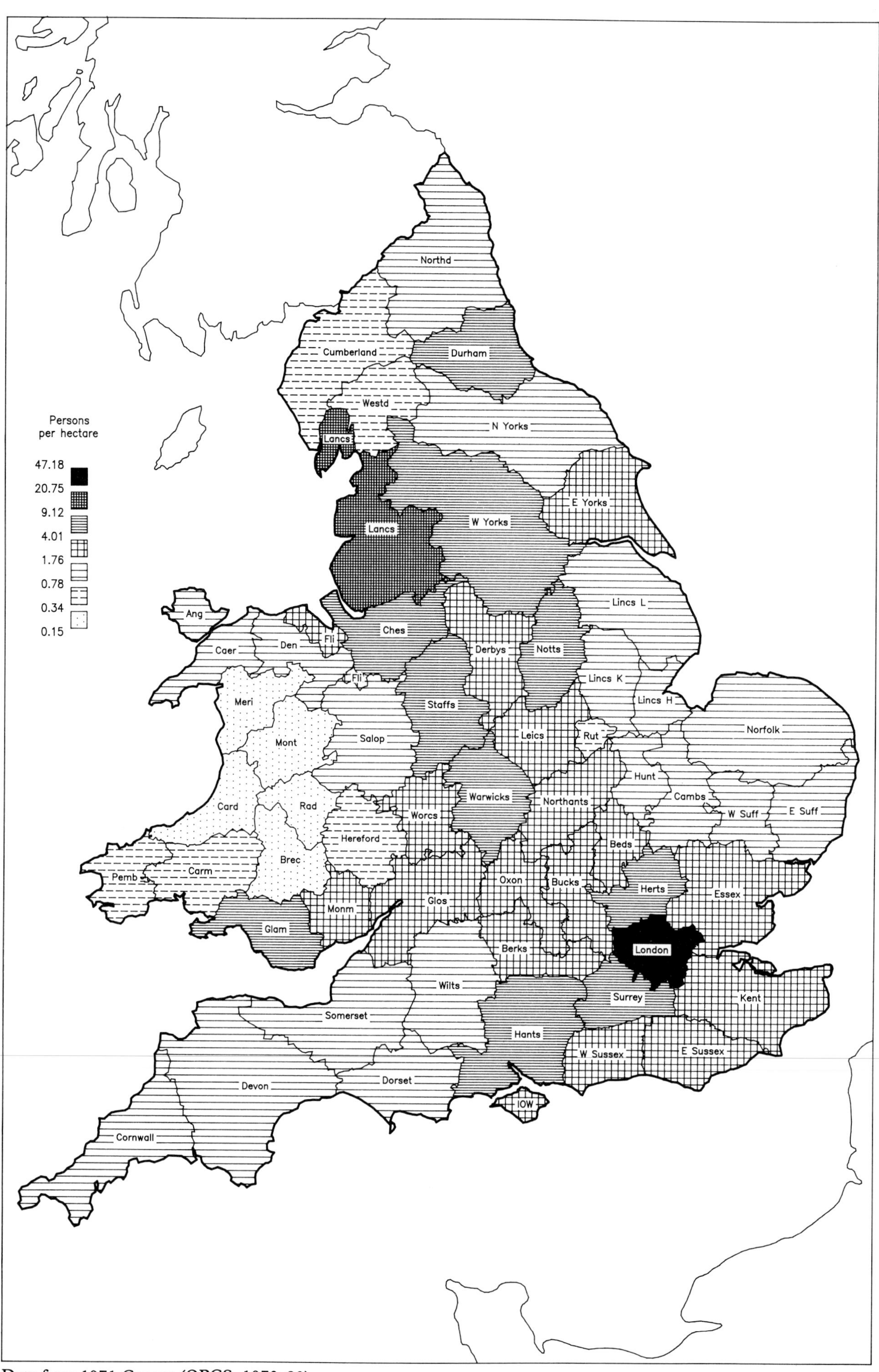

Data from 1971 Census (OPCS, 1972–83)

MAP E3 MEAN AGE AT FIRST BIRTH WITHIN MARRIAGE, WOMEN AGED 50–54, ENGLAND AND WALES, 1971.

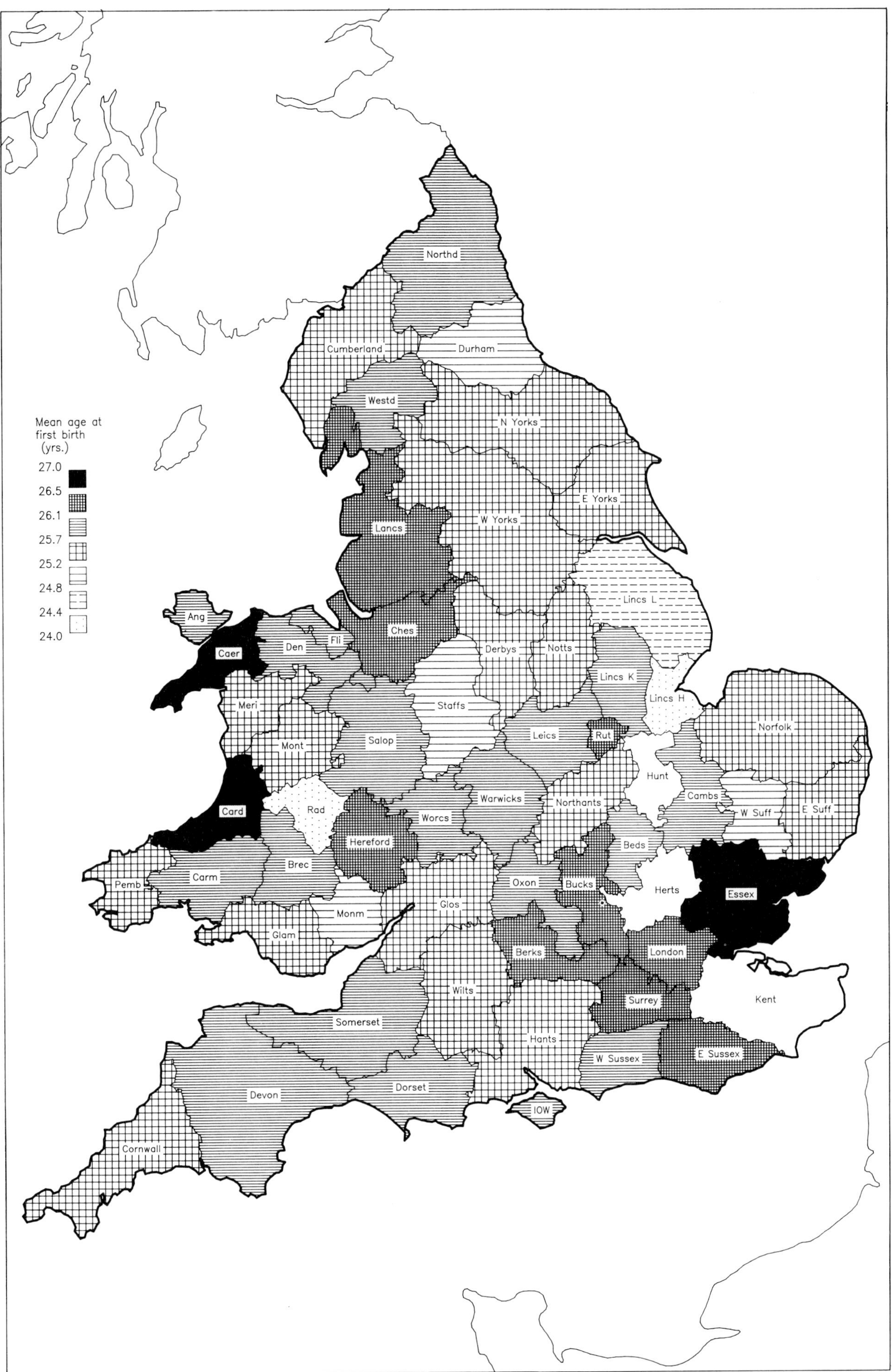

Data calculated from 1971 Census tabulations (OPCS, unpublished)

MAP E4 AVERAGE HEIGHT OF MEN, ENGLAND AND WALES, DATA FROM 1958 AND 1970.

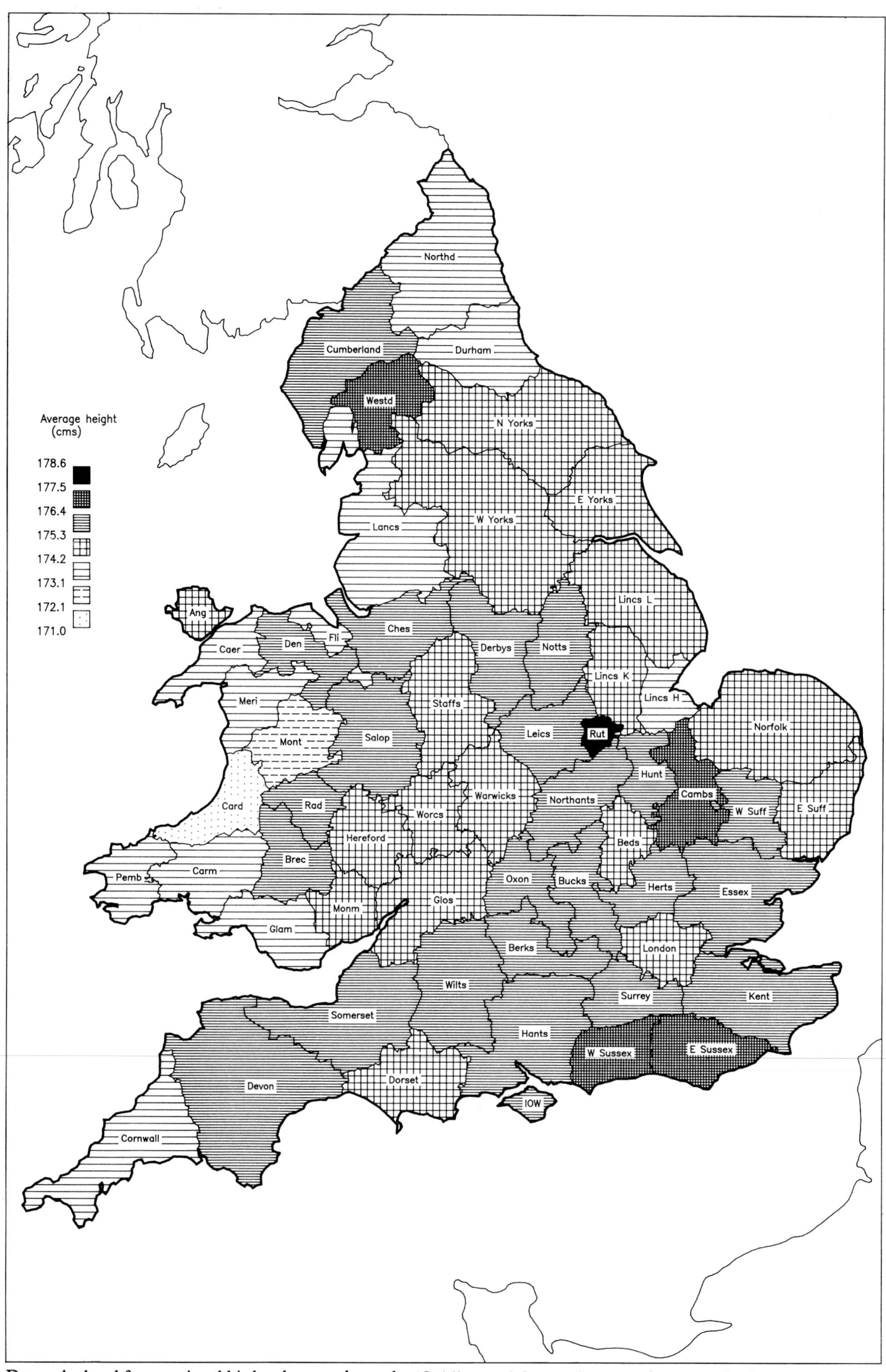

Data calculated from national birth cohort study results (Golding and Osmond, personal communication)

MAP E5 AVERAGE HEIGHT OF WOMEN, ENGLAND AND WALES, DATA FROM 1958 AND 1970.

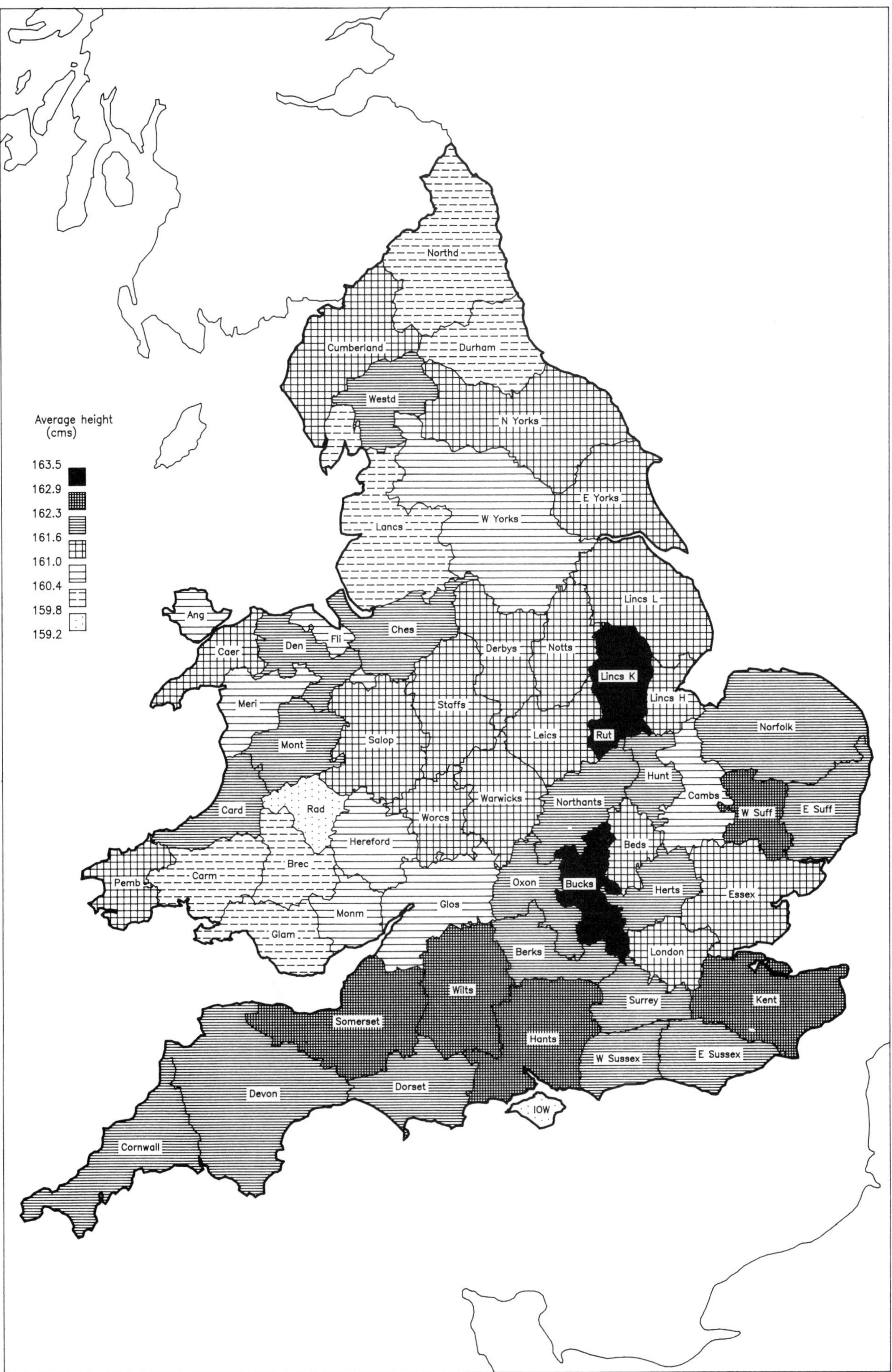

Data calculated from national birth cohort study results (Golding & Osmond, personal communication)

MAP E6 ESTIMATED PERCENTAGE OF POPULATION OF INDIAN SUBCONTINENT ETHNICITY, ENGLAND AND WALES, 1981.

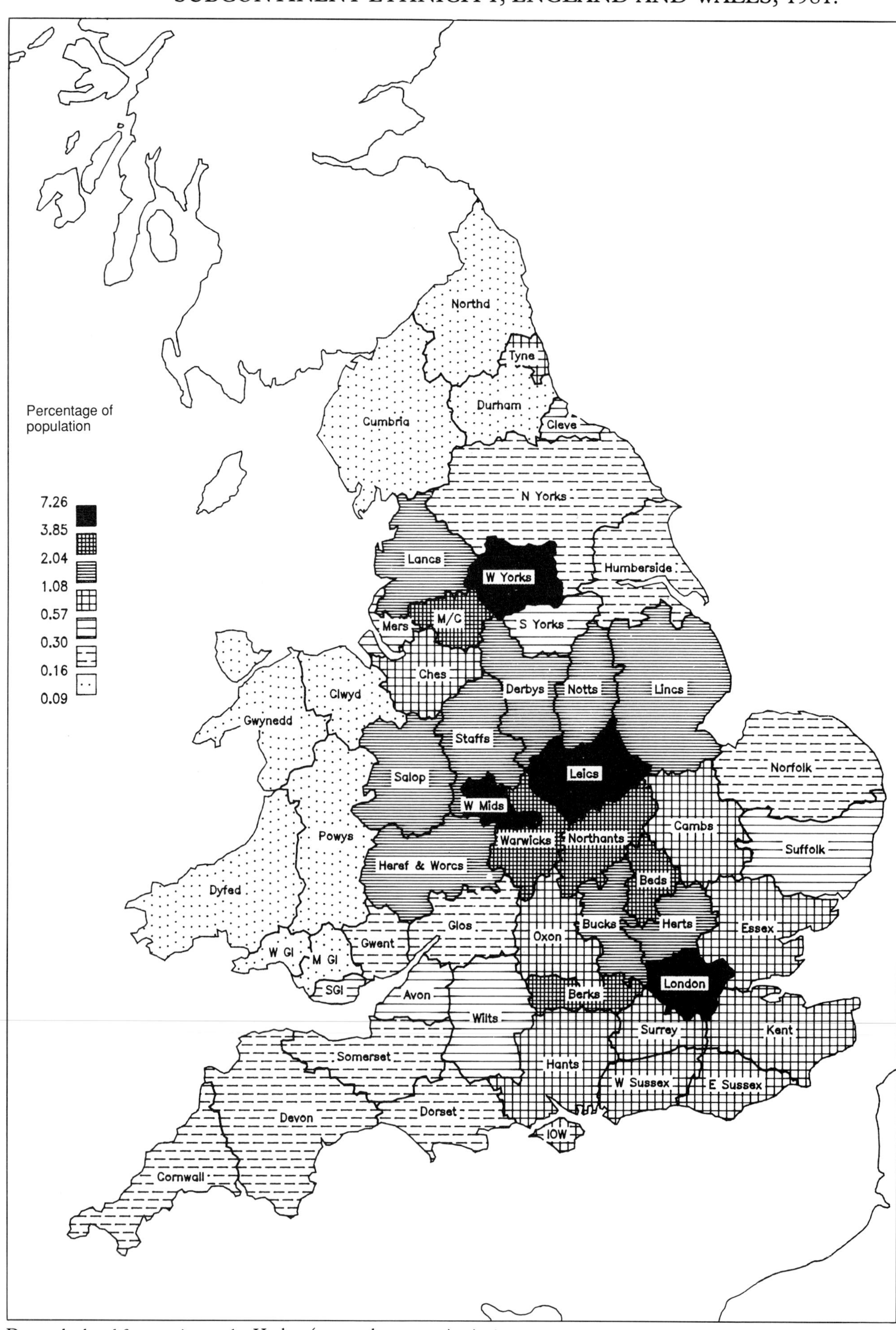

Data calculated from estimates by Haskey (personal communication)

MAP E7 ESTIMATED PERCENTAGE OF POPULATION OF WEST INDIAN ETHNICITY, ENGLAND AND WALES, 1981.

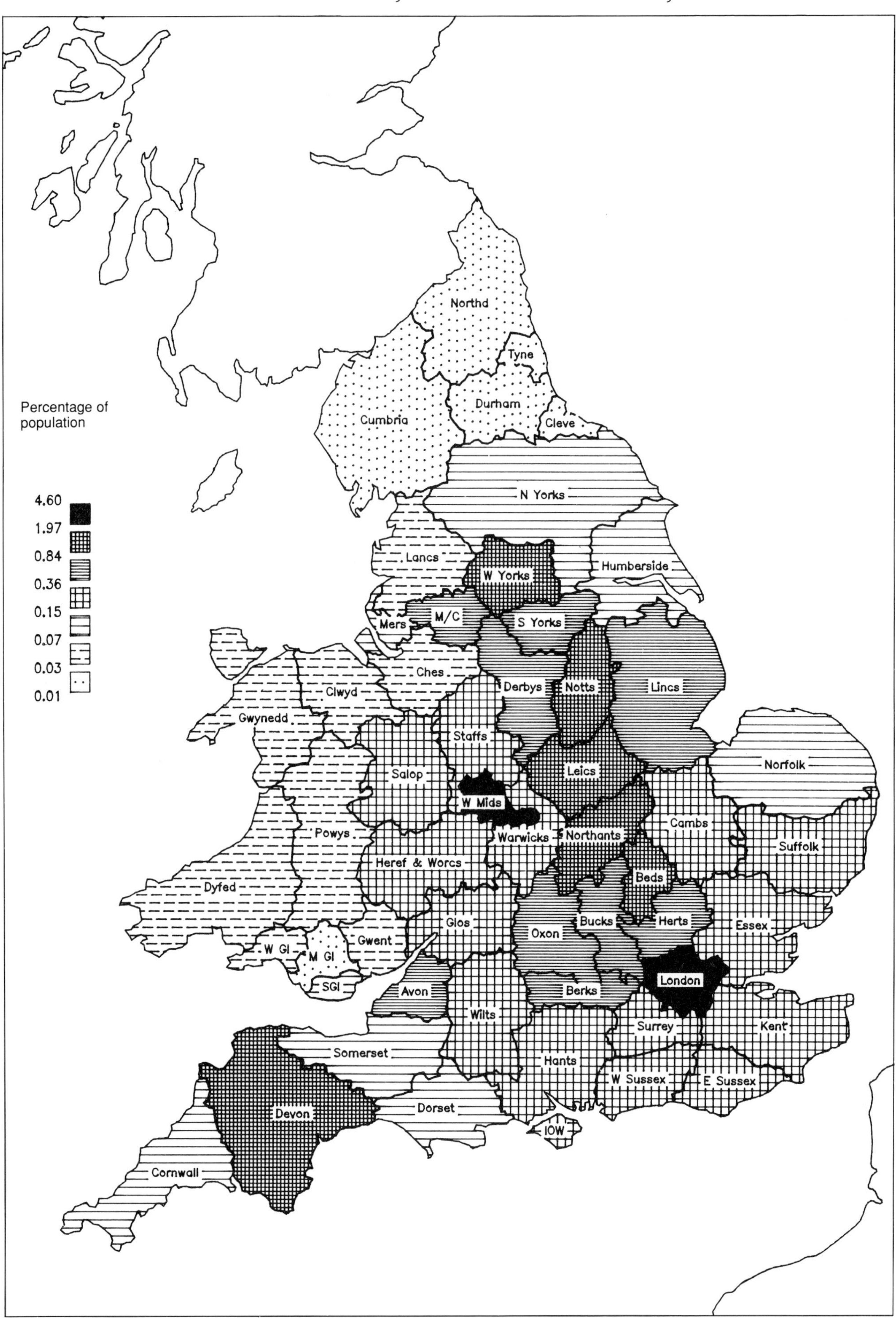

Data calculated from estimates by Haskey (personal communication)

MAP E8 MEAN INDOOR RADON CONCENTRATIONS, ENGLAND AND WALES, 1981–5.

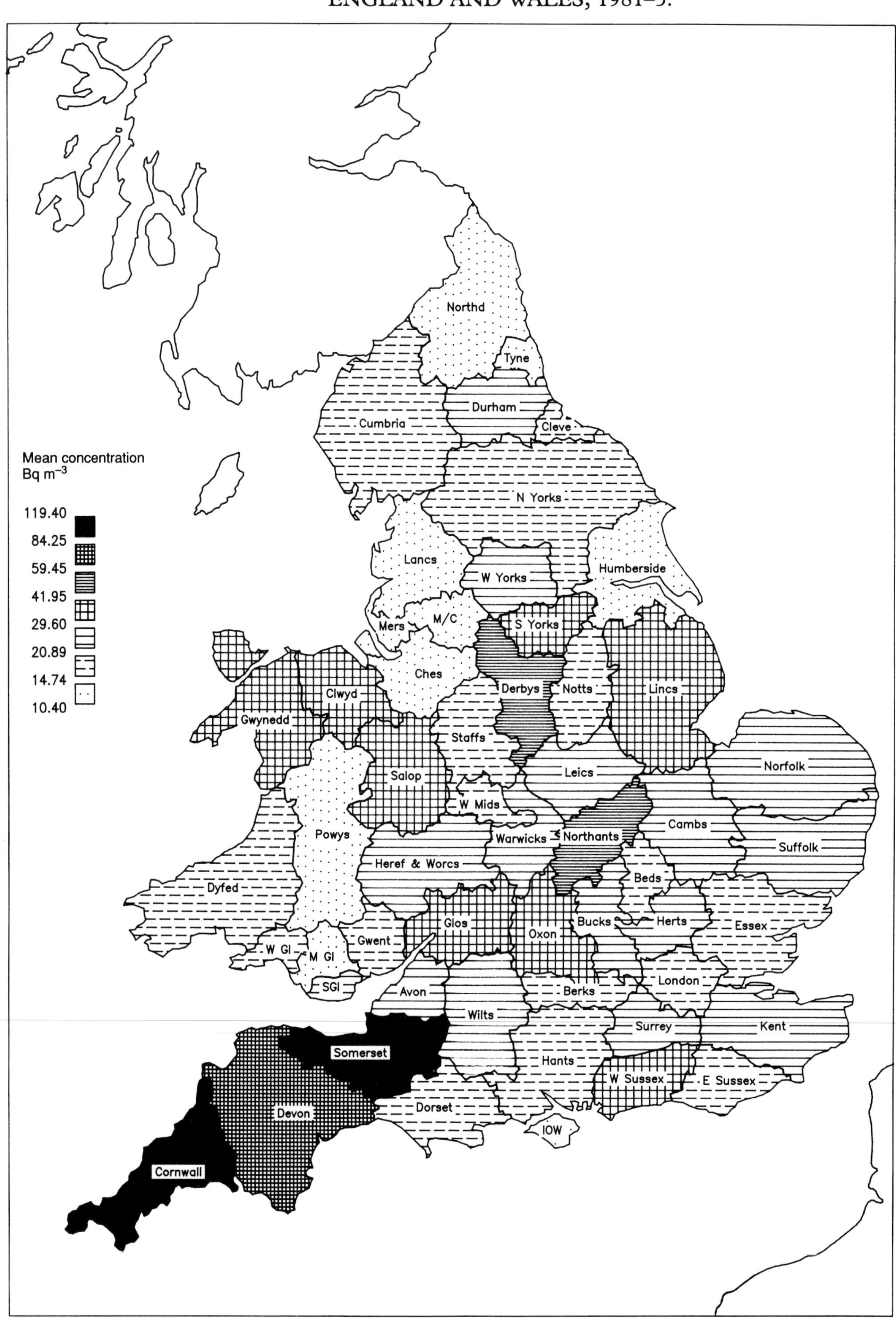

Data from Wrixon *et al.* (1988)

MAP E9 NUCLEAR ESTABLISHMENTS IN ENGLAND, WALES AND SOUTHERN SCOTLAND.

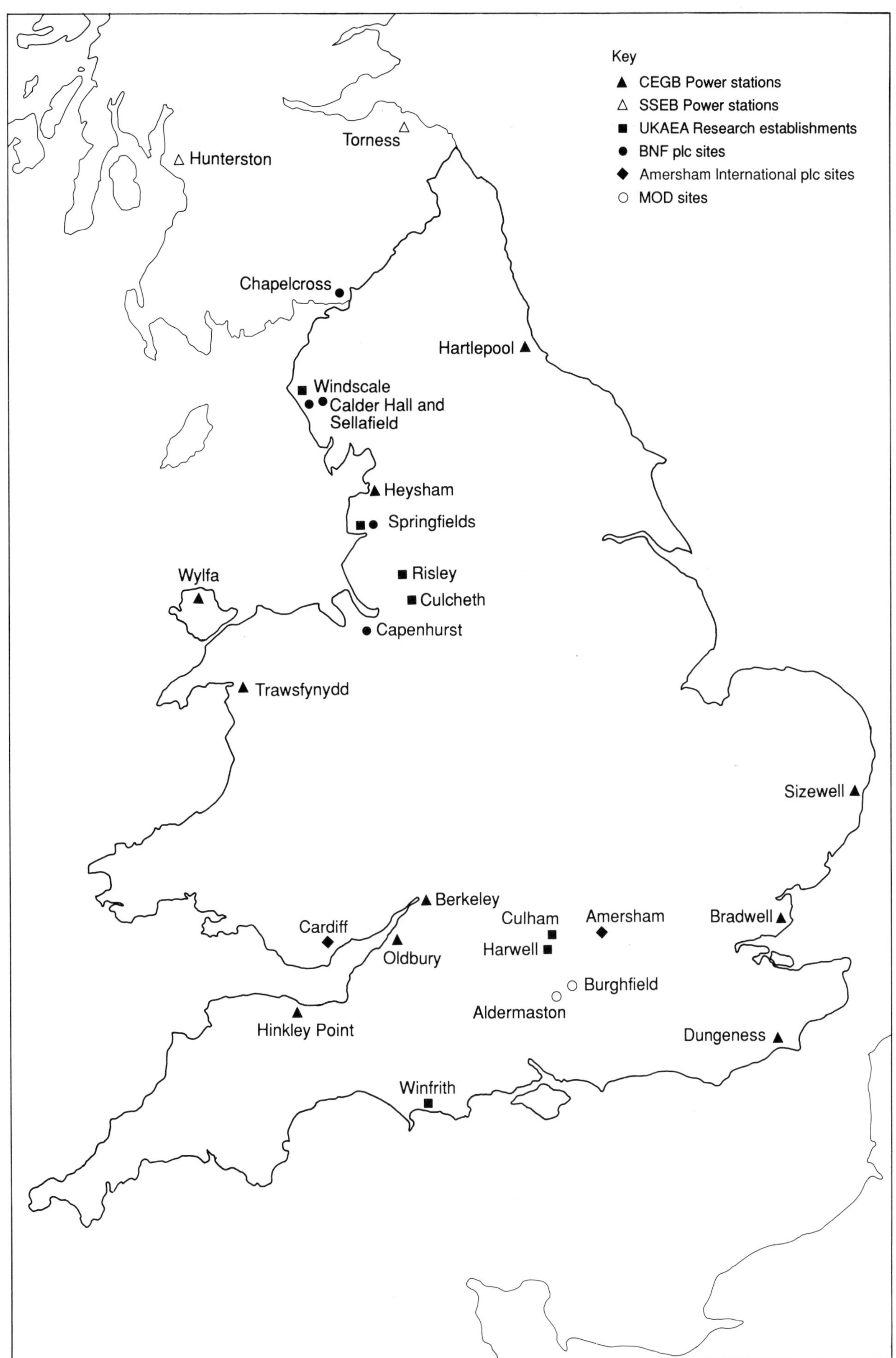

Adapted from Cook-Mozaffari *et al.* (1987)

MAP E10 MEAN PARITY OF WOMEN AGED 35–39, ENGLAND AND WALES, 1971.

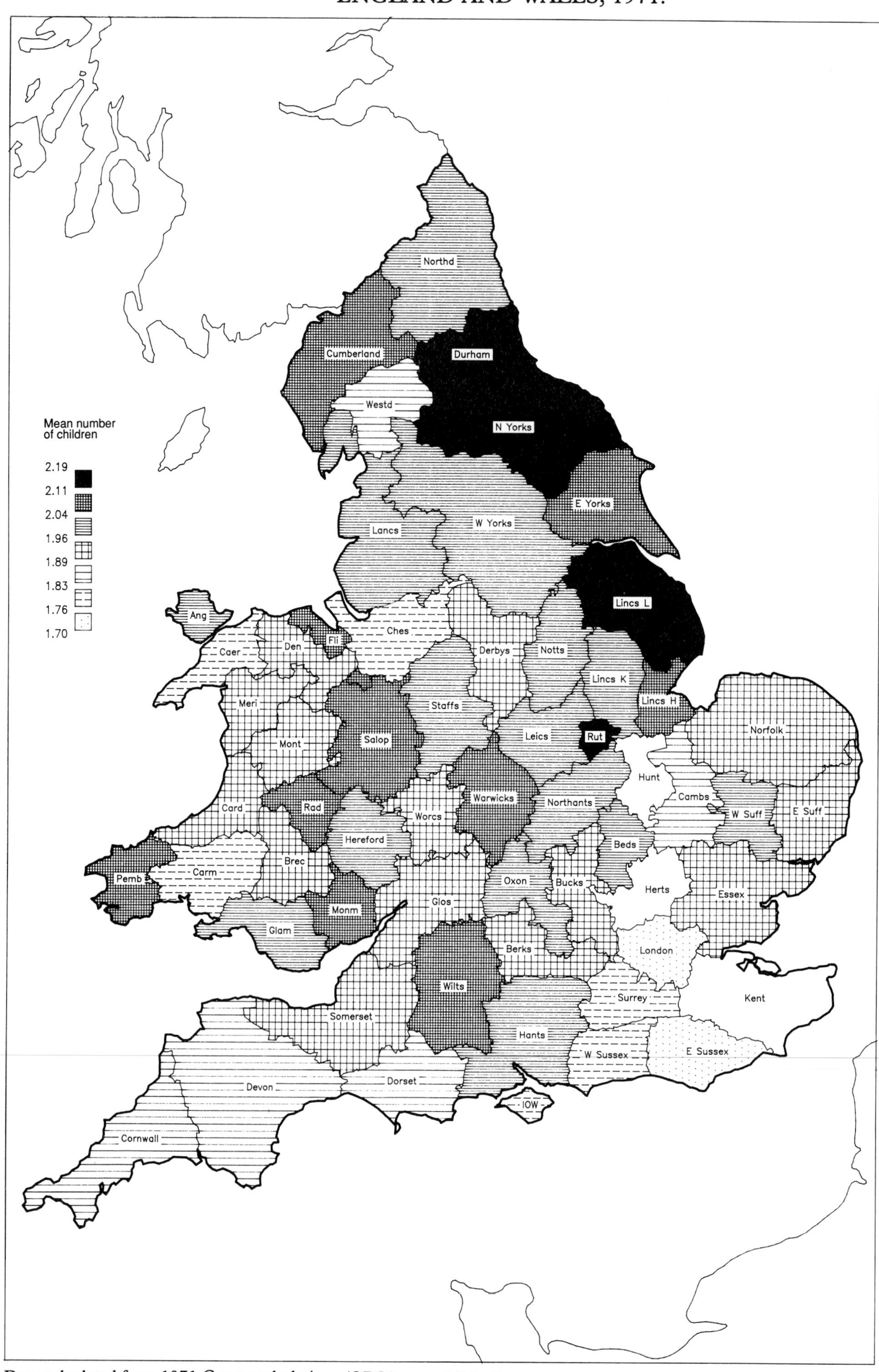

Data calculated from 1971 Census tabulations (OPCS, unpublished)

MAP E11 POPULATION MOBILITY*, AGES 1–14, ENGLAND AND WALES, 1971.

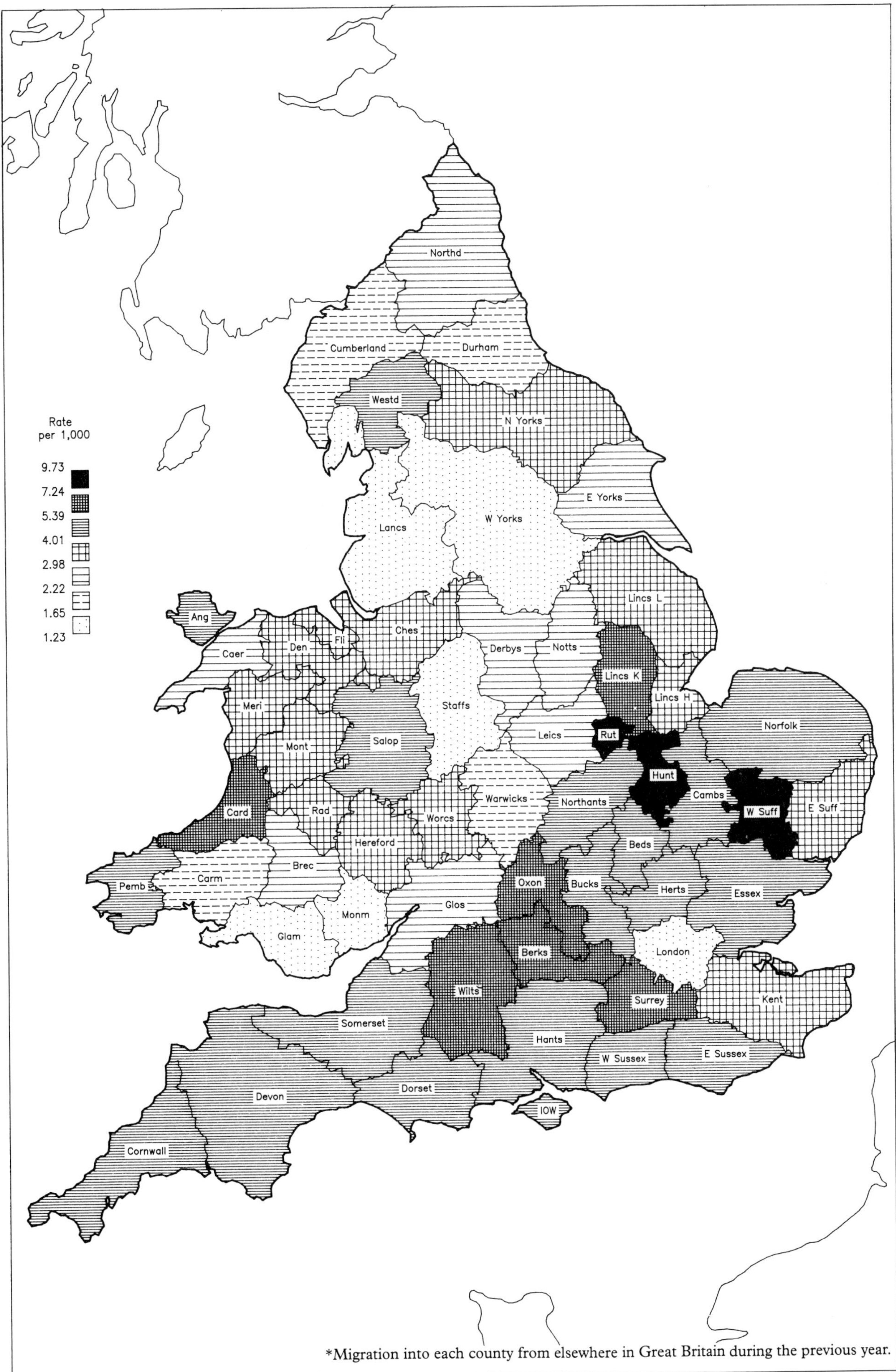

*Migration into each county from elsewhere in Great Britain during the previous year.

Data calculated from 1971 Census tabulations (OPCS, unpublished)

MAP E12 POSTNEONATAL MORTALITY RATES, ENGLAND AND WALES, 1950.

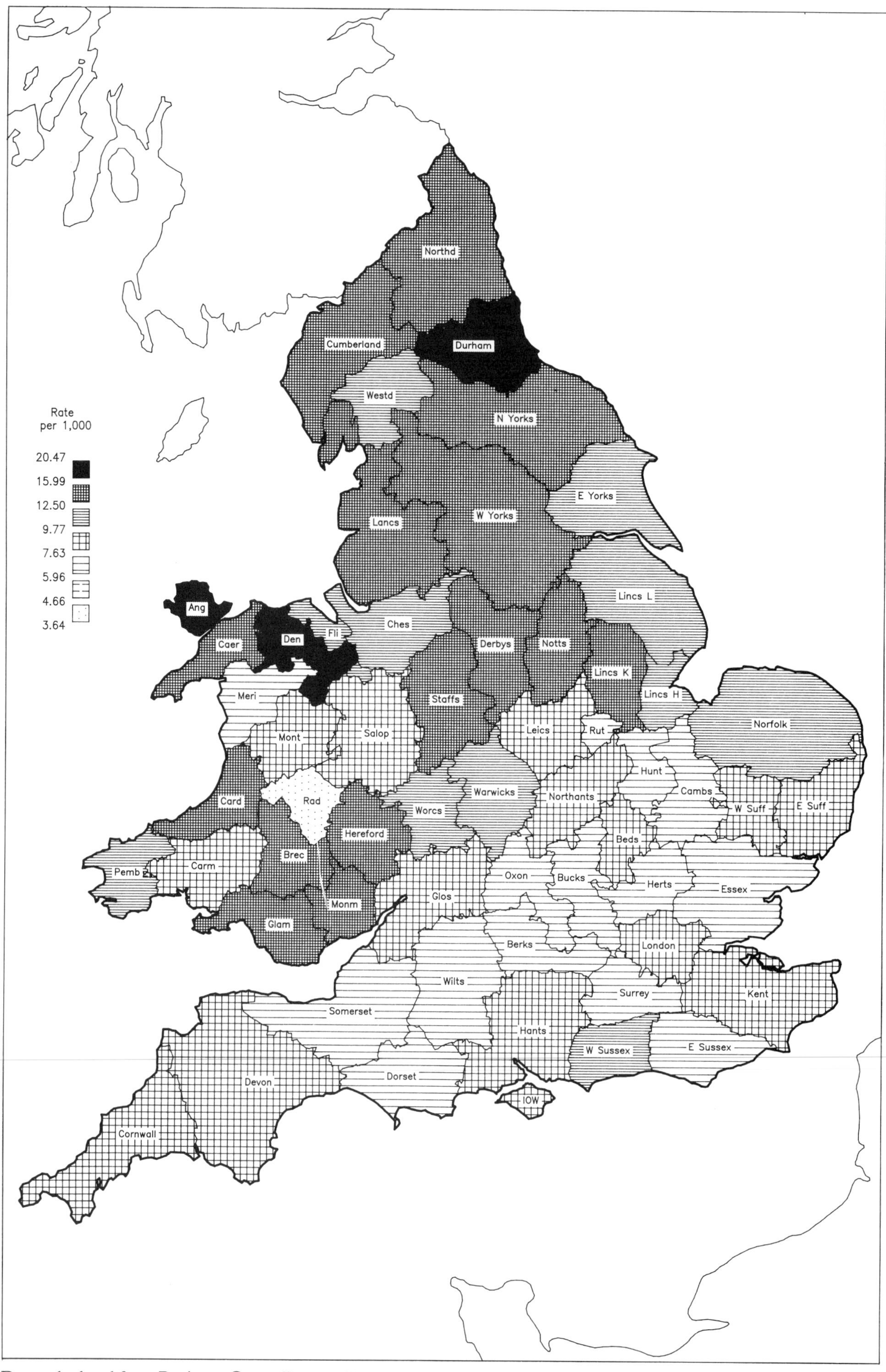

Data calculated from Registrar General's mortality statistics (General Register Office, 1952)

MAP E13 MEAN DAILY HOURS OF BRIGHT SUNSHINE, ENGLAND AND WALES, 1953–73.

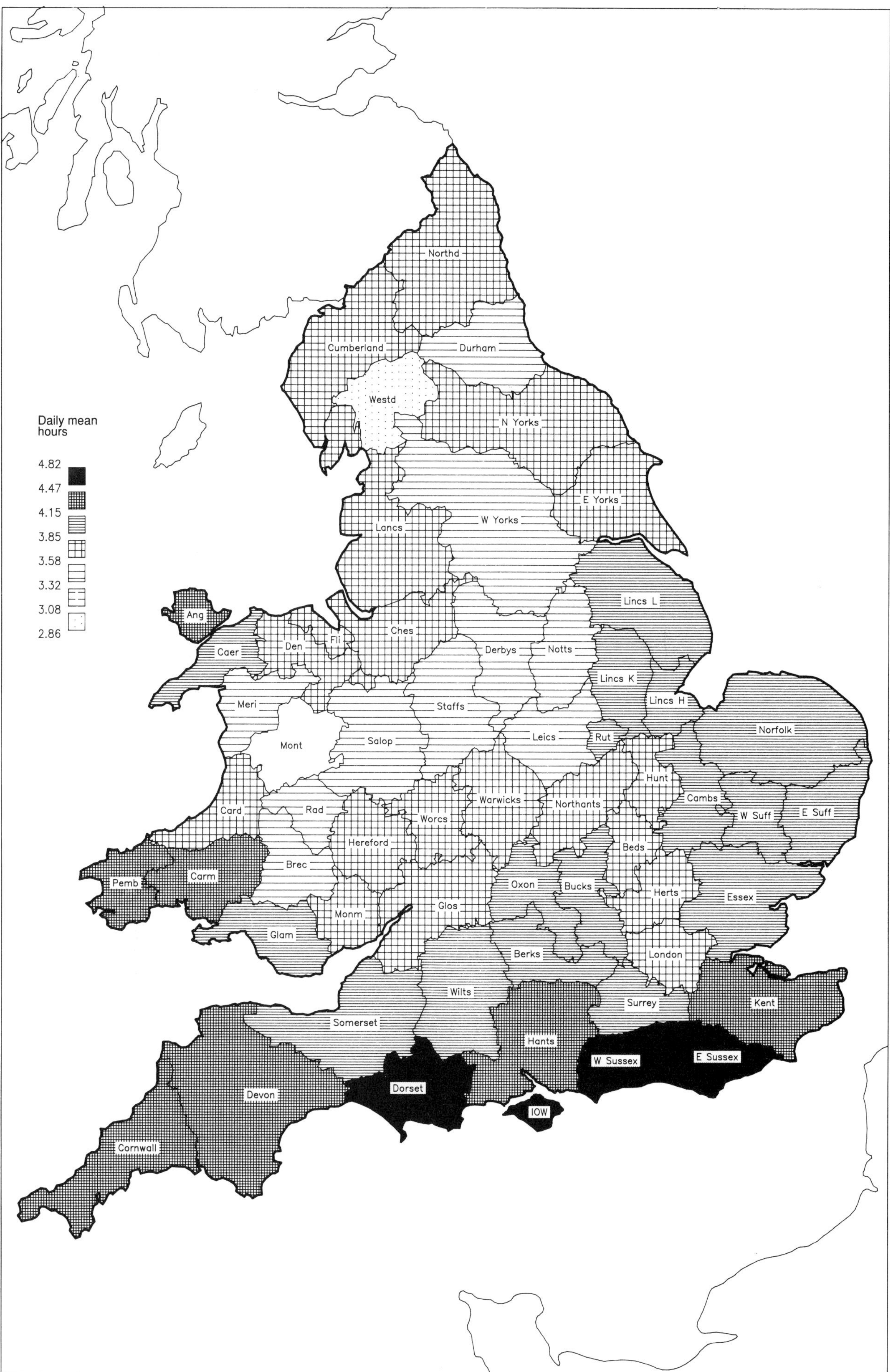

Data calculated from Meteorological Office measurements (Meteorological Office, 1954, 1959, 1964, 1969, 1974)

Maps of cancer mortality in England and Wales, 1921–30. From Stocks (1936, 1937, 1939)

MAP S1 CANCER OF OESOPHAGUS IN MALES AGES 25–65, 1921–30. STANDARDIZED MORTALITY RATIOS

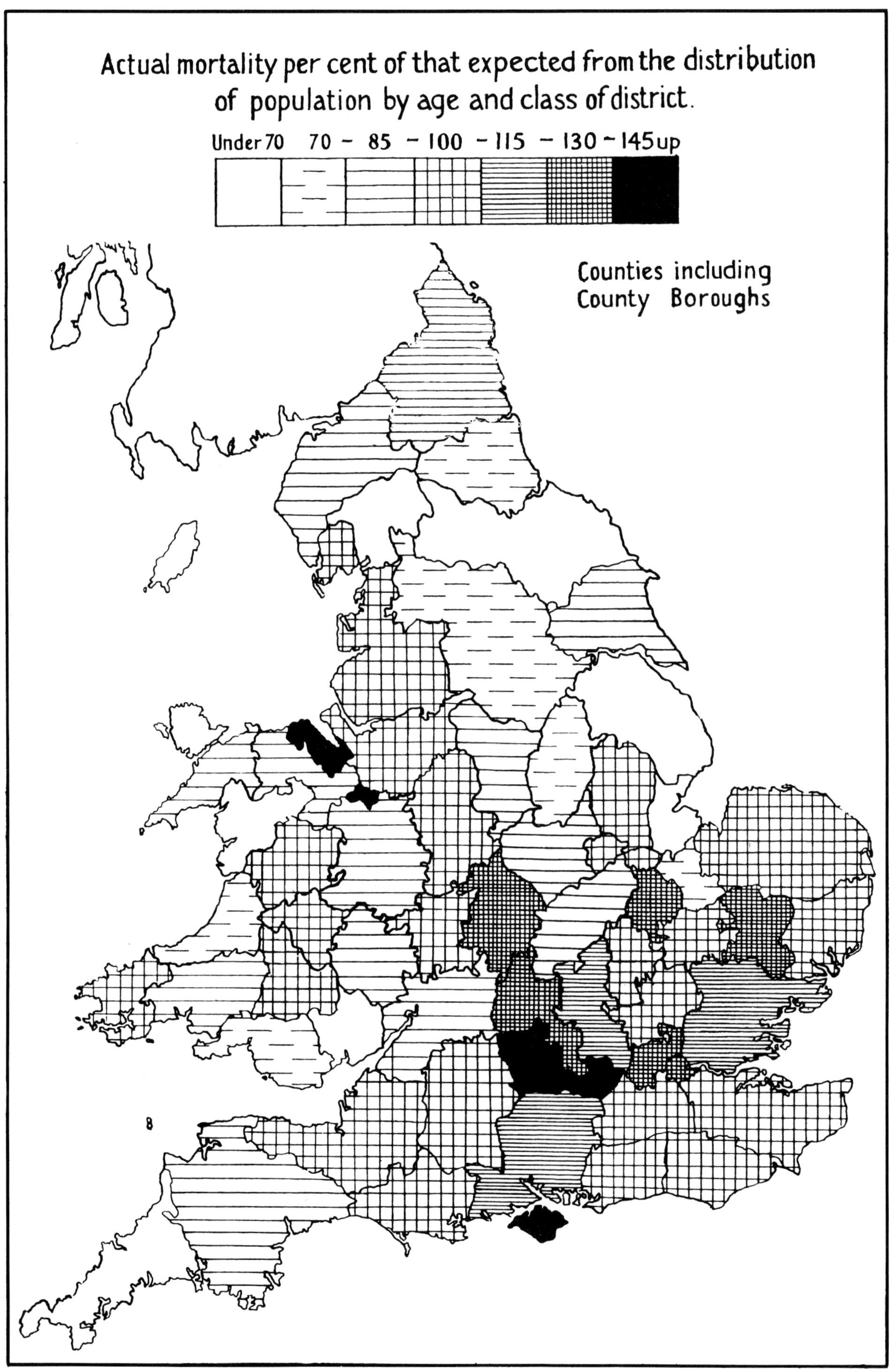

From Stocks (1936).

MAP S2 CANCER OF STOMACH IN FEMALES AGES 25+, 1921–30. STANDARDIZED MORTALITY RATIOS

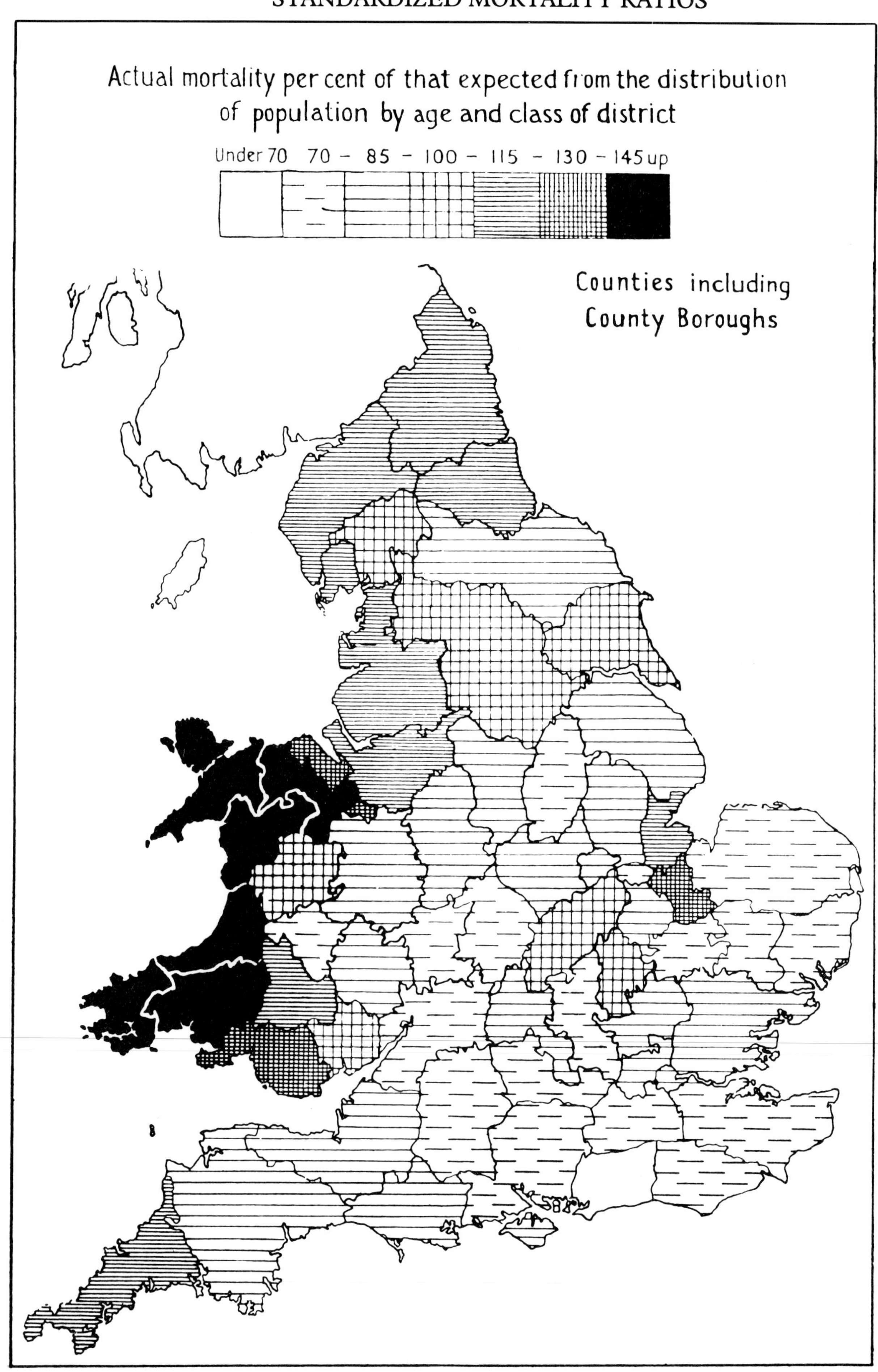

From Stocks (1936).

MAP S3 CANCER OF LARYNX IN MALES AGES 25+, 1921–30. STANDARDIZED MORTALITY RATIOS

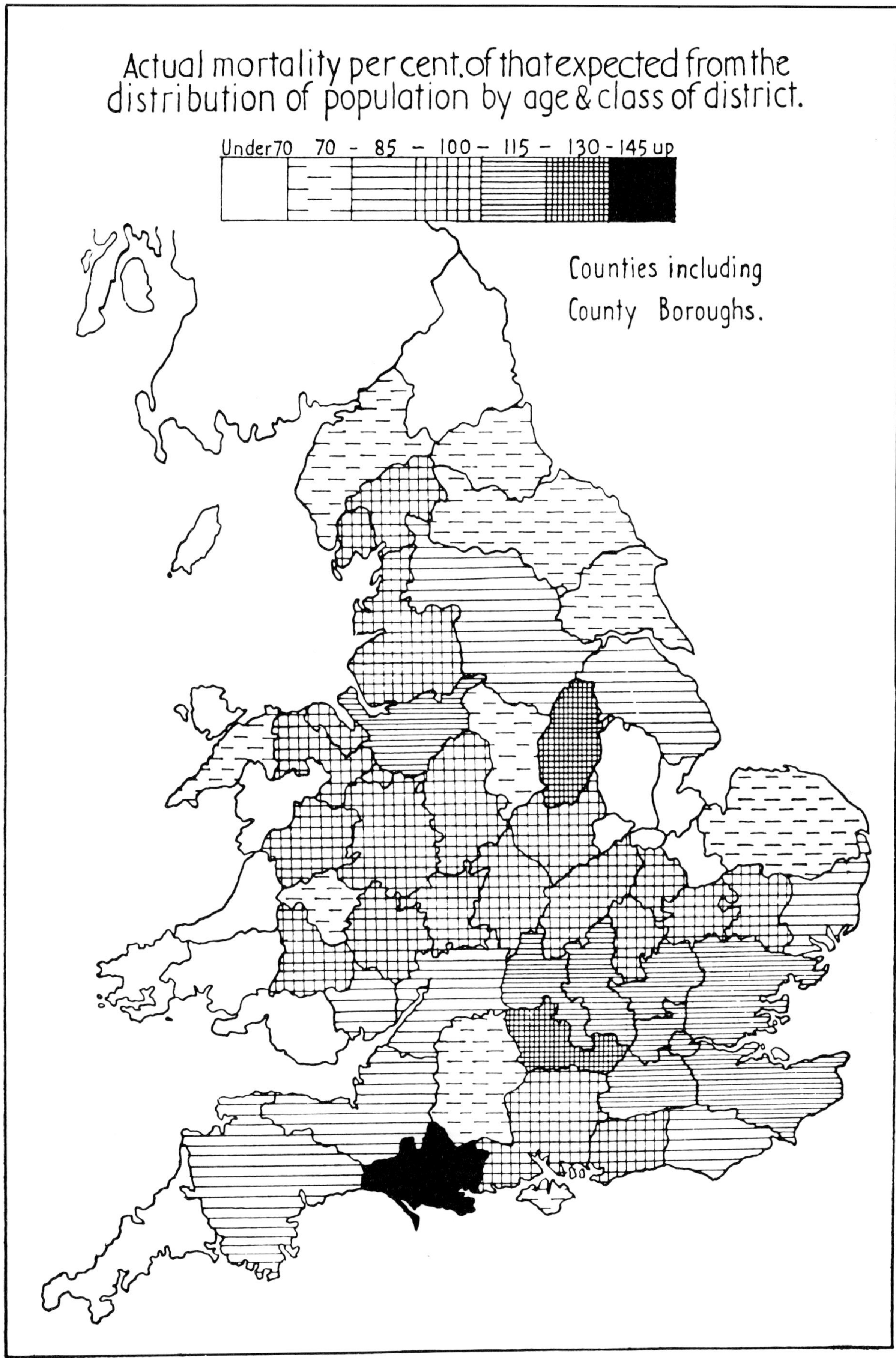

From Stocks (1937).

MAP S4 CANCER OF LUNG IN MALES AGES 25+, 1921–30. STANDARDIZED MORTALITY RATIOS

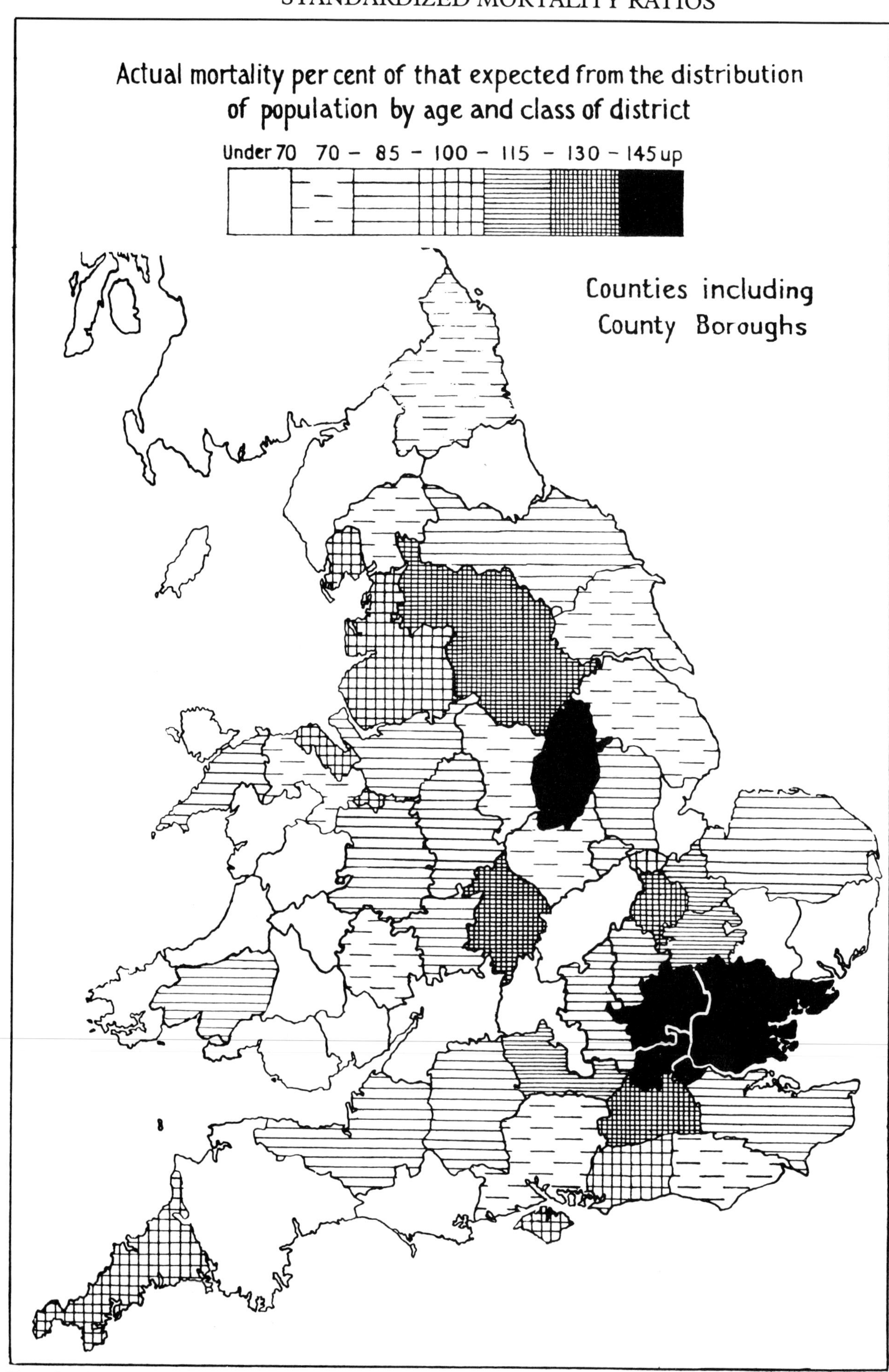

From Stocks (1936).

MAP S5 CANCER OF LUNG IN FEMALES AGE 25+, 1921–30. STANDARDIZED MORTALITY RATIOS

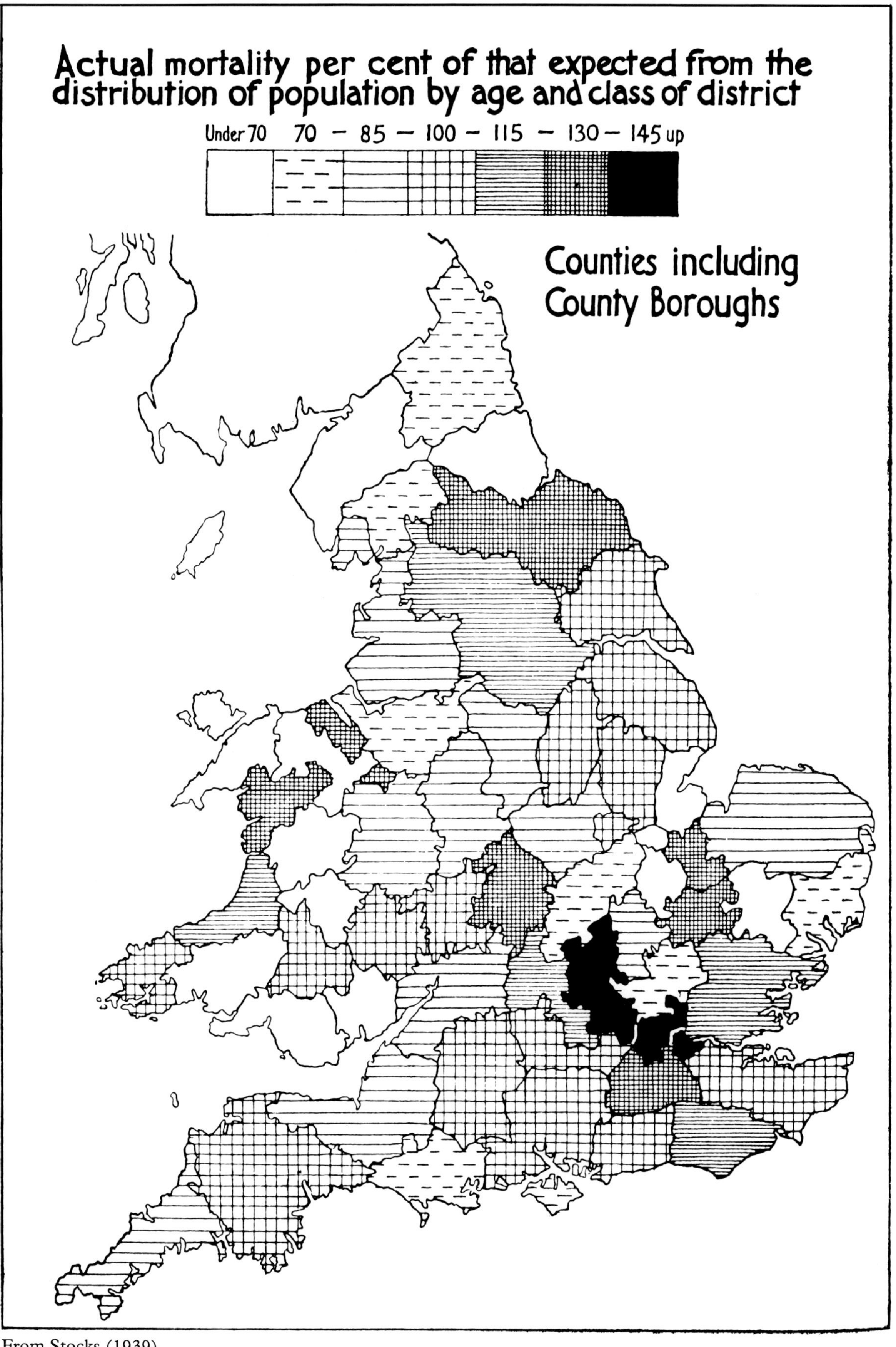

From Stocks (1939).

MAP S6 CANCER OF BREAST IN FEMALES AGES 25–65, 1921–30. STANDARDIZED MORTALITY RATIOS

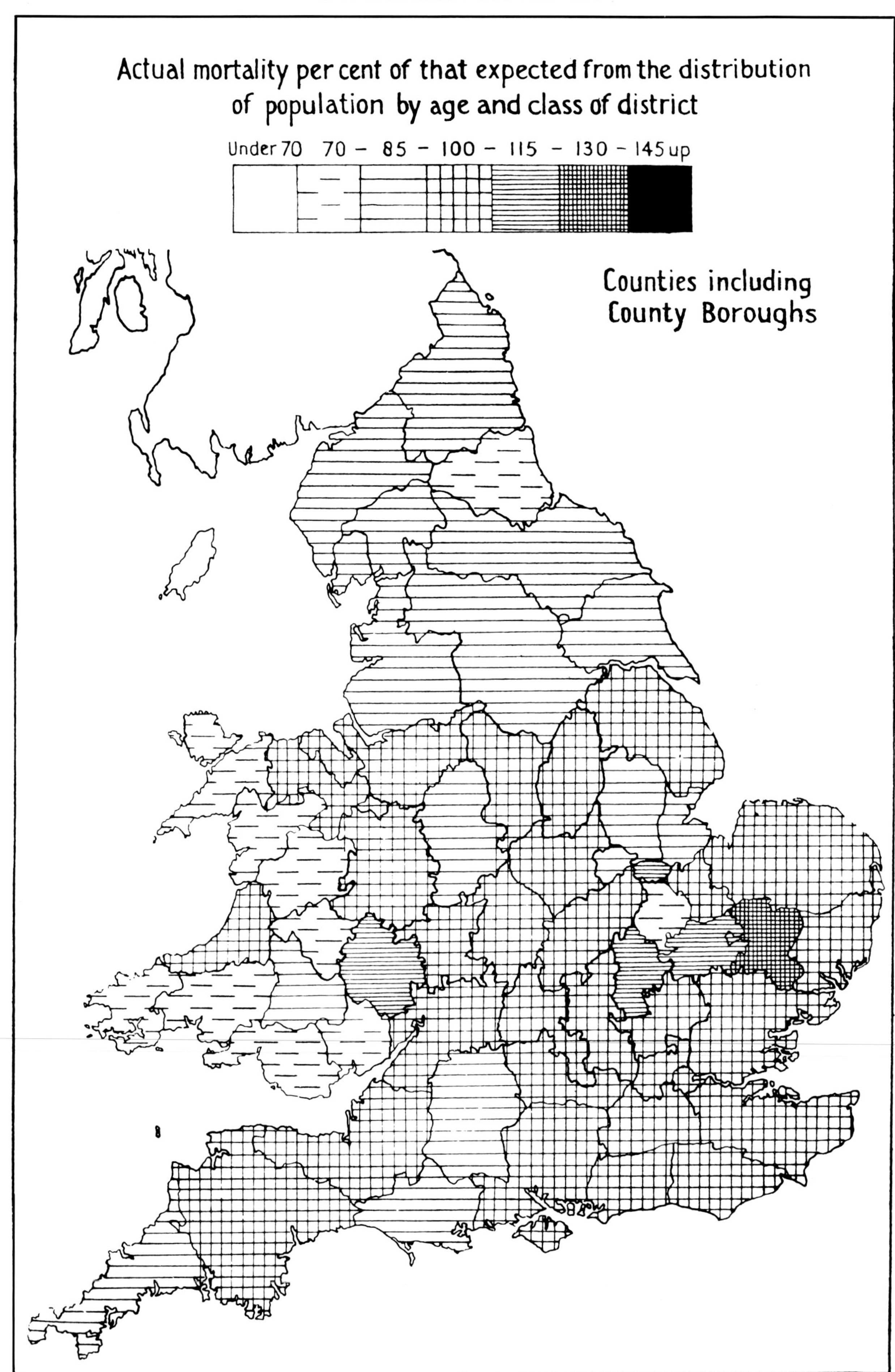

From Stocks (1936).

MAP S7 CANCER OF OVARY AGES 25+, 1921–30.
STANDARDIZED MORTALITY RATIOS

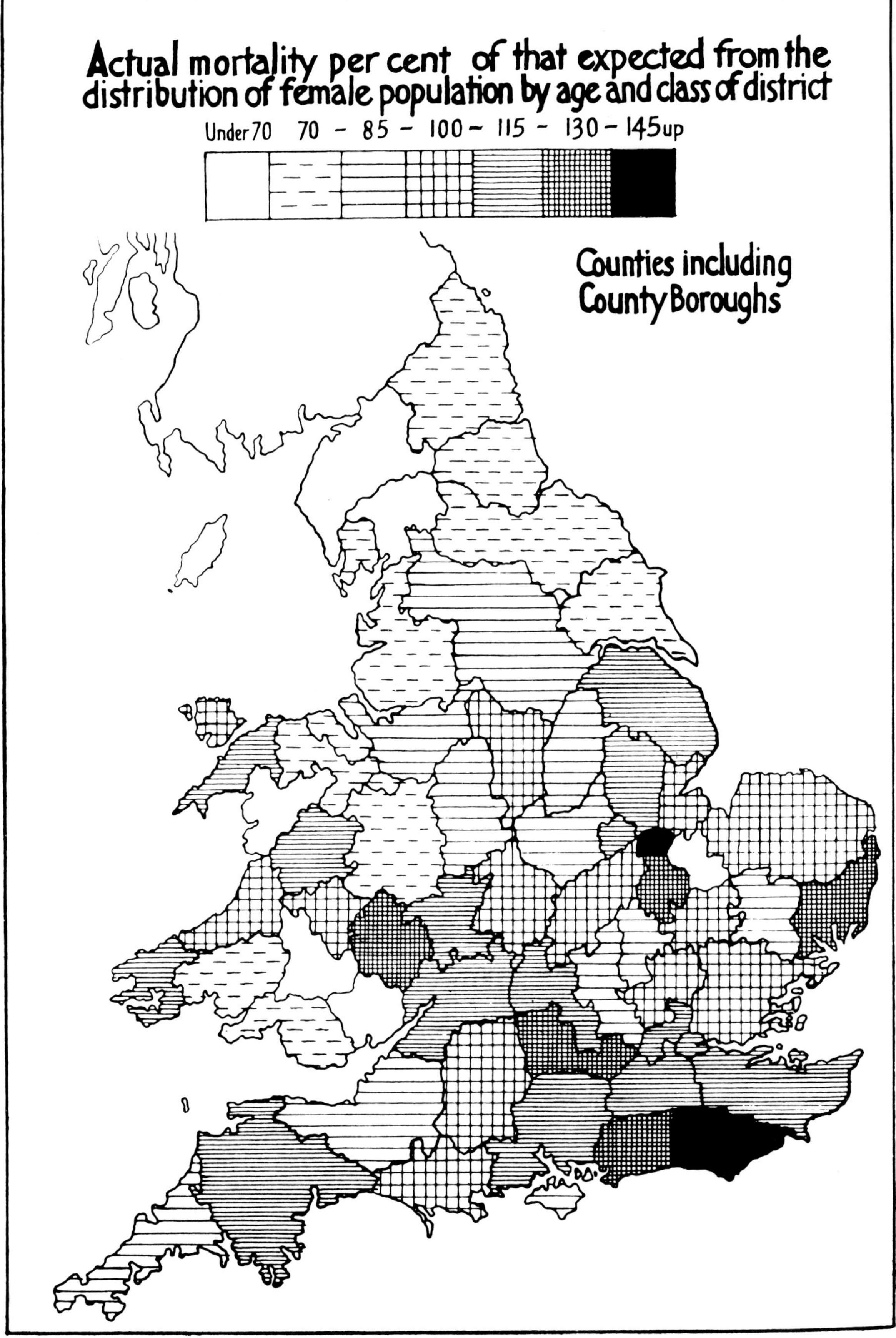

From Stocks (1939).

MAP S8 CANCER OF VAGINA AND VULVA AGES 25+, 1921–30. STANDARDIZED MORTALITY RATIOS

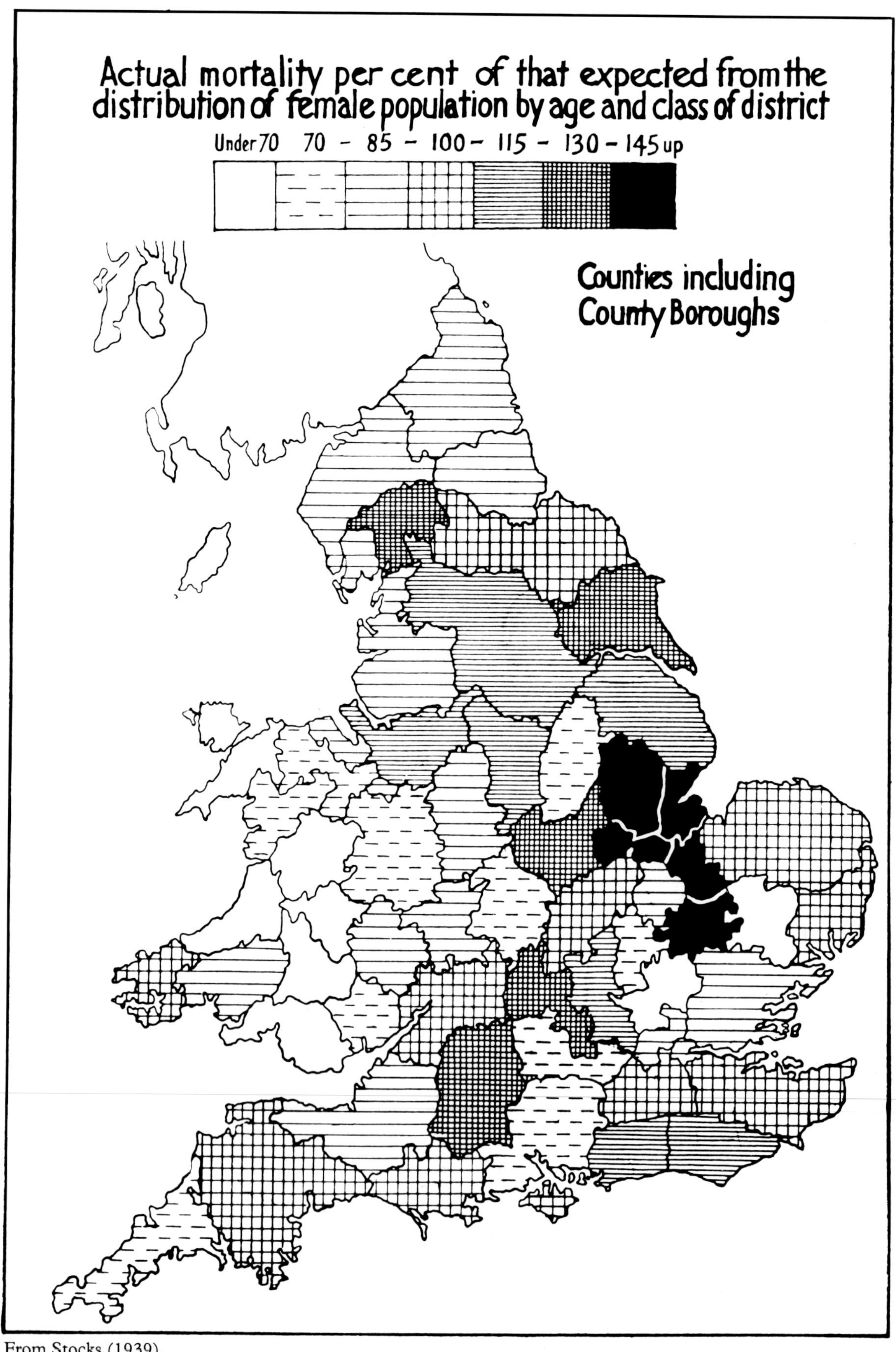

From Stocks (1939).

MAP S9 CANCER OF BLADDER IN MALES AGES 25+, 1921–30. STANDARDIZED MORTALITY RATIOS

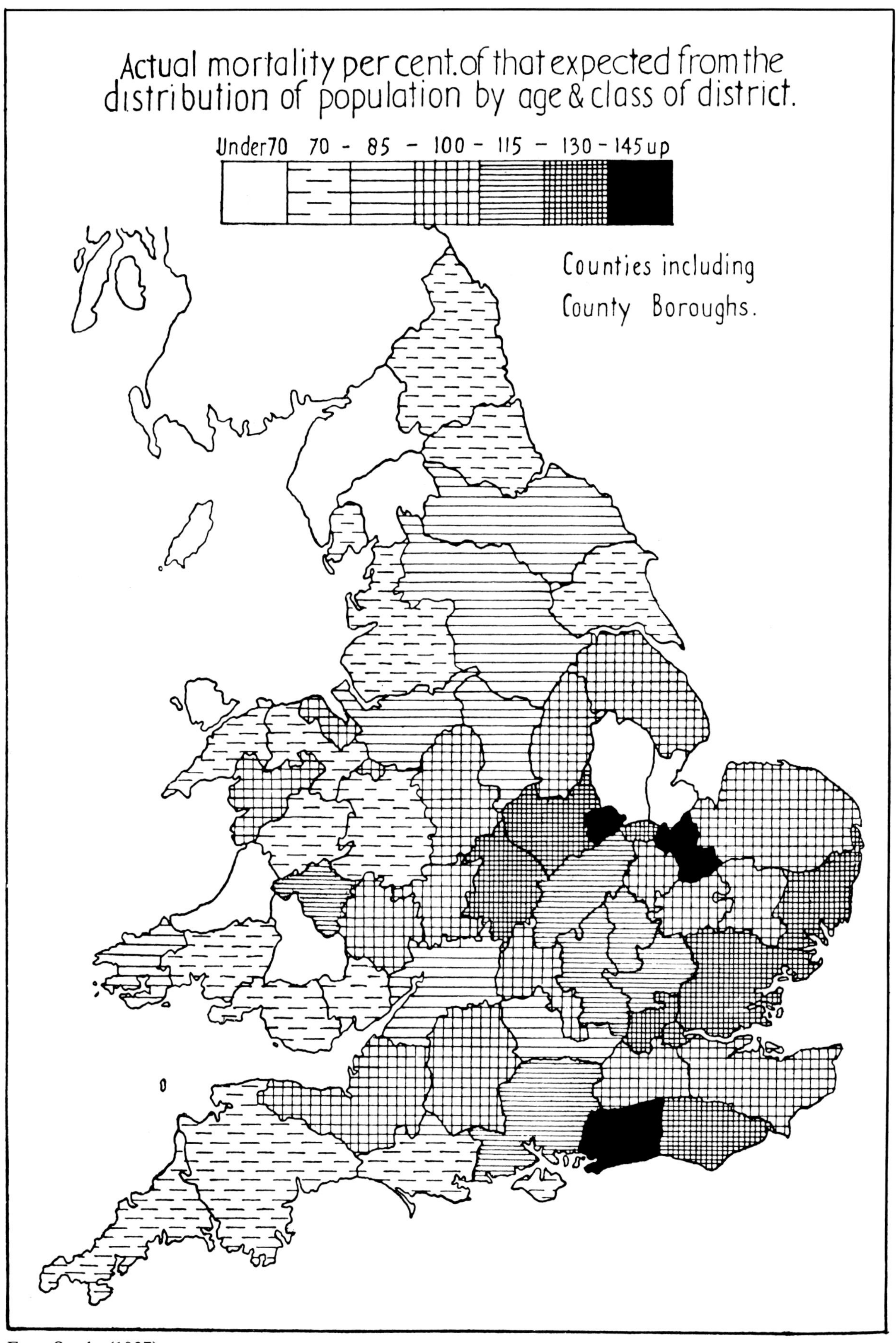

From Stocks (1937).

Maps of cancer incidence in England and Wales, 1968–85*

* Childhood leukaemia, 1966–83.

MAP 1 CANCER OF LIP, MALES, 1968–85

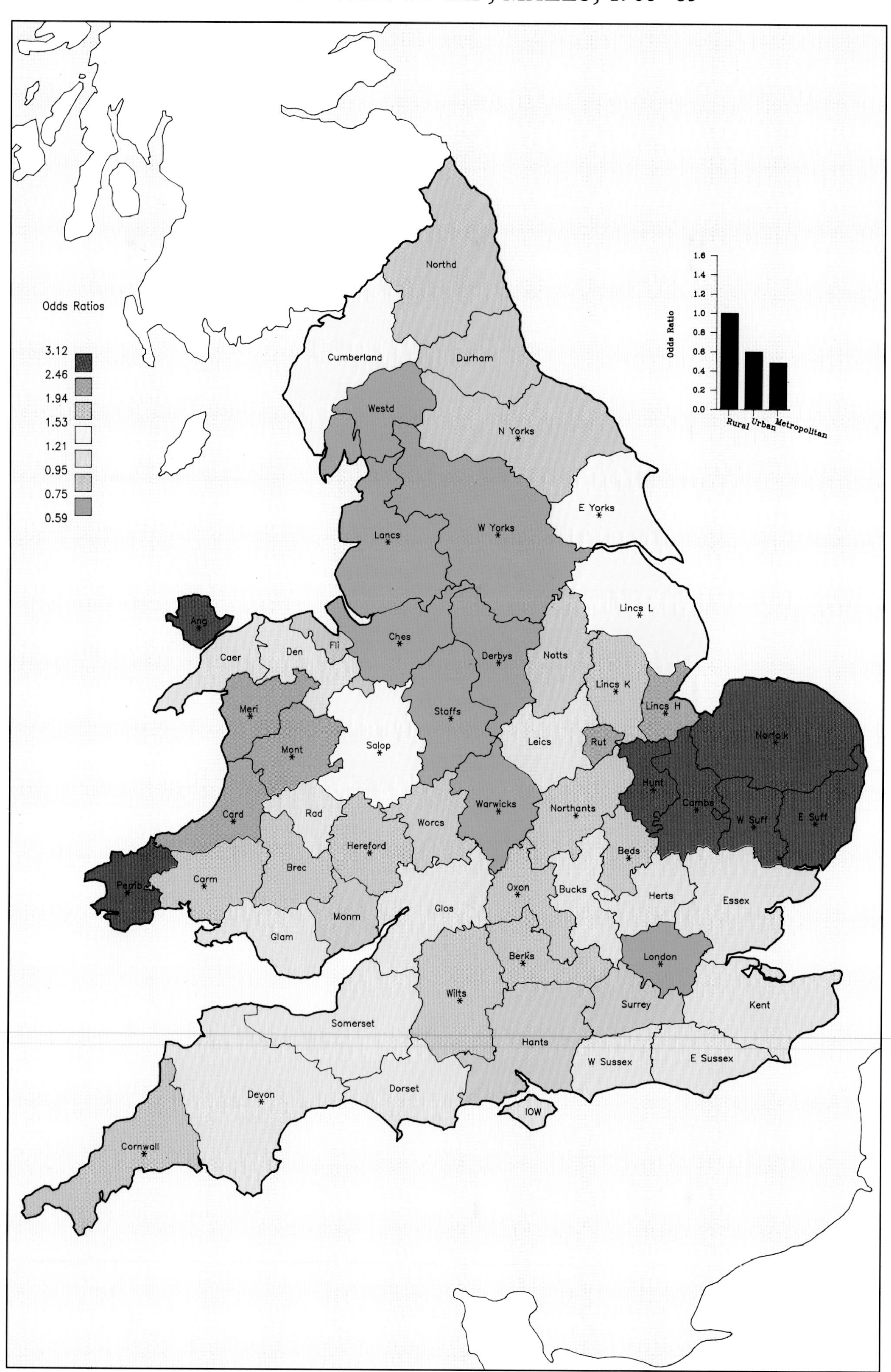

*p<0.05

MAP 2 CANCER OF LIP, FEMALES, 1968–85

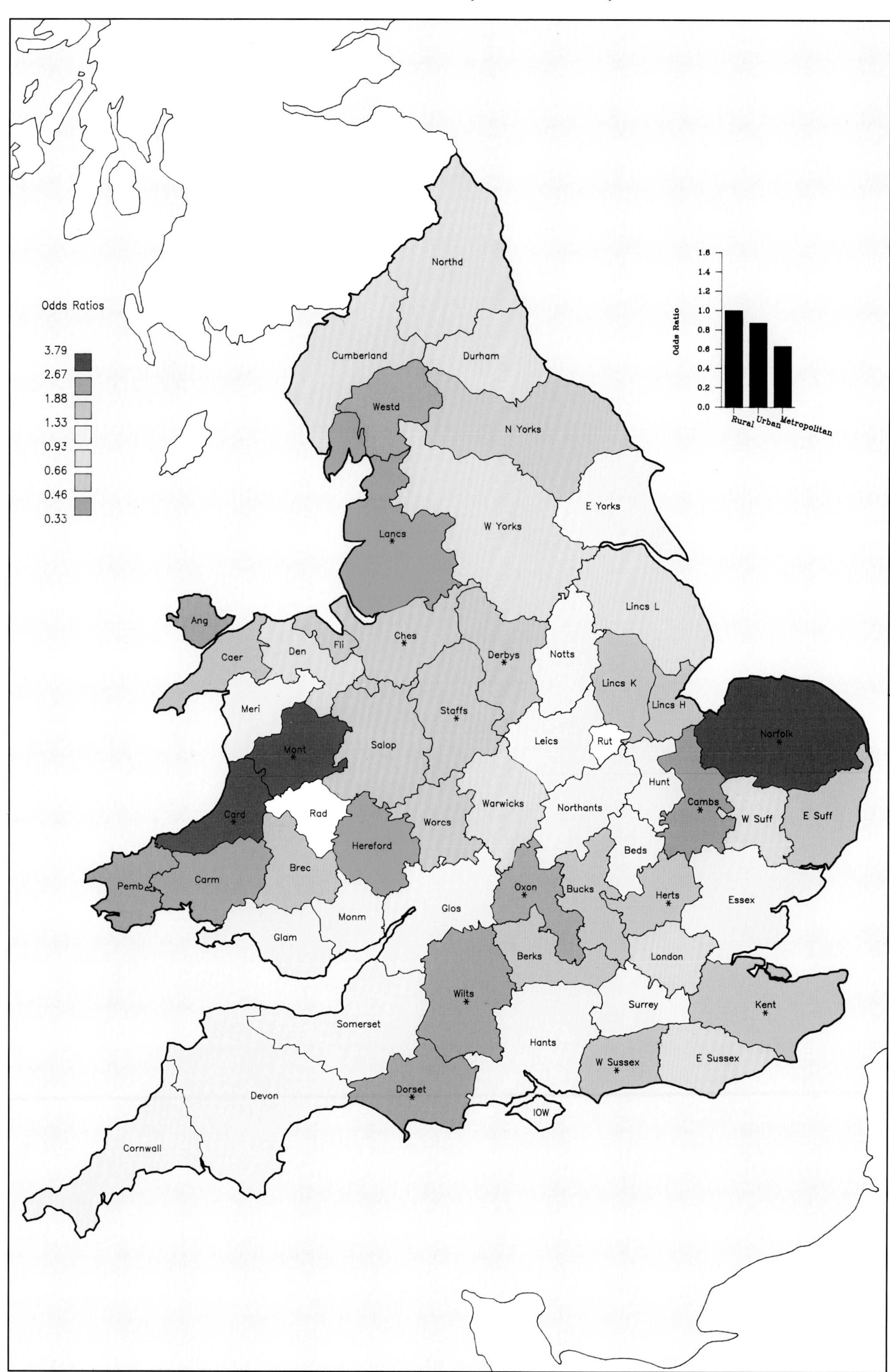

*p<0.05

In counties coloured white, no cases occurred during the period

MAP 3 CANCER OF SALIVARY GLANDS, MALES, 1968–85

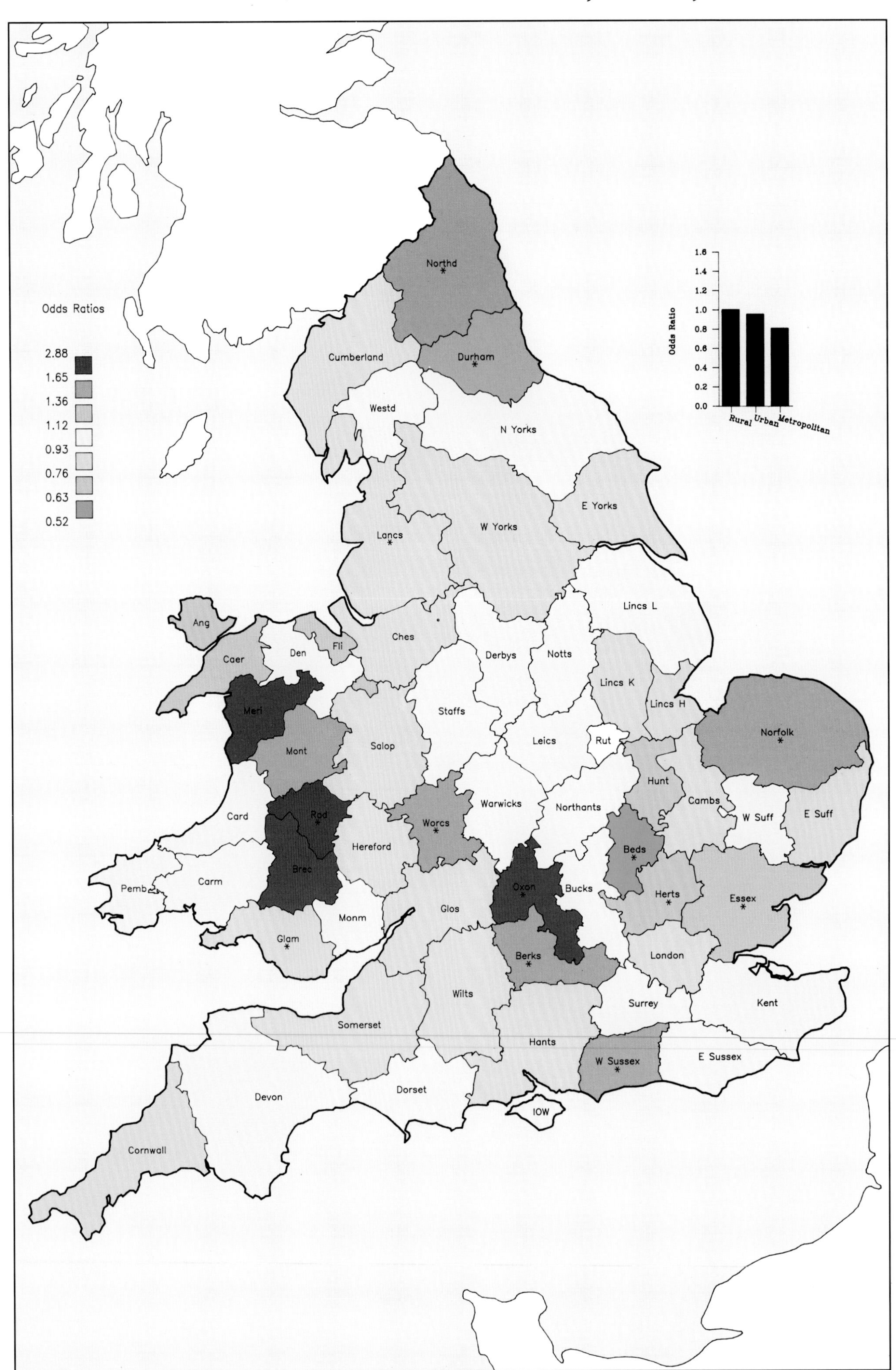

*p<0.05

In counties coloured white, no cases occurred during the period

MAP 4 CANCER OF SALIVARY GLANDS, FEMALES, 1968–85

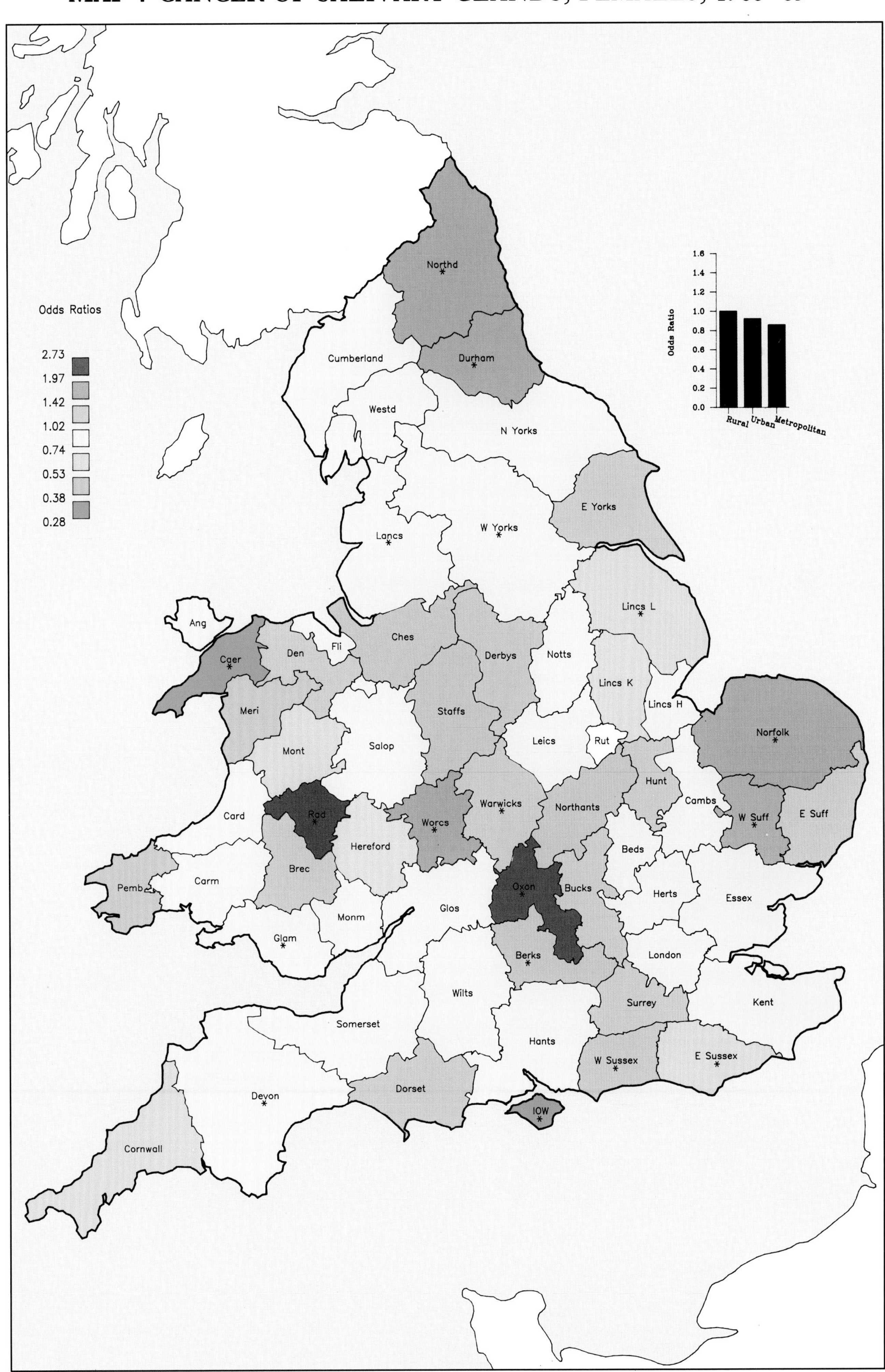

*p<0.05

In counties coloured white, no cases occurred during the period

MAP 5 CANCER OF TONGUE, MALES, 1968–85

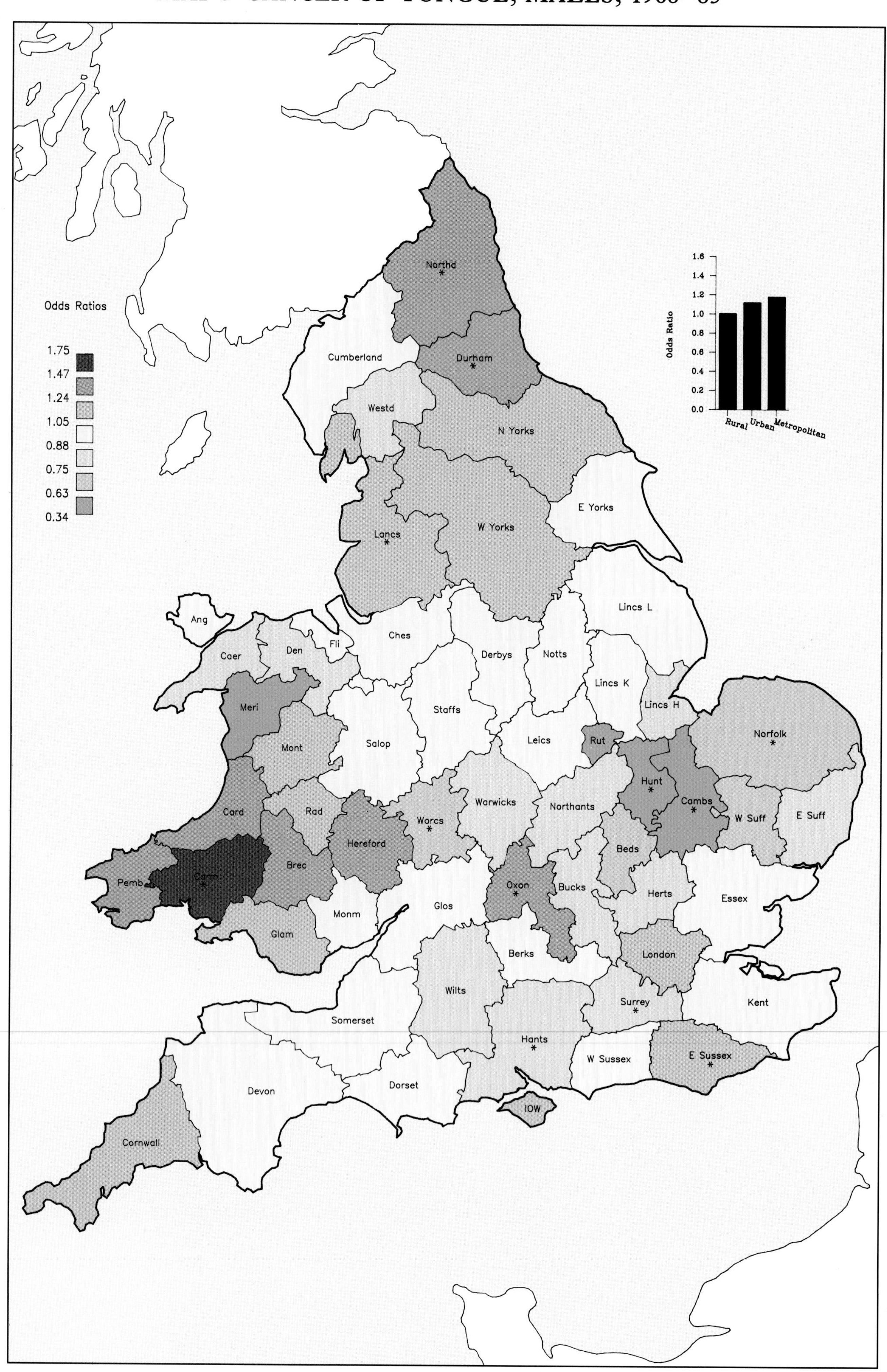

*p<0.05

MAP 6 CANCER OF MOUTH, MALES, 1968–85

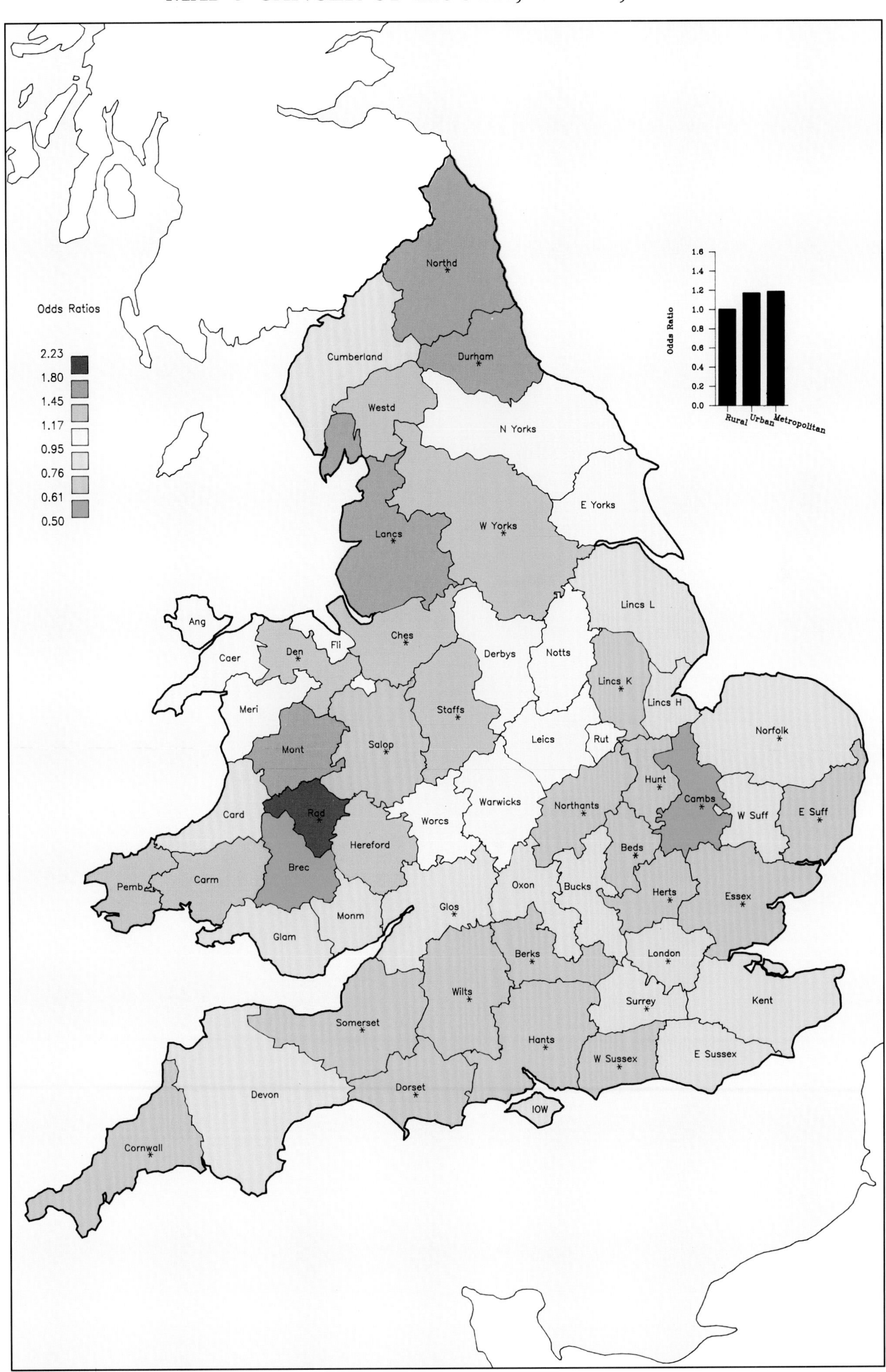

*p<0.05

MAP 7 CANCER OF PHARYNX, MALES, 1968–85

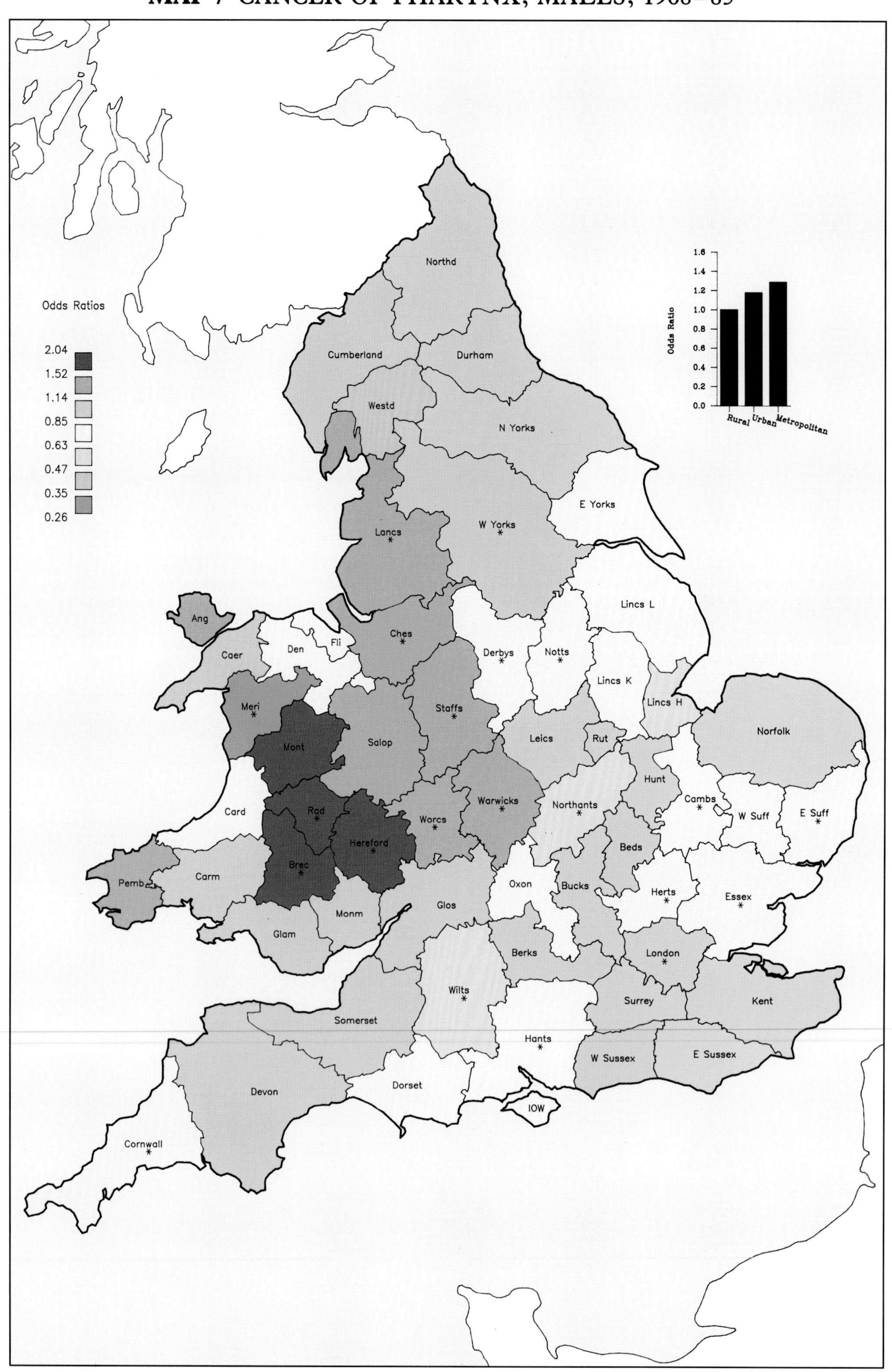

$^{*}p<0.05$

MAP 8 CANCERS OF TONGUE, MOUTH, AND PHARYNX, FEMALES, 1968–85

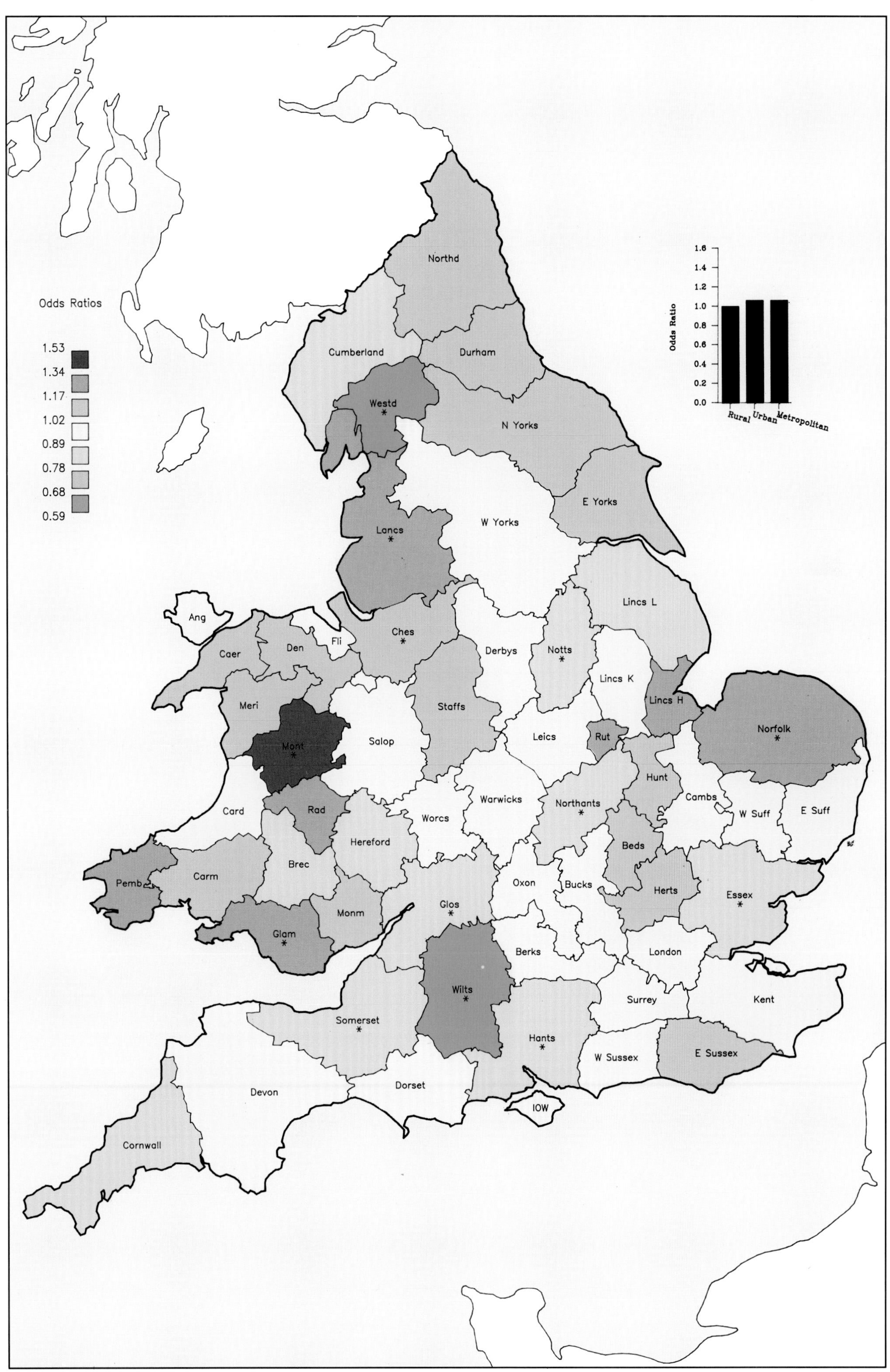

⋆p<0.05

MAP 9 CANCER OF NASOPHARYNX, MALES, 1968–85

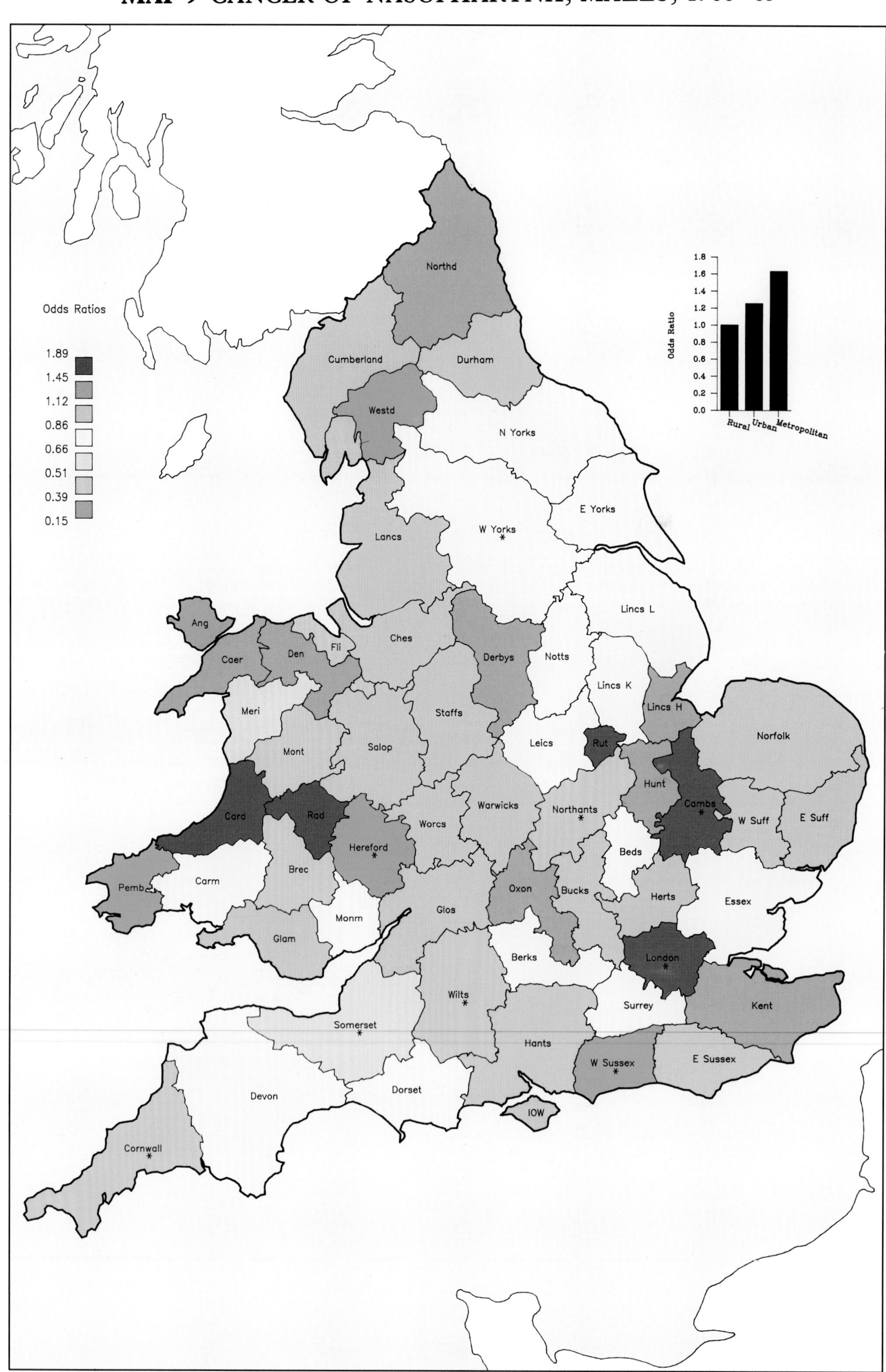

*p<0.05

MAP 10 CANCER OF NASOPHARYNX, FEMALES, 1968–85

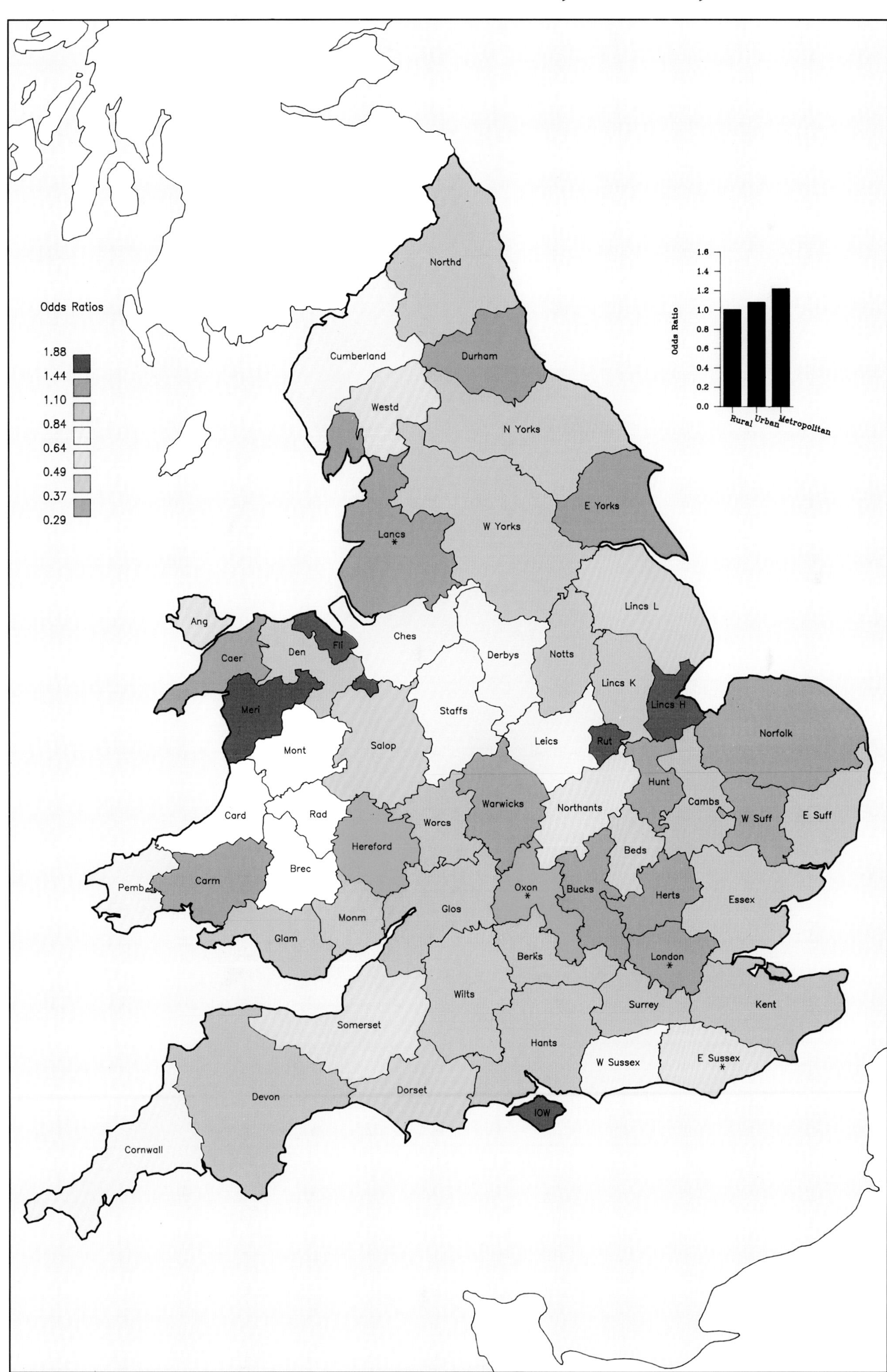

*p<0.05

In counties coloured white, no cases occurred during the period

MAP 11 CANCER OF OESOPHAGUS, MALES, 1968–85

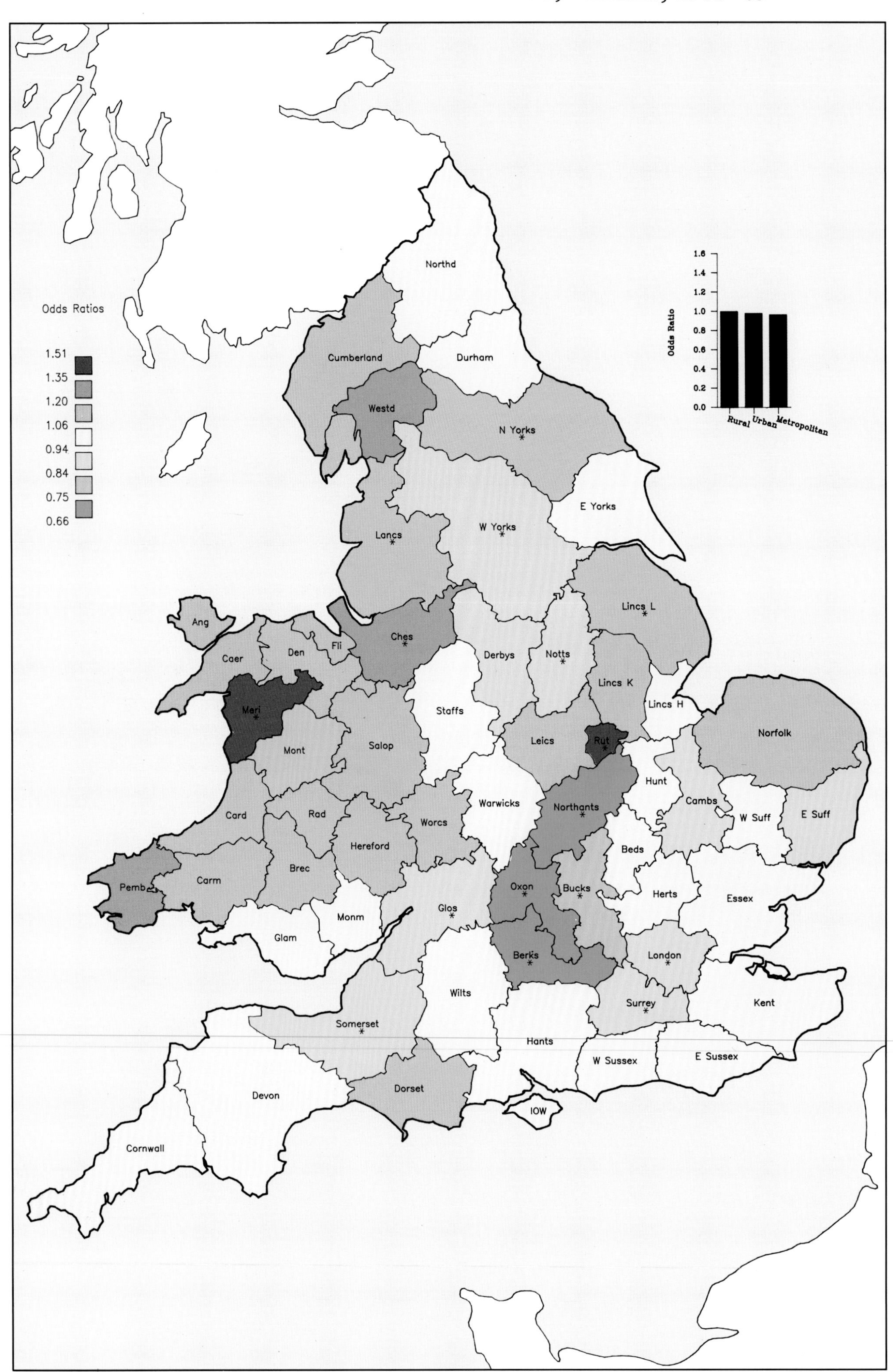

*p<0.05

MAP 12 CANCER OF OESOPHAGUS, FEMALES, 1968–85

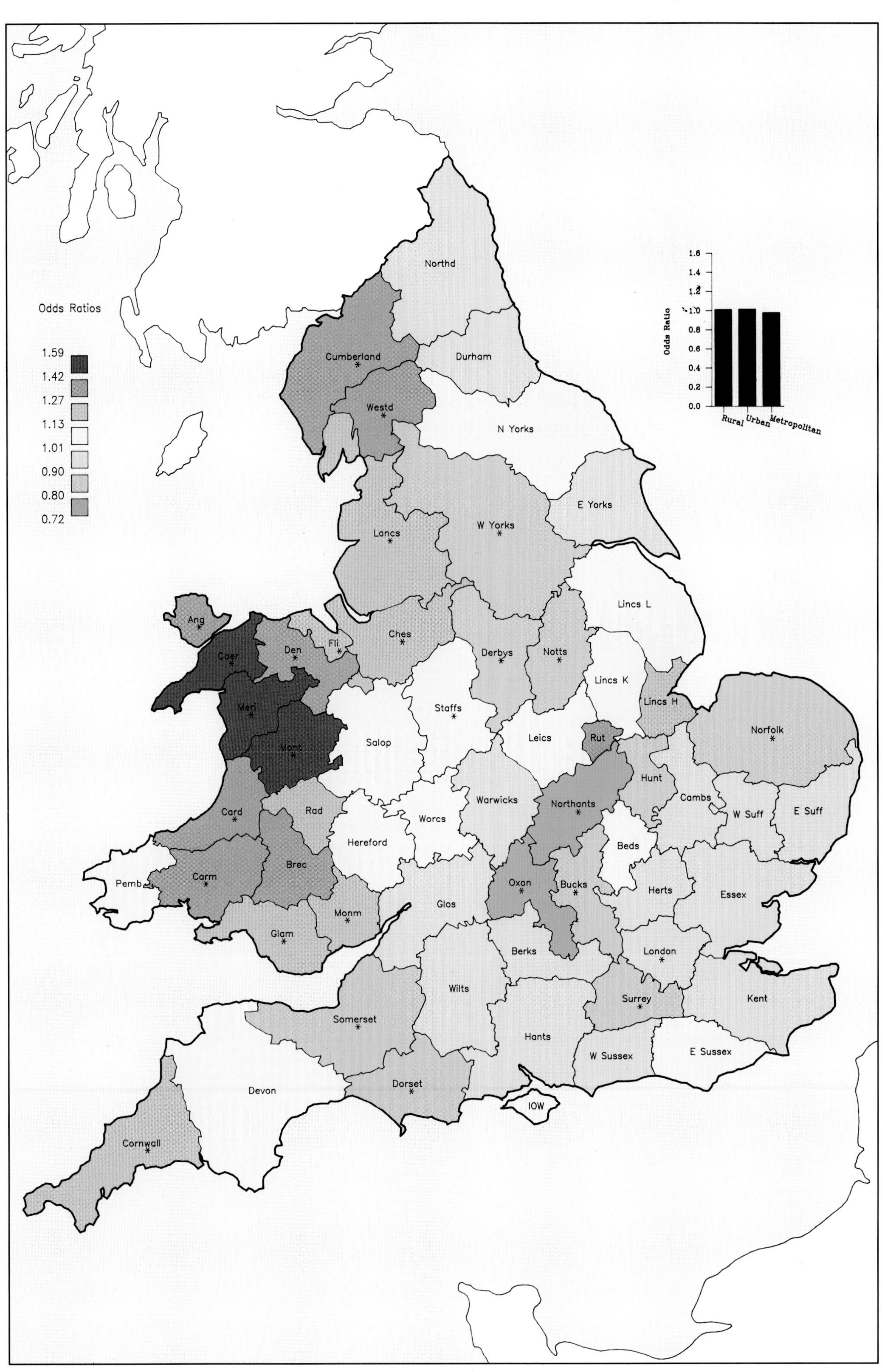

*p<0.05

MAP 13 CANCER OF STOMACH, MALES, 1968–85

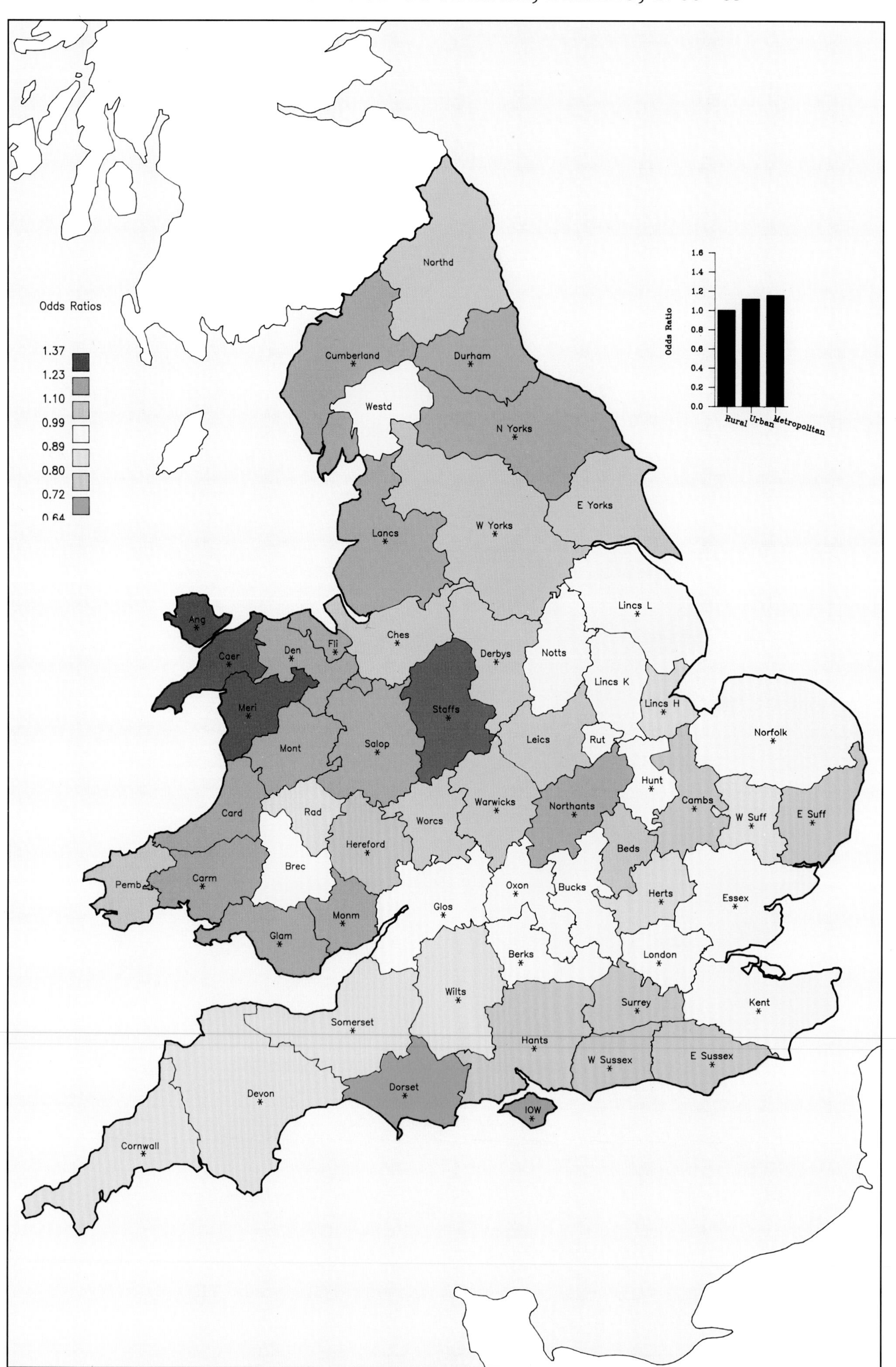

*$p<0.05$

MAP 14 CANCER OF STOMACH, FEMALES, 1968–85

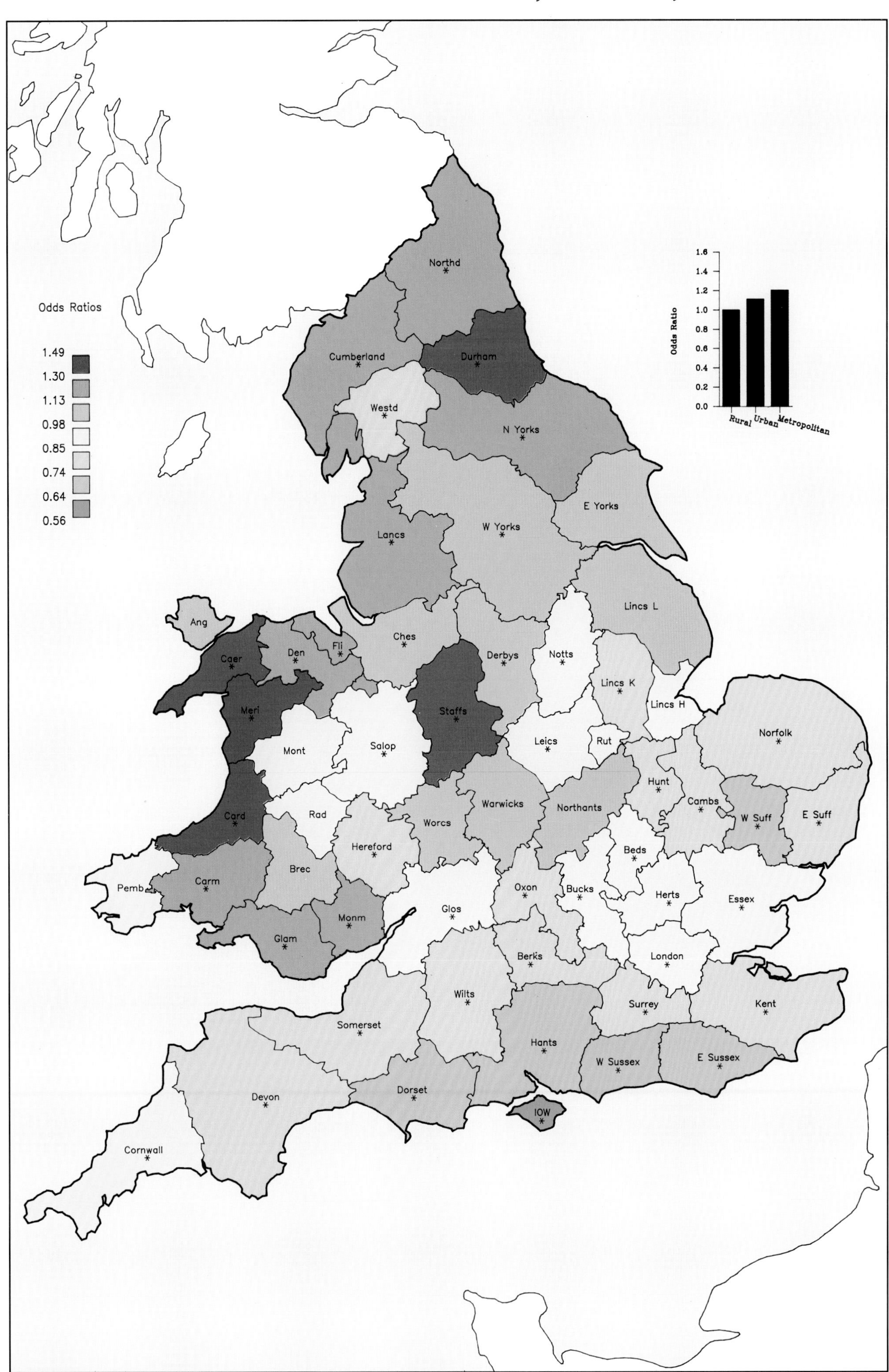

*p<0.05

MAP 15 CANCERS OF COLON AND RECTUM, MALES, 1968–85

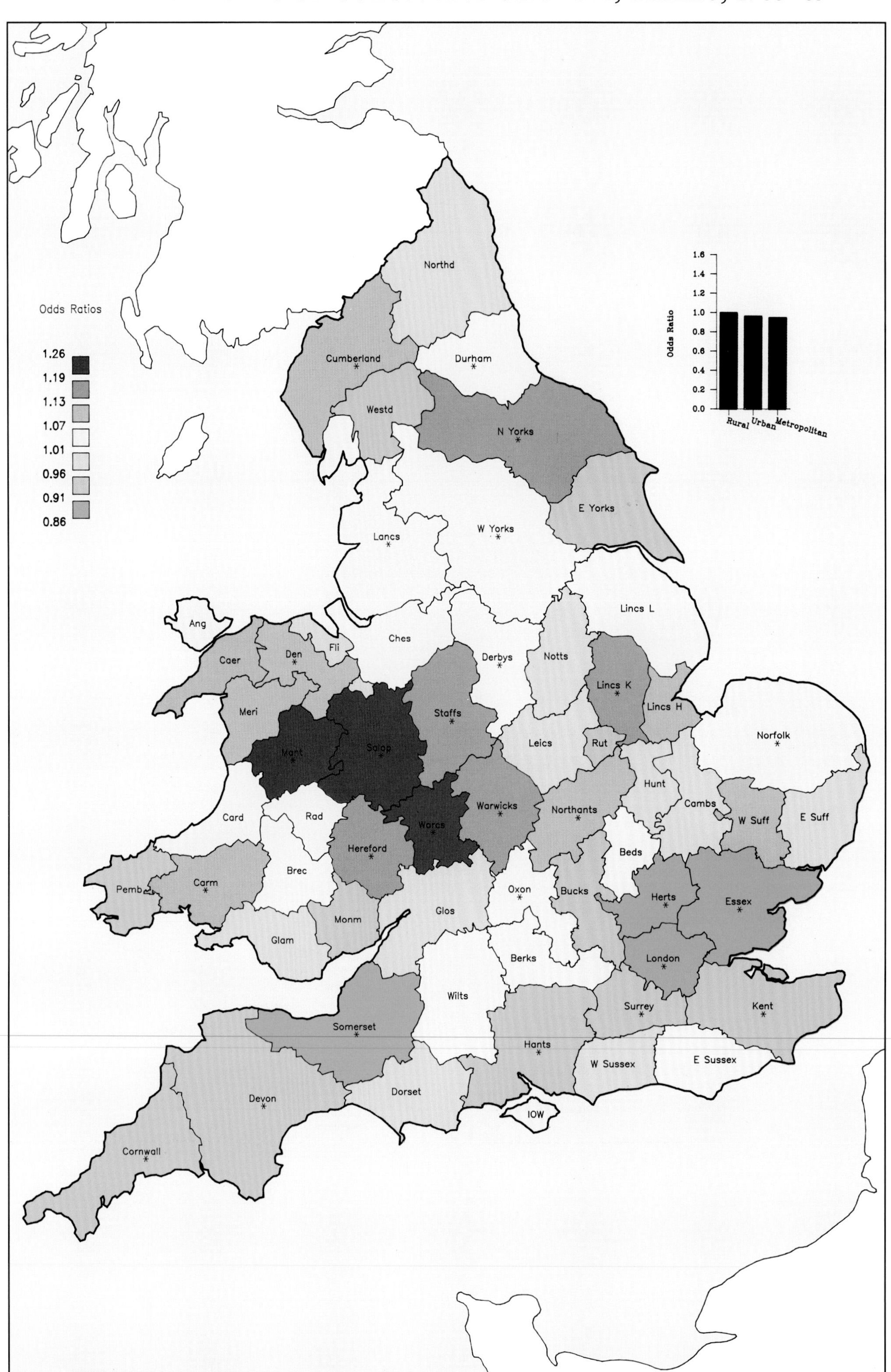

*p<0.05

MAP 16 CANCERS OF COLON AND RECTUM, FEMALES, 1968–85

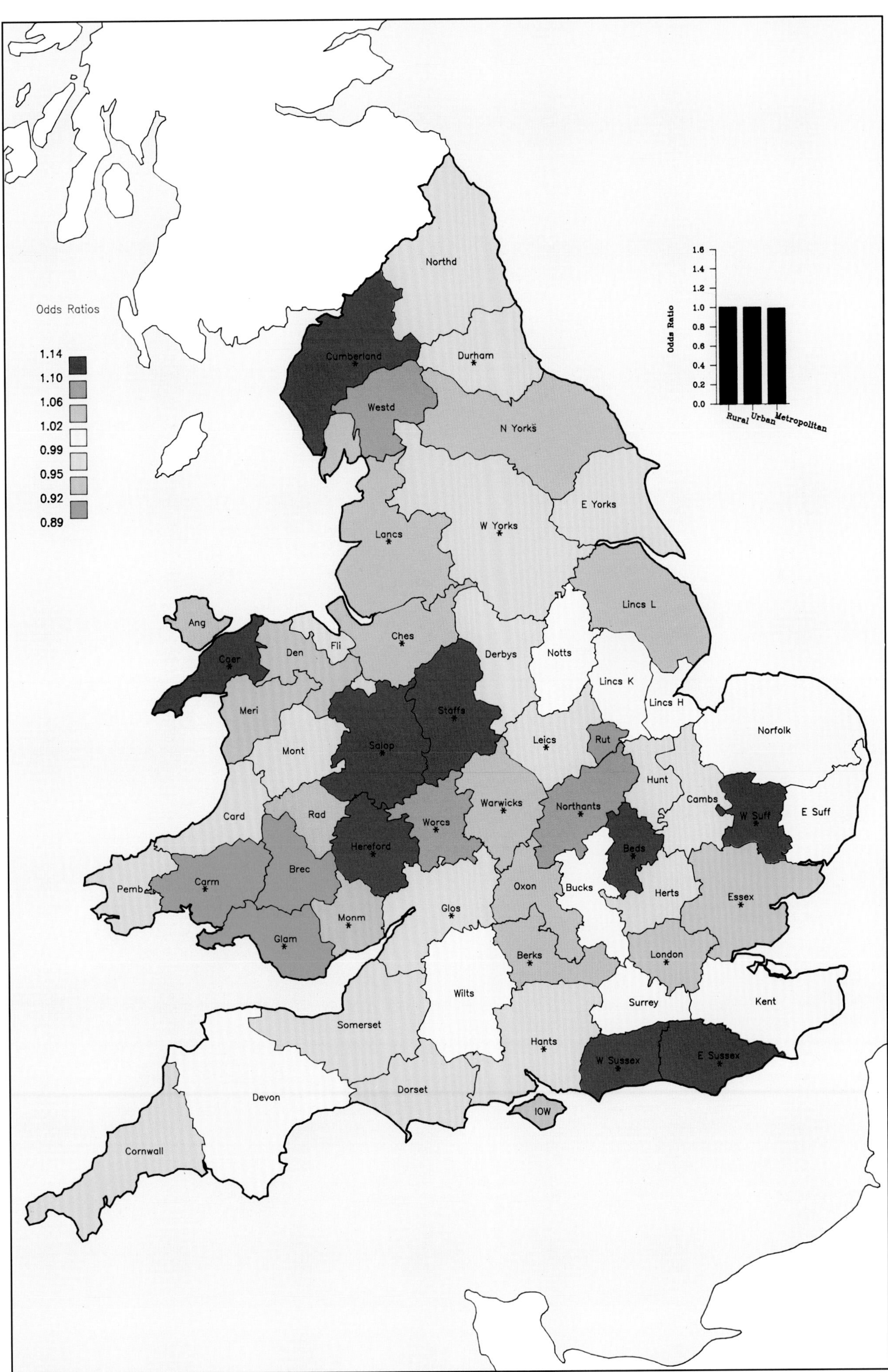

*p<0.05

MAP 17 CANCER OF LIVER, MALES, 1968–85

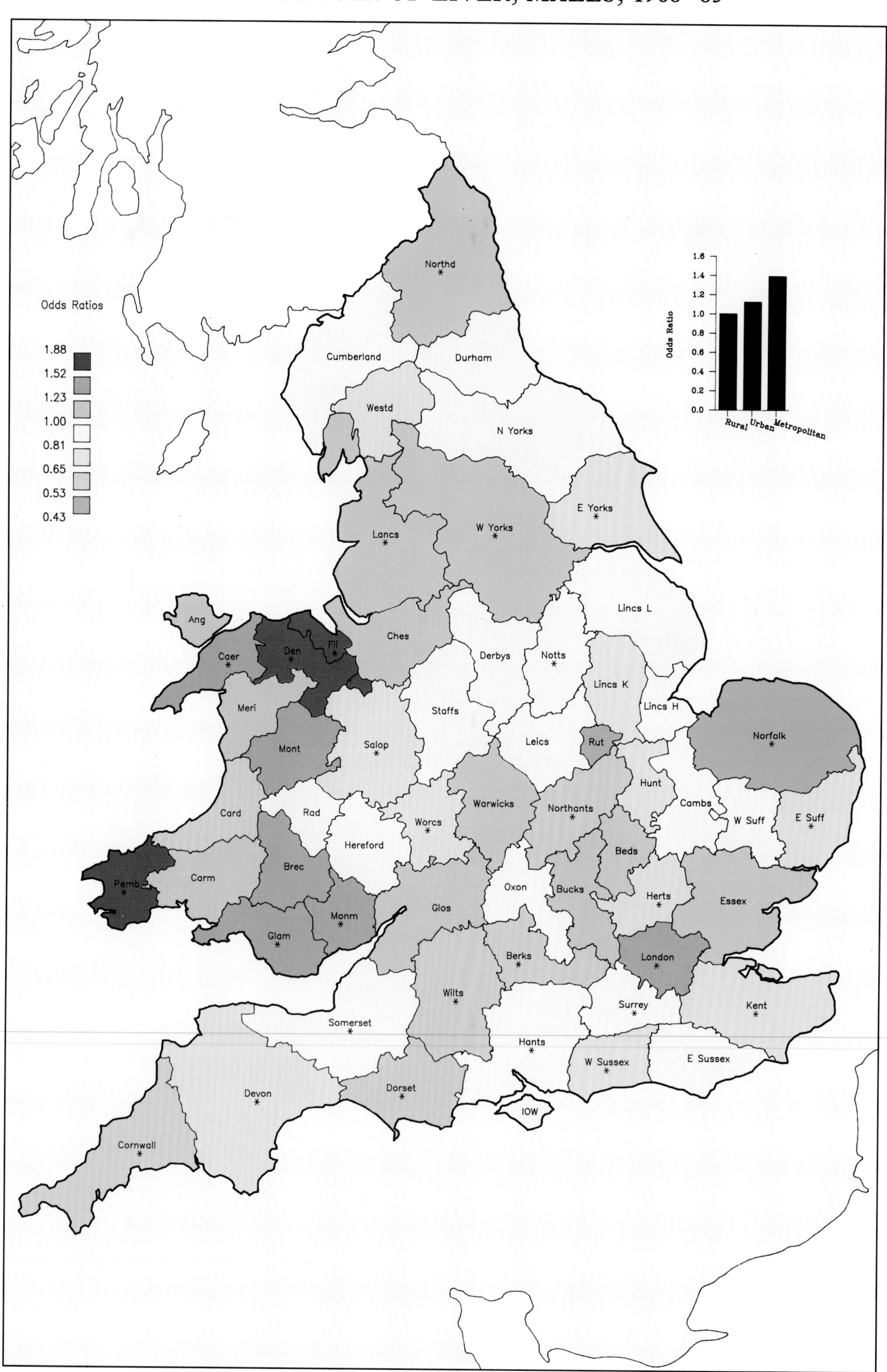

*p<0.05

MAP 18 CANCER OF LIVER, FEMALES, 1968–85

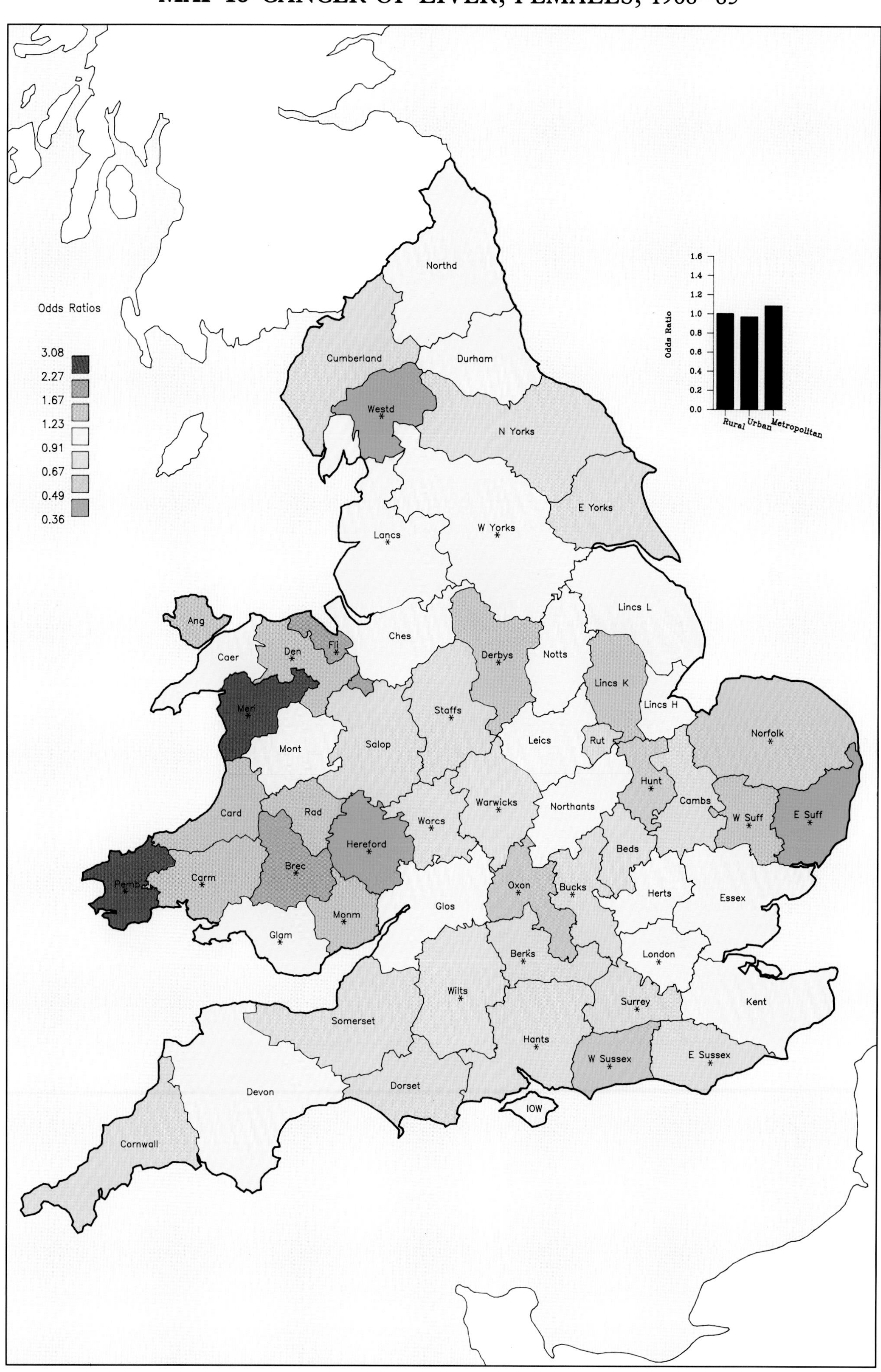

*p<0.05

MAP 19 CANCER OF GALLBLADDER, MALES, 1968–85

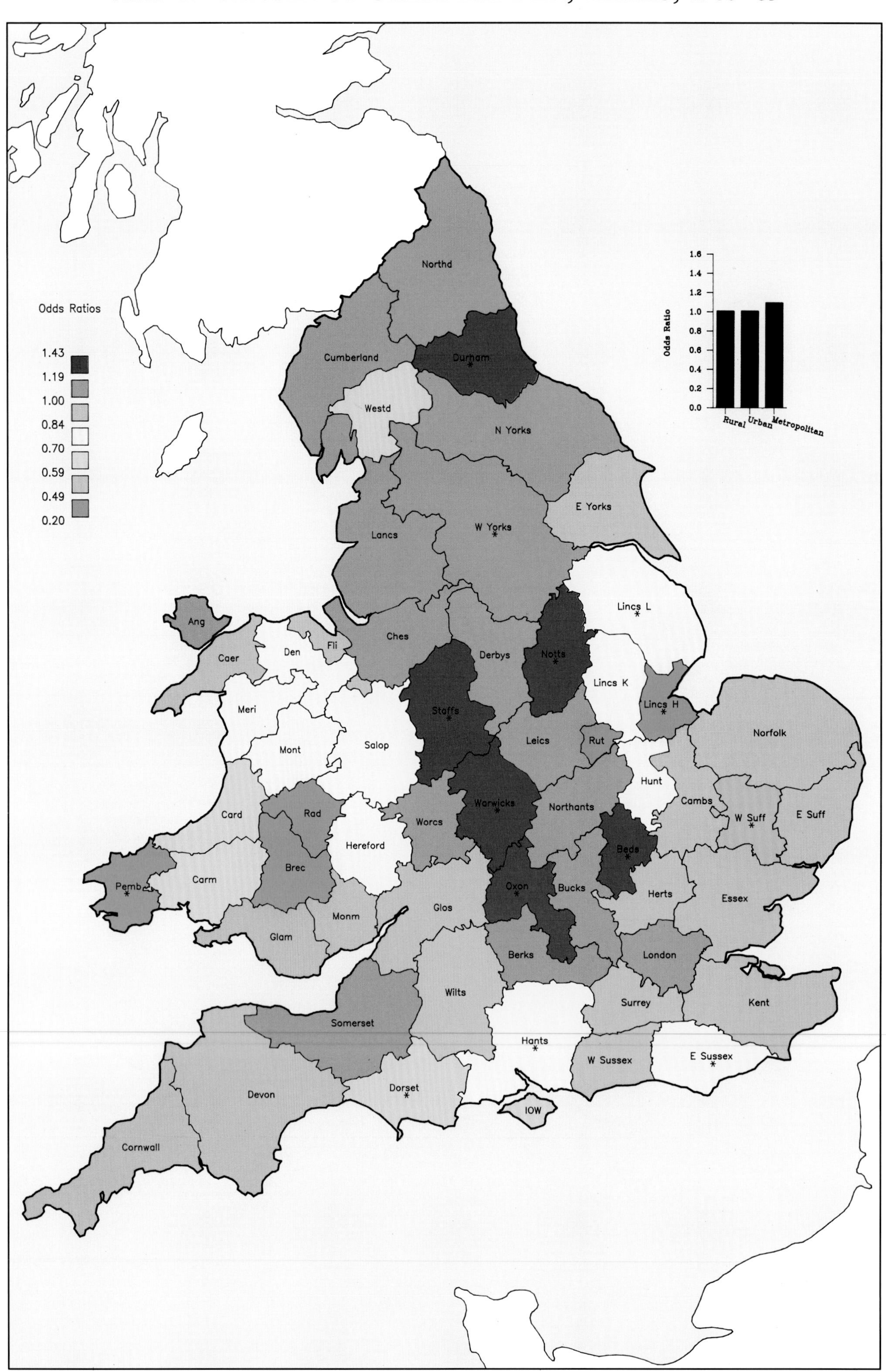

*p<0.05

MAP 20 CANCER OF GALLBLADDER, FEMALES, 1968–85

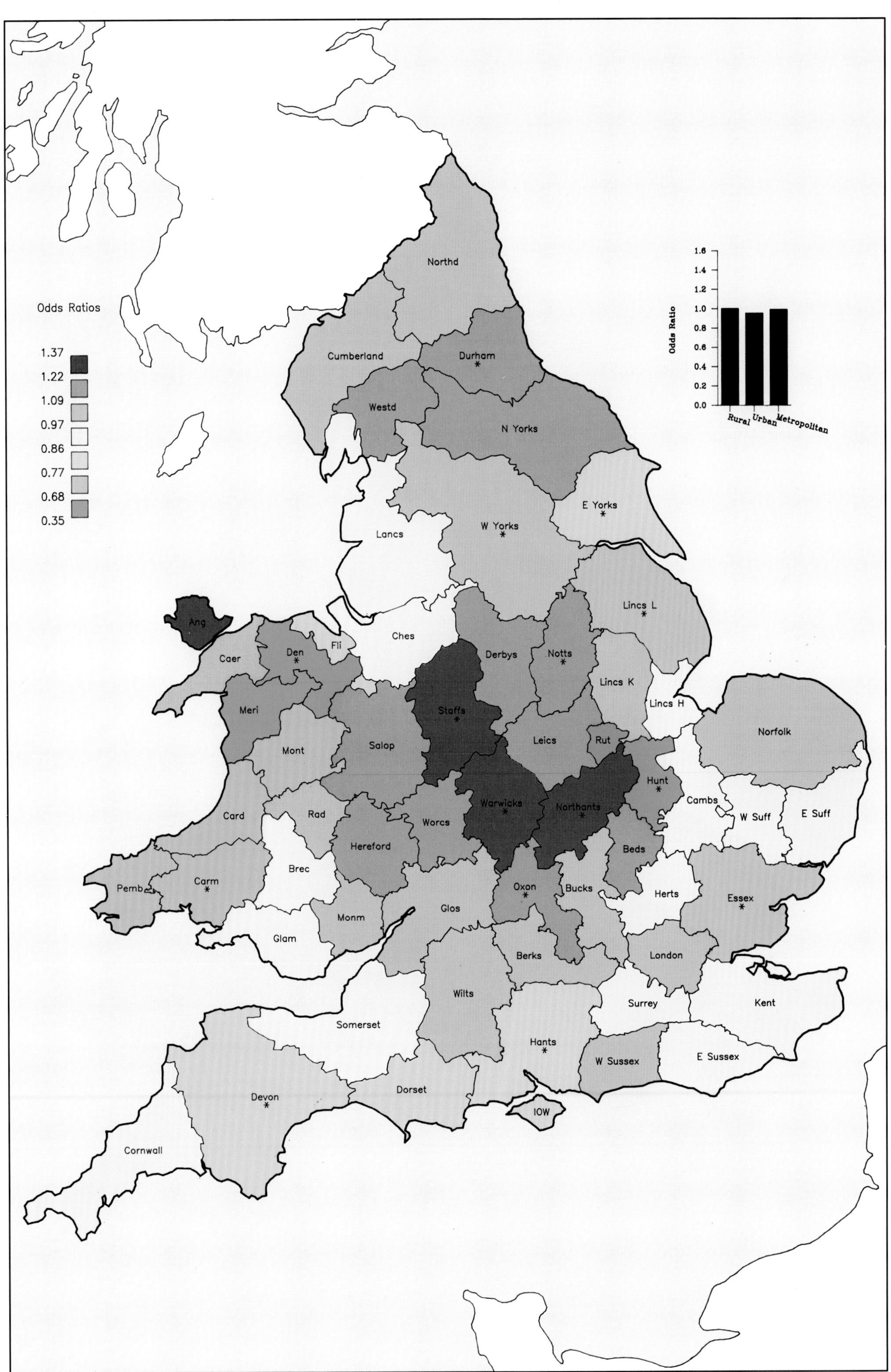

*$p<0.05$

MAP 21 CANCER OF PANCREAS, MALES, 1968–85

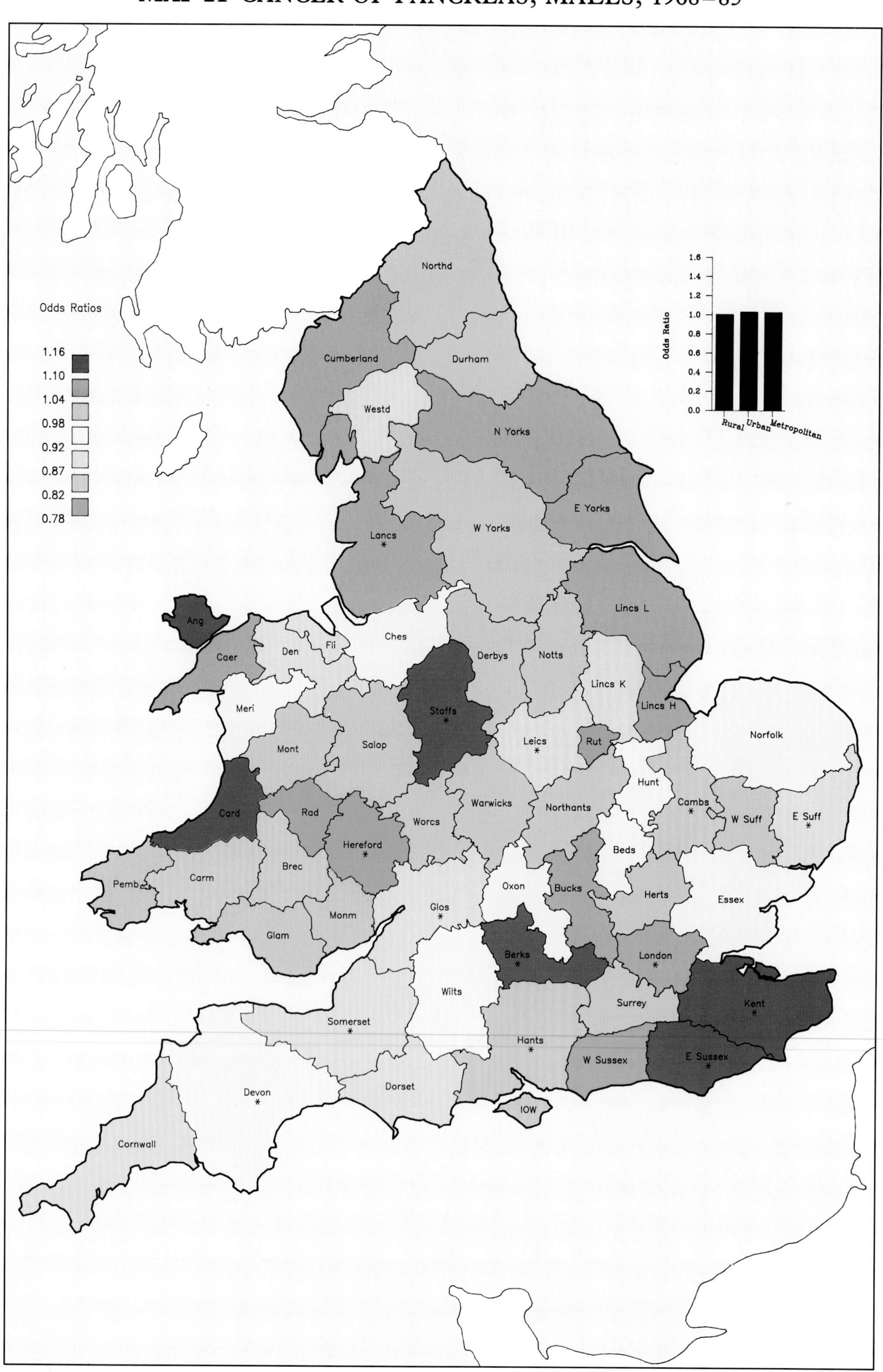

*p<0.05

MAP 22 CANCER OF PANCREAS, FEMALES, 1968–85

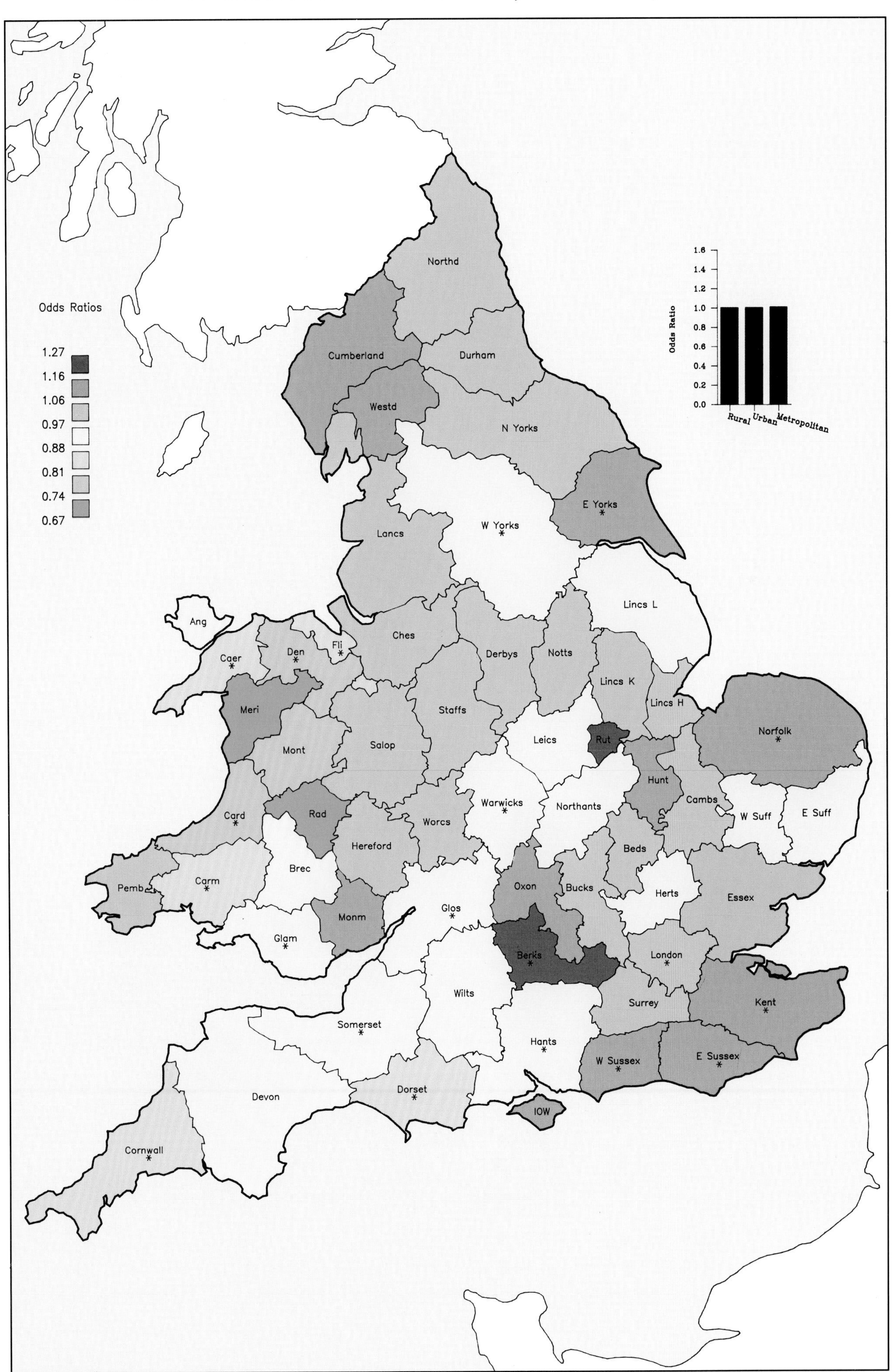

*p<0.05

MAP 23 CANCERS OF NOSE, EAR, AND NASAL SINUSES, MALES, 1968–85

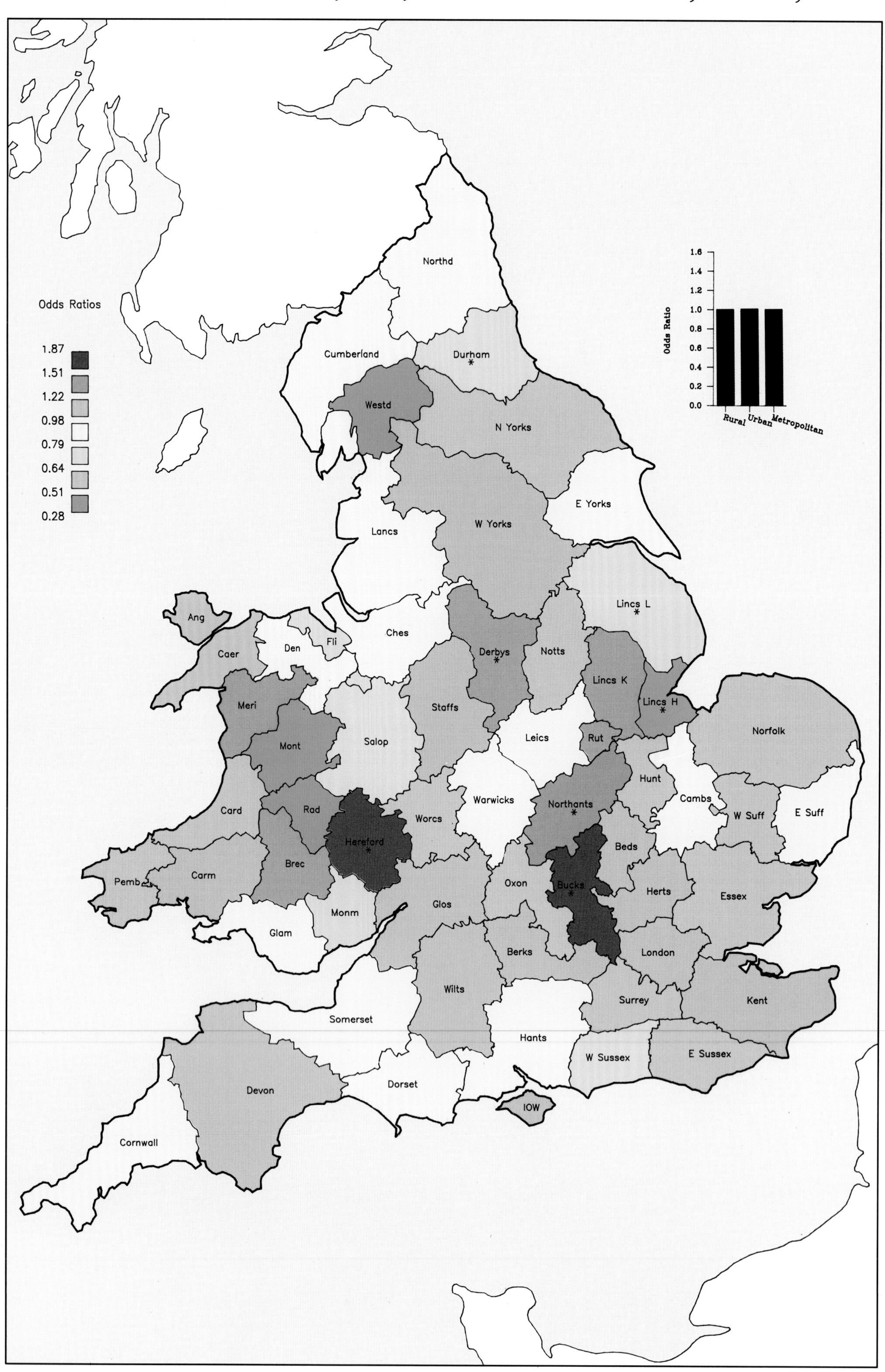

*p<0.05

MAP 24 CANCERS OF NOSE, EAR, AND NASAL SINUSES, FEMALES, 1968–85

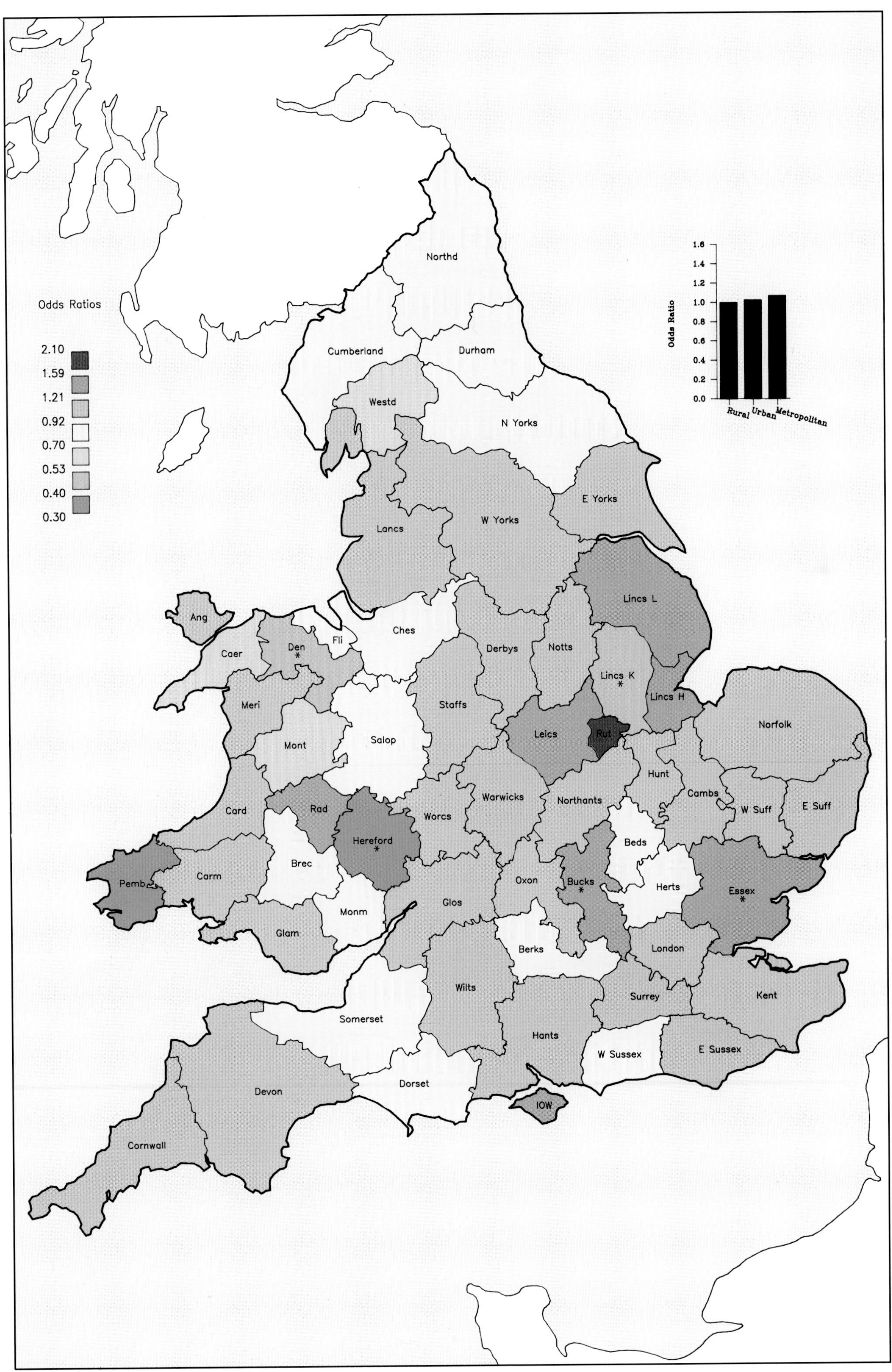

*p<0.05

MAP 25 CANCER OF LARYNX, MALES, 1968–85

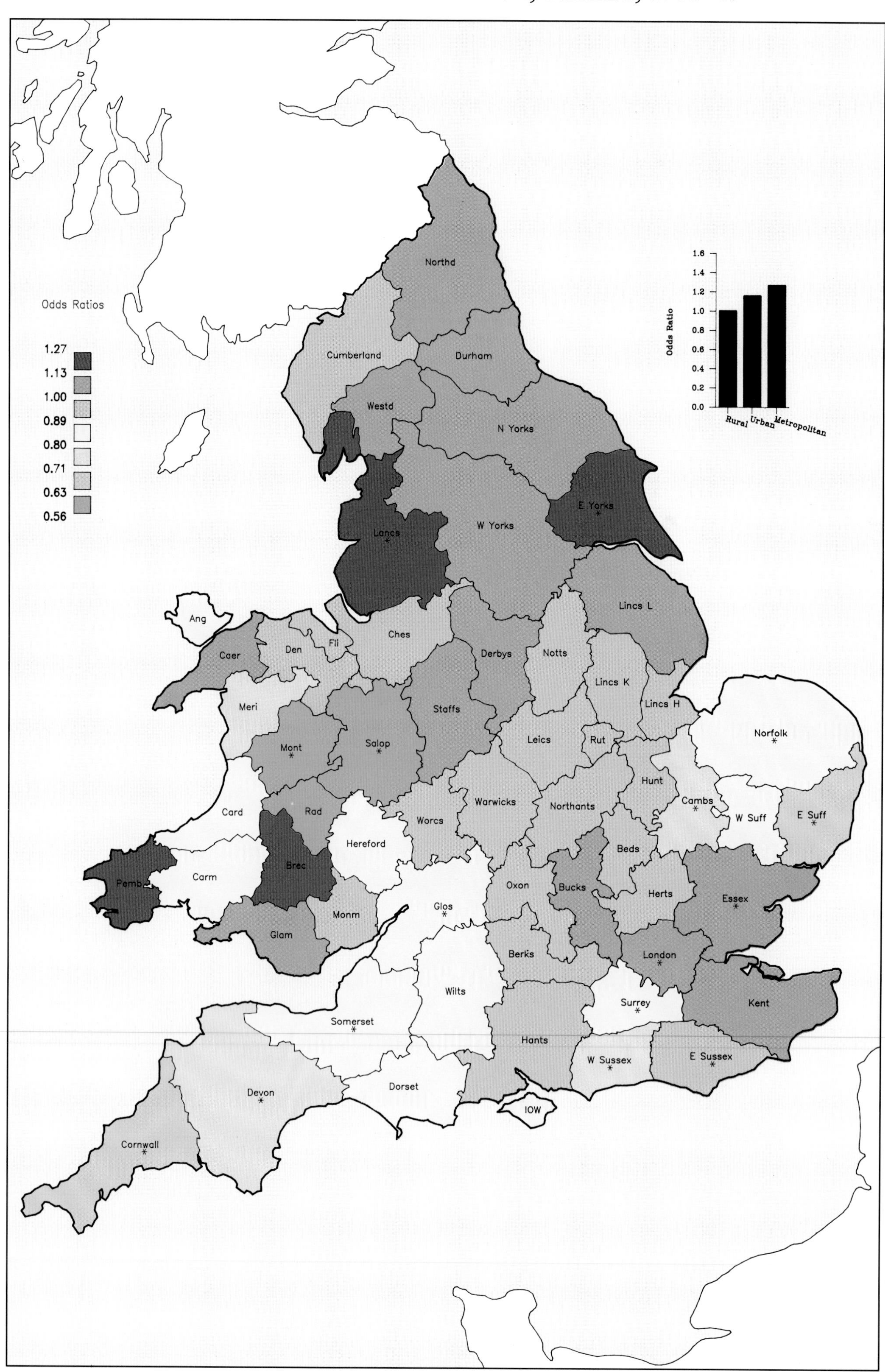

*p<0.05

MAP 26 CANCER OF LARYNX, FEMALES, 1968–85

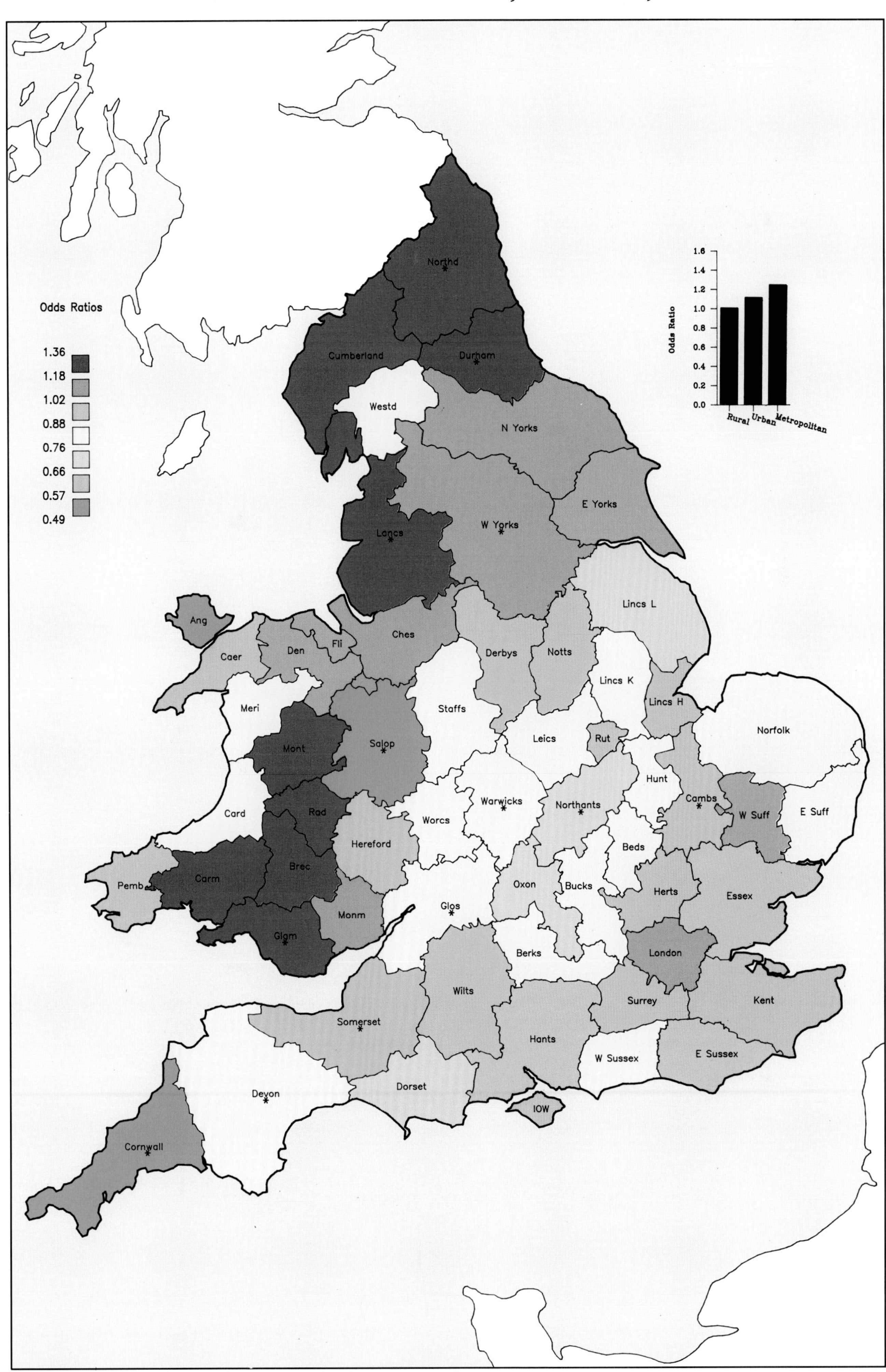

*p<0.05

MAP 27 CANCER OF LUNG, MALES, AGES 0–44, 1968–85

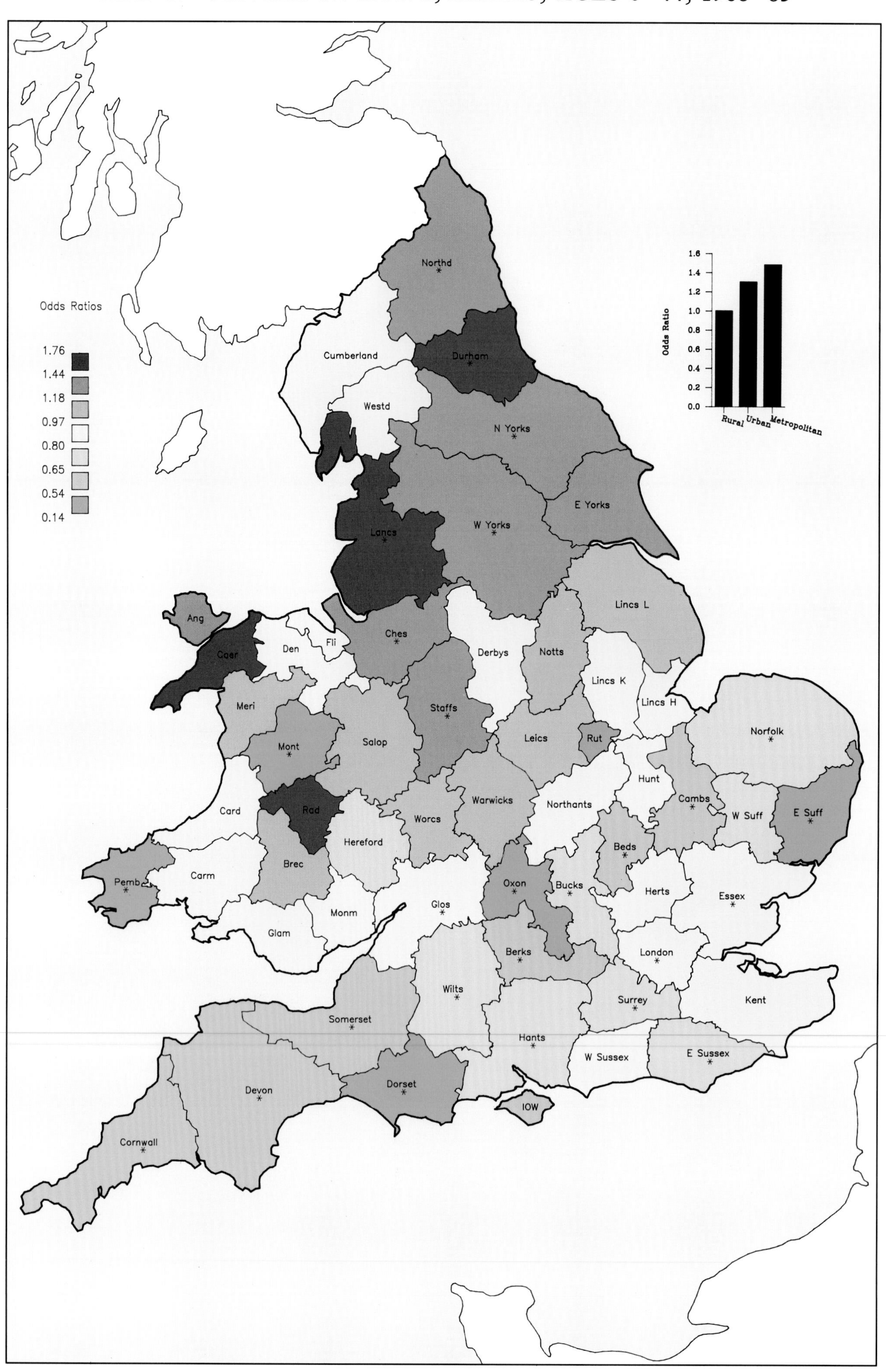

*p<0.05

MAP 28 CANCER OF LUNG, FEMALES, AGES 0–44, 1968–85

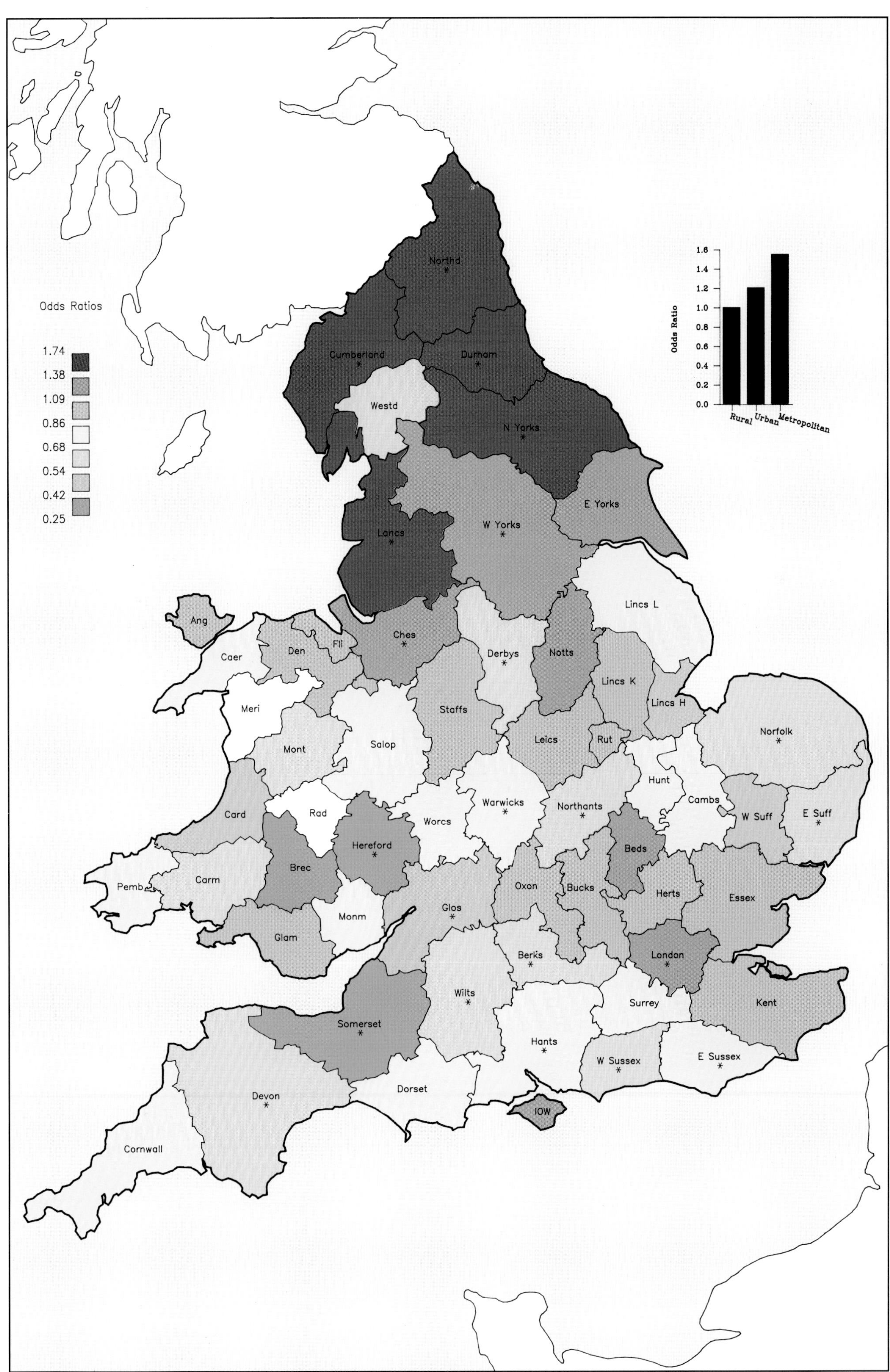

*p<0.05

In counties coloured white, no cases occurred during the period

MAP 29 CANCER OF LUNG, MALES, AGES 45+, 1968–85

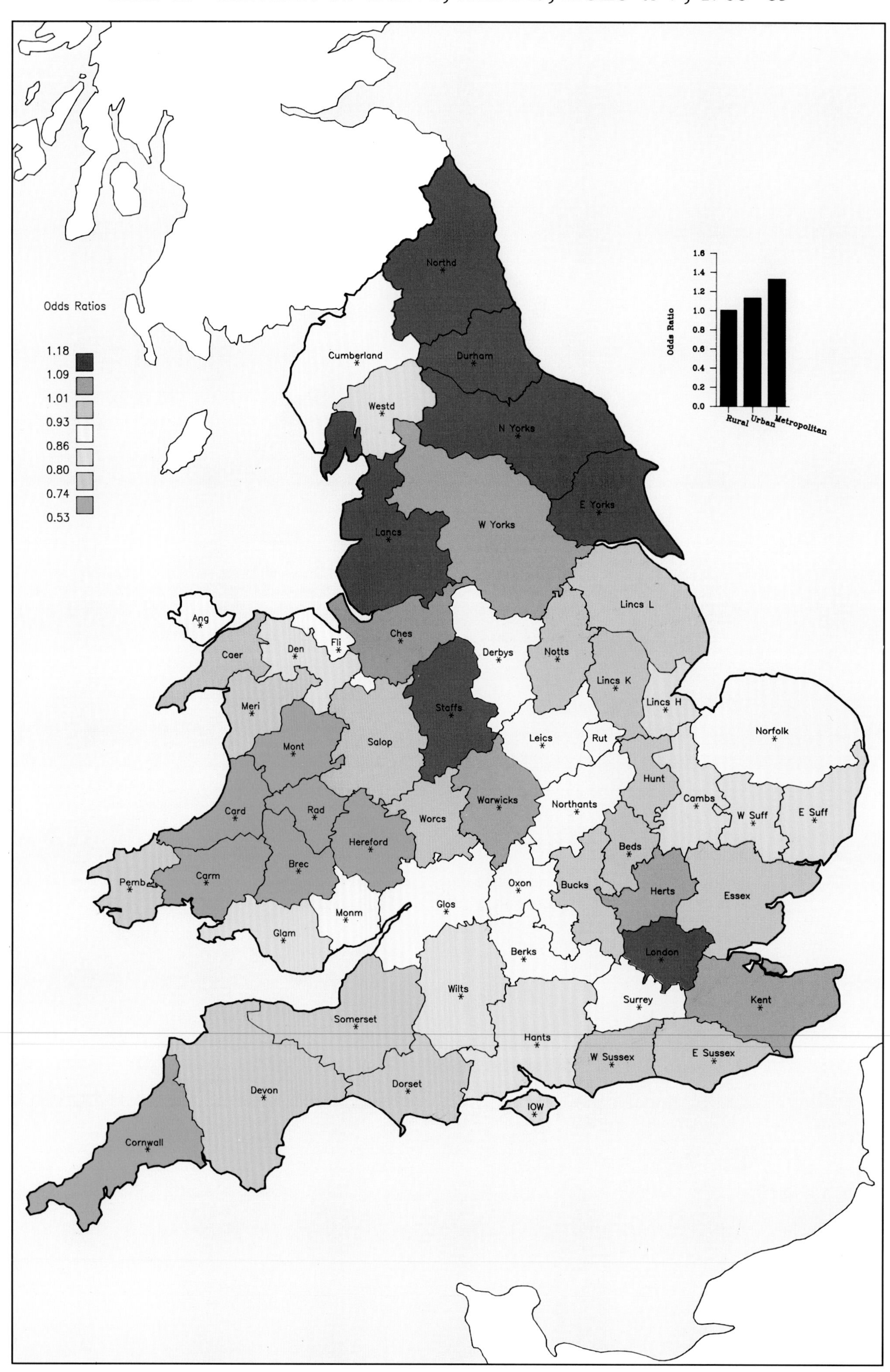

*p<0.05

MAP 30 CANCER OF LUNG, FEMALES, AGES 45+, 1968–85

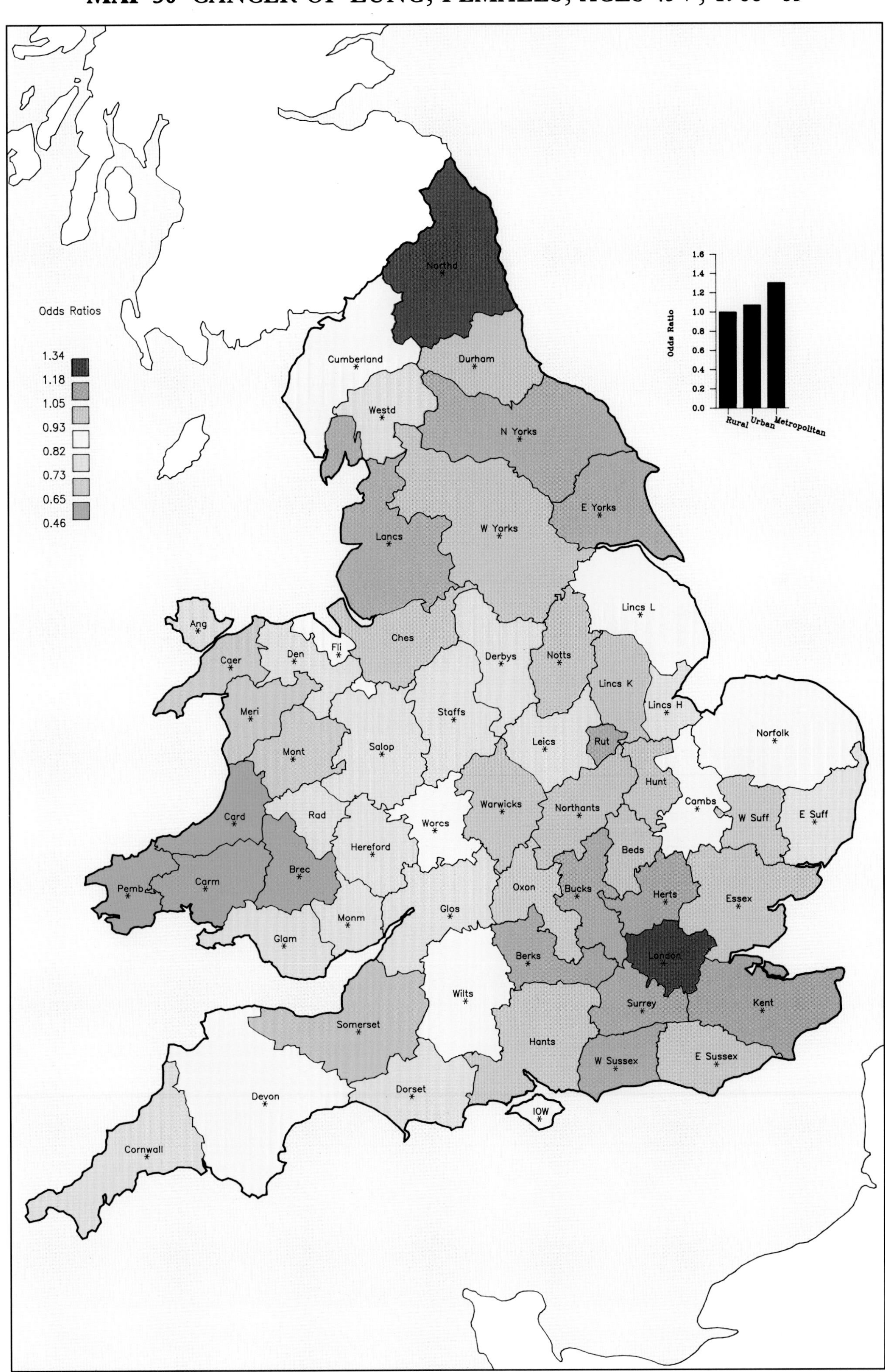

*p<0.05

MAP 31 CANCER OF PLEURA, MALES, 1968–85

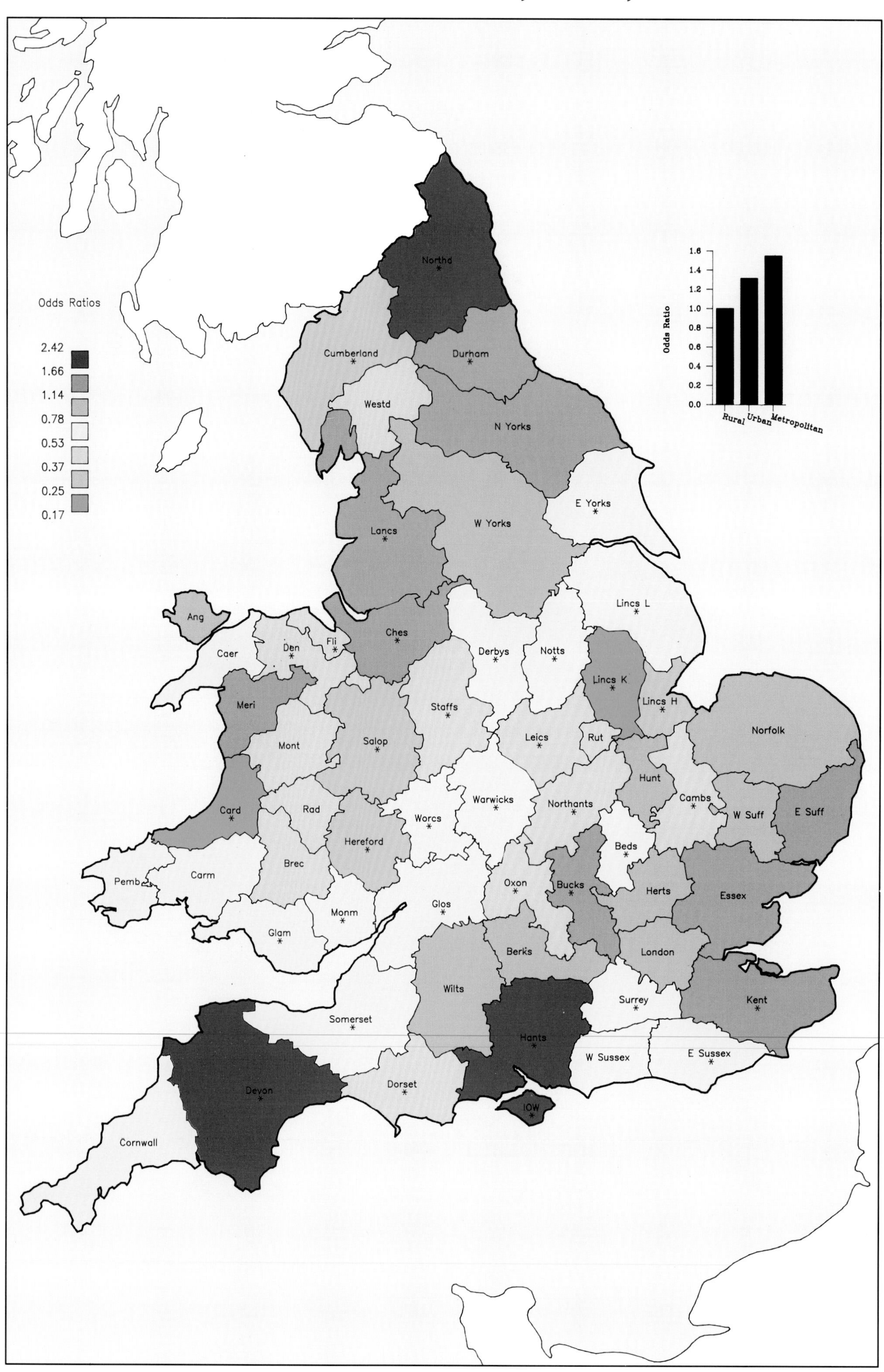

*p<0.05

MAP 32 CANCER OF PLEURA, FEMALES, 1968–85

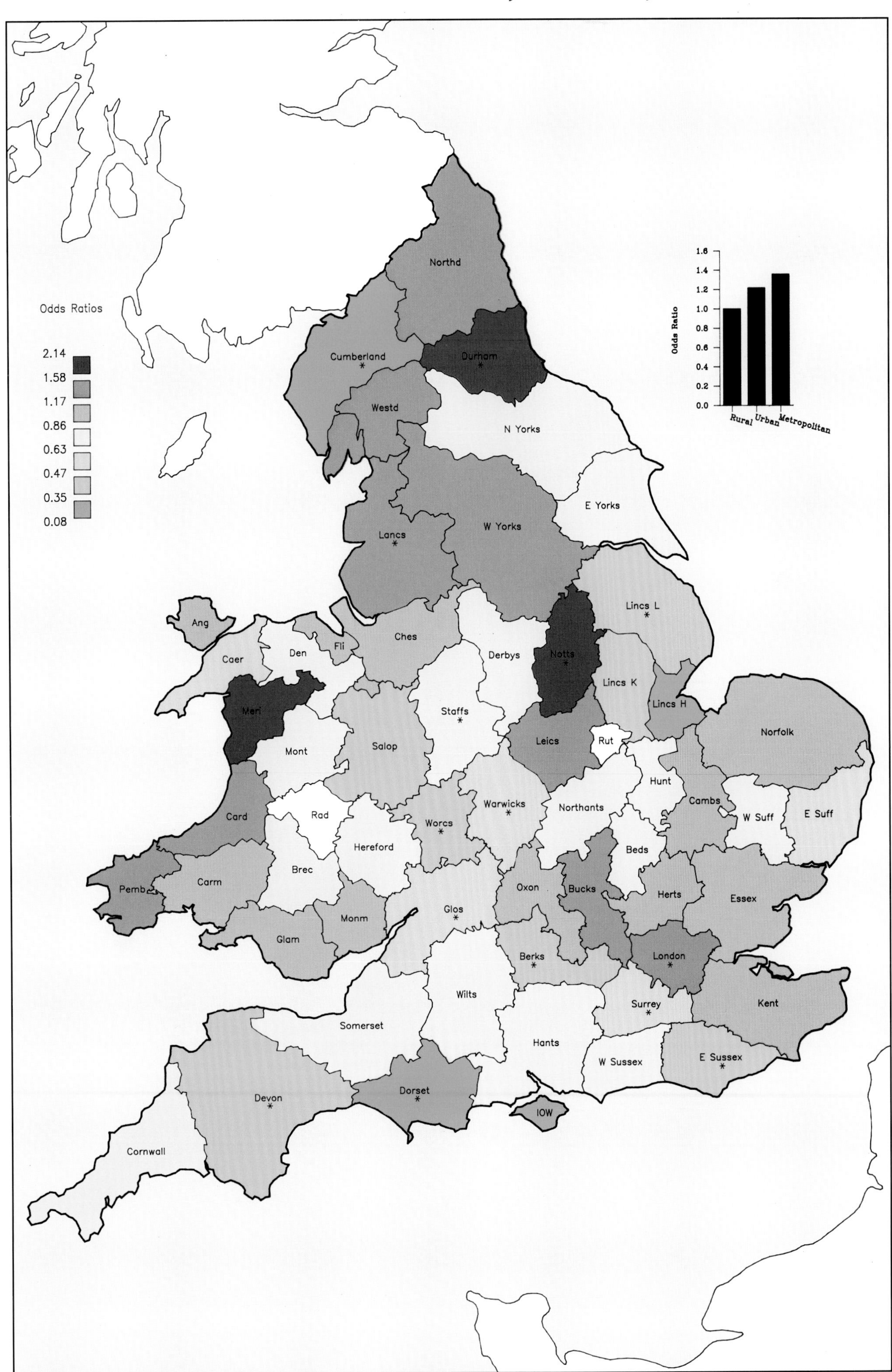

*p<0.05

In counties coloured white, no cases occurred during the period

MAP 33 CANCER OF BONE, MALES, AGES 0–24, 1968–85

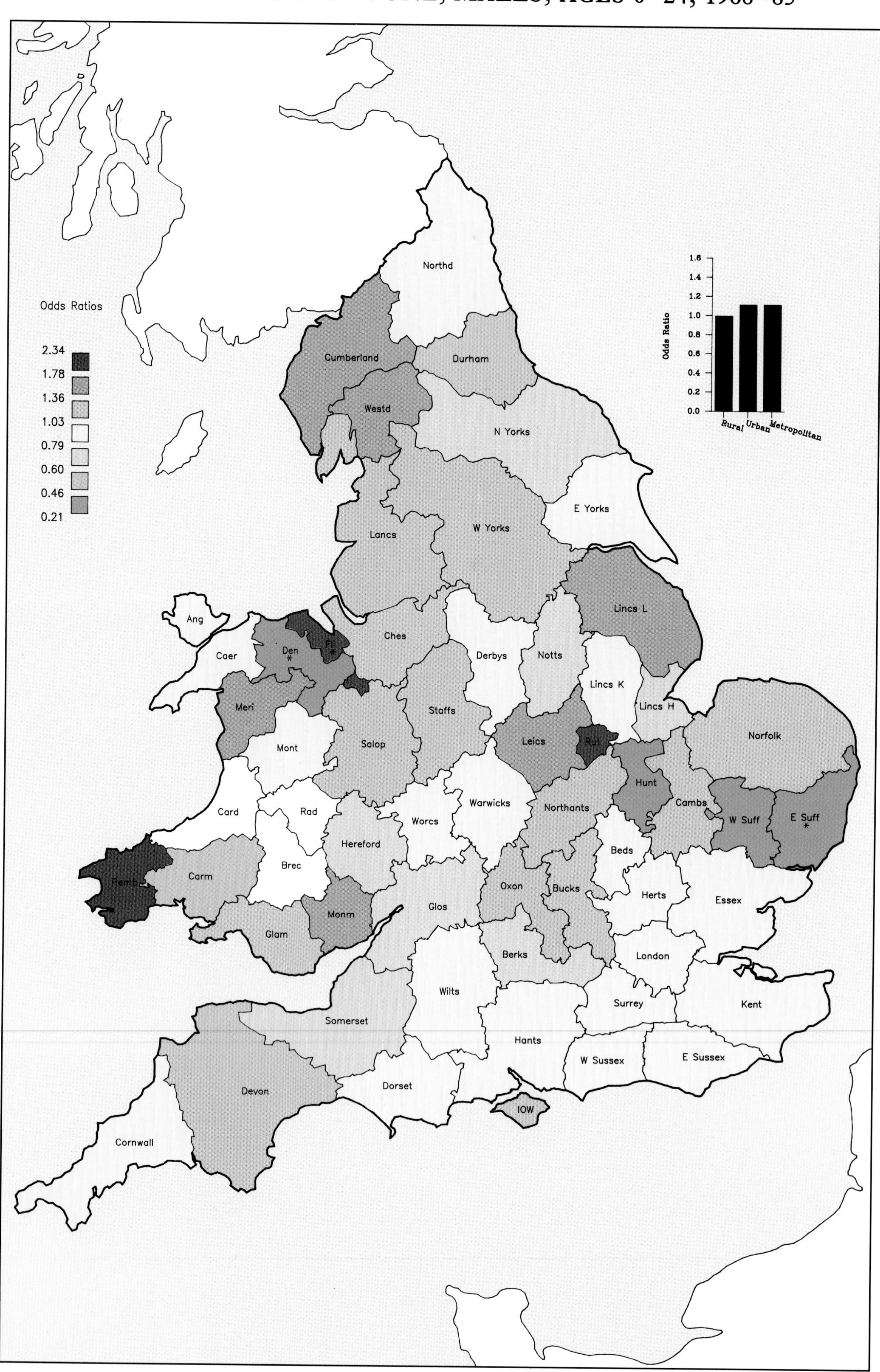

*p<0.05

In counties coloured white, no cases occurred during the period

MAP 34 CANCER OF BONE, FEMALES, AGES 0–24, 1968–85

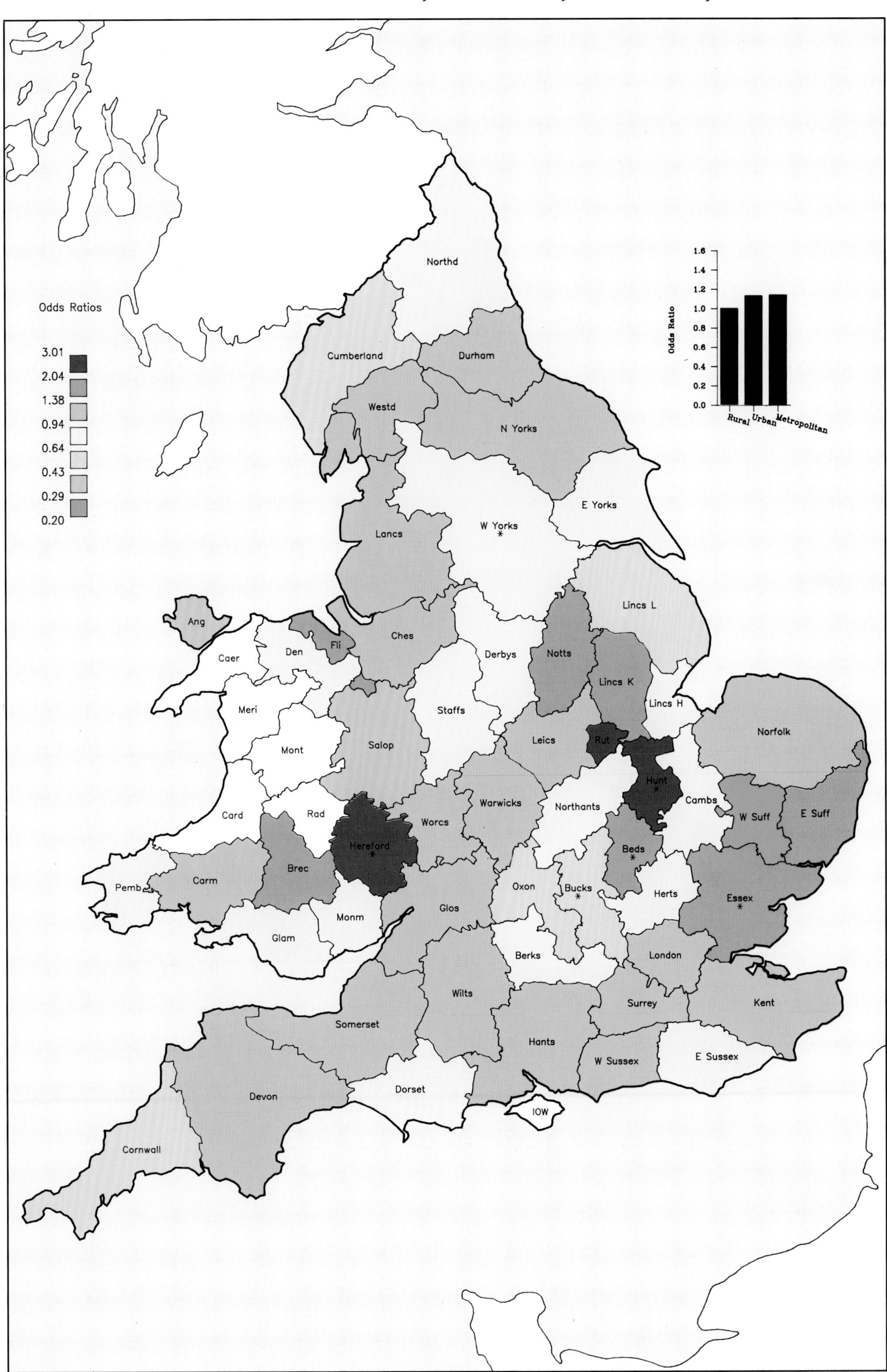

*p<0.05

In counties coloured white, no cases occurred during the period

MAP 35 CANCER OF BONE, MALES, AGES 25+, 1968–85

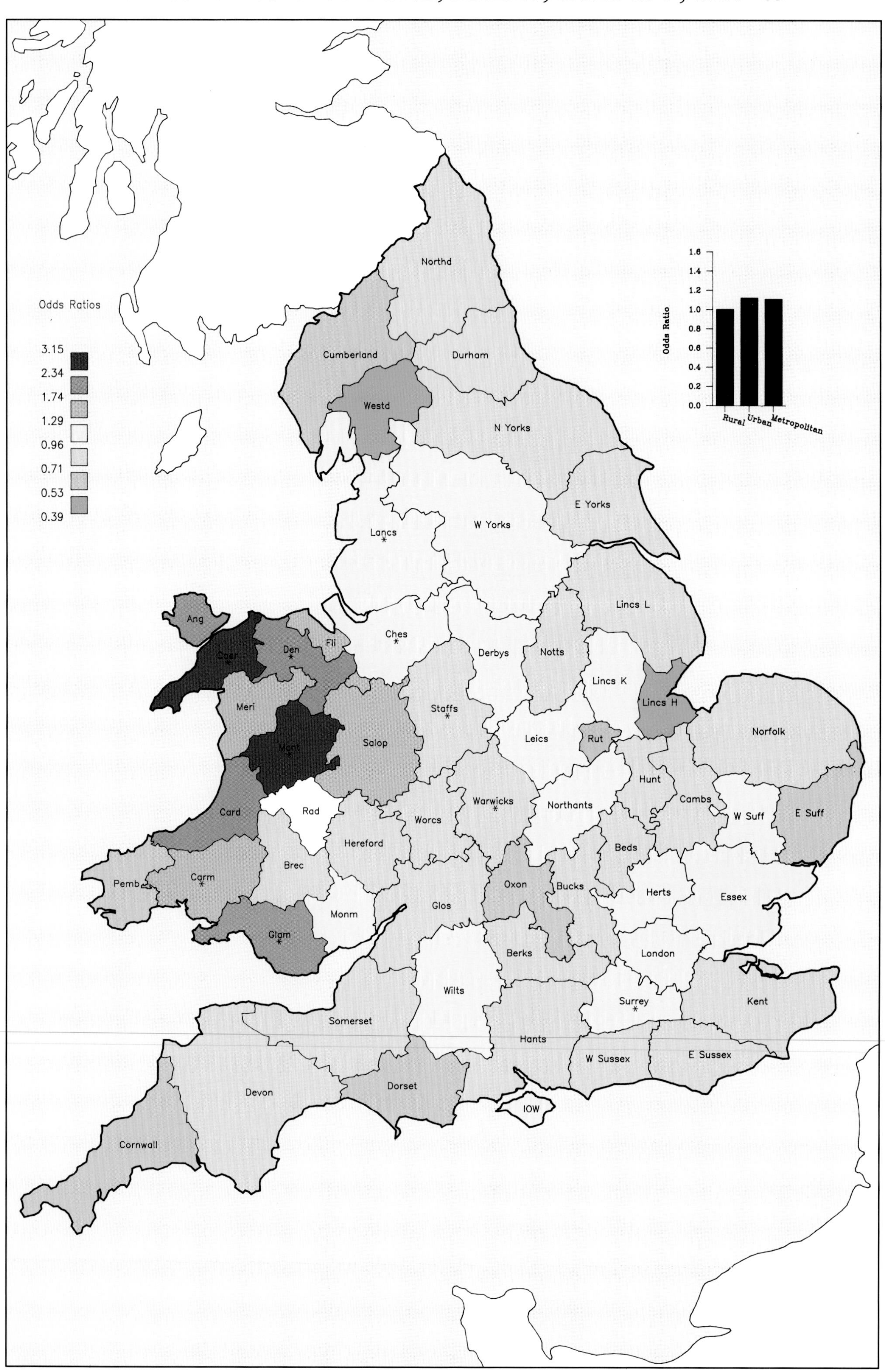

*p<0.05

In counties coloured white, no cases occurred during the period

MAP 36 CANCER OF BONE, FEMALES, AGES 25+, 1968–85

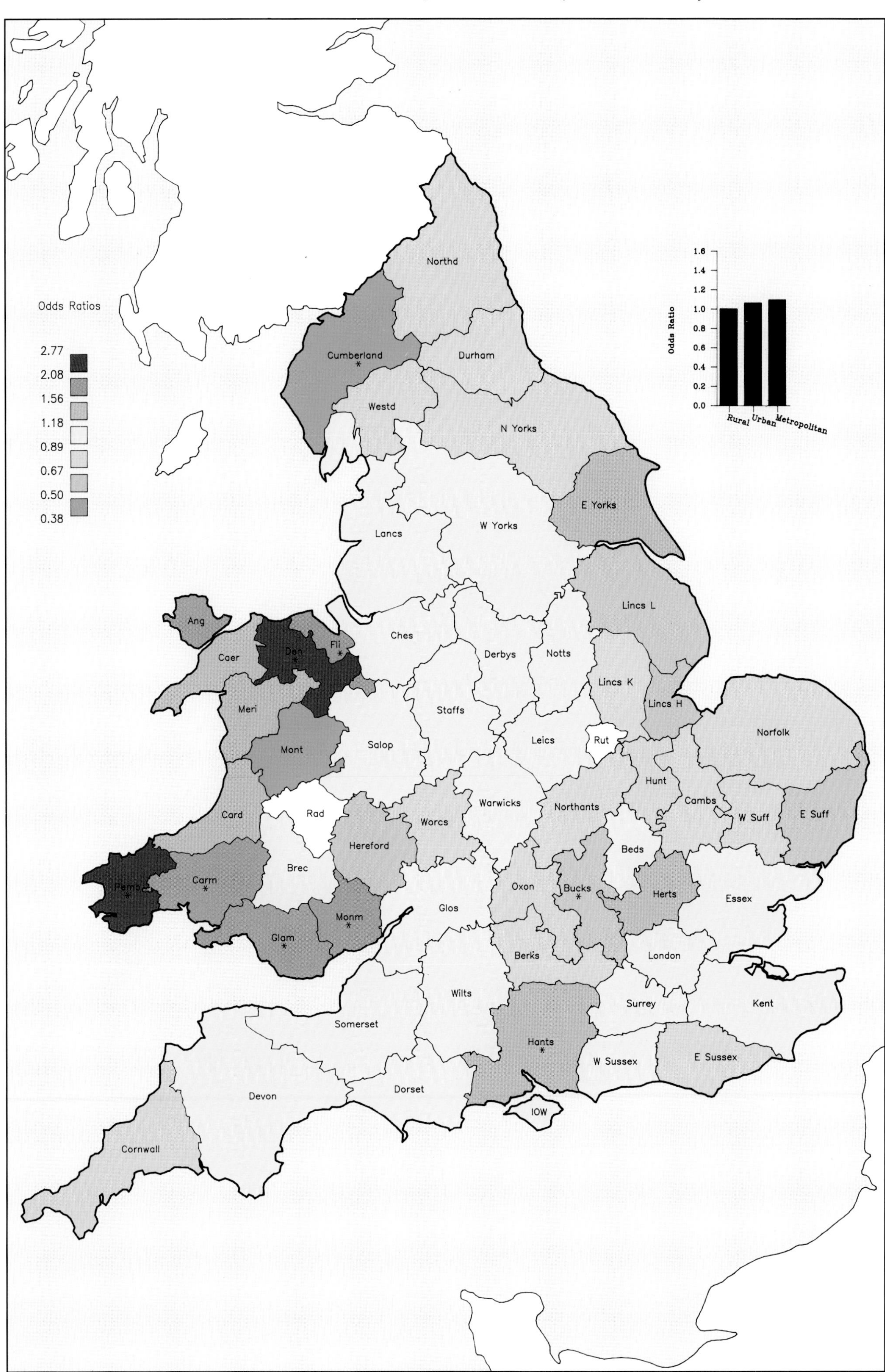

*p<0.05

In counties coloured white, no cases occurred during the period

MAP 37 CANCER OF SOFT TISSUES, MALES, 1968–85

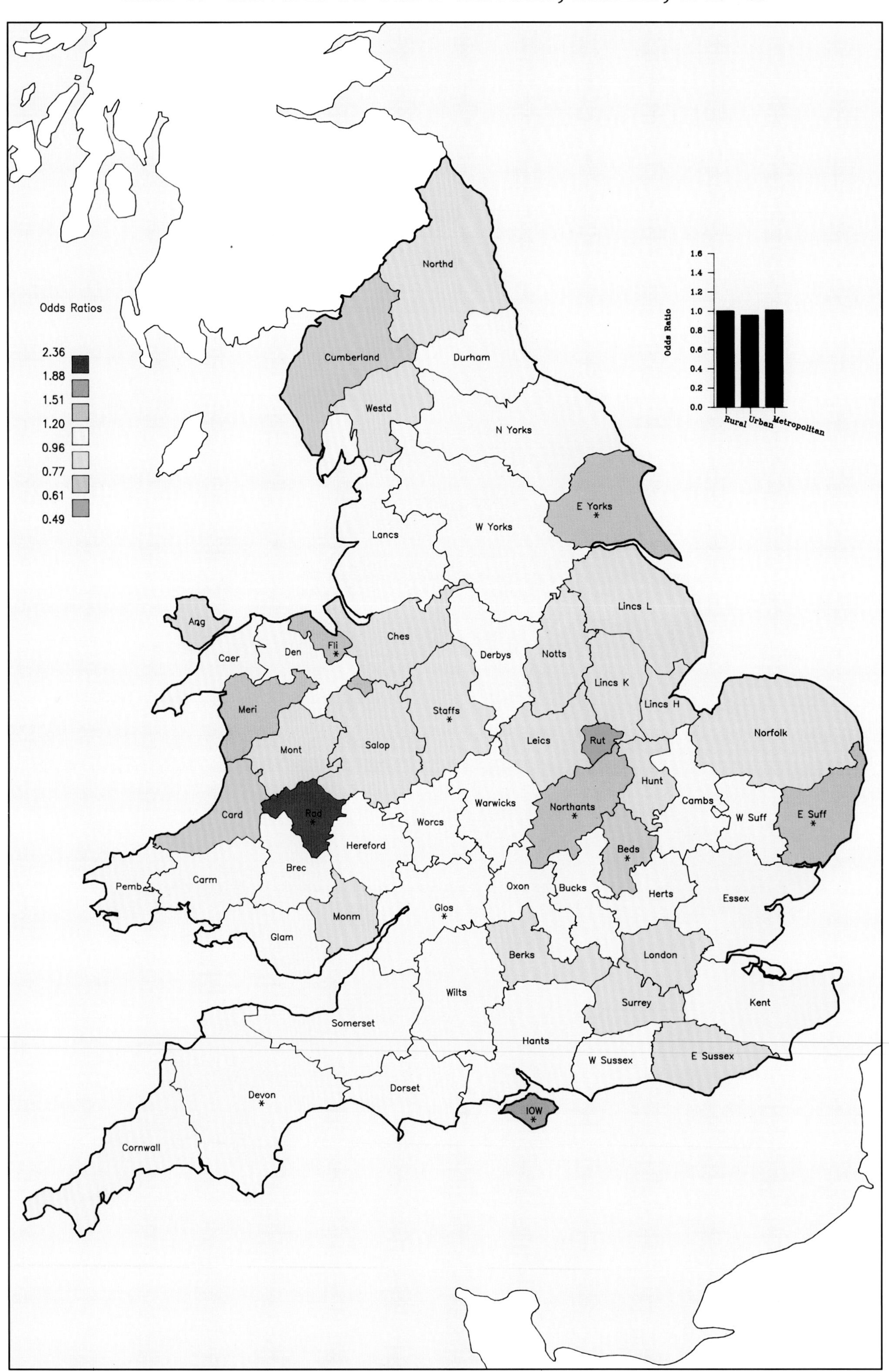

*p<0.05

MAP 38 CANCER OF SOFT TISSUES, FEMALES, 1968–85

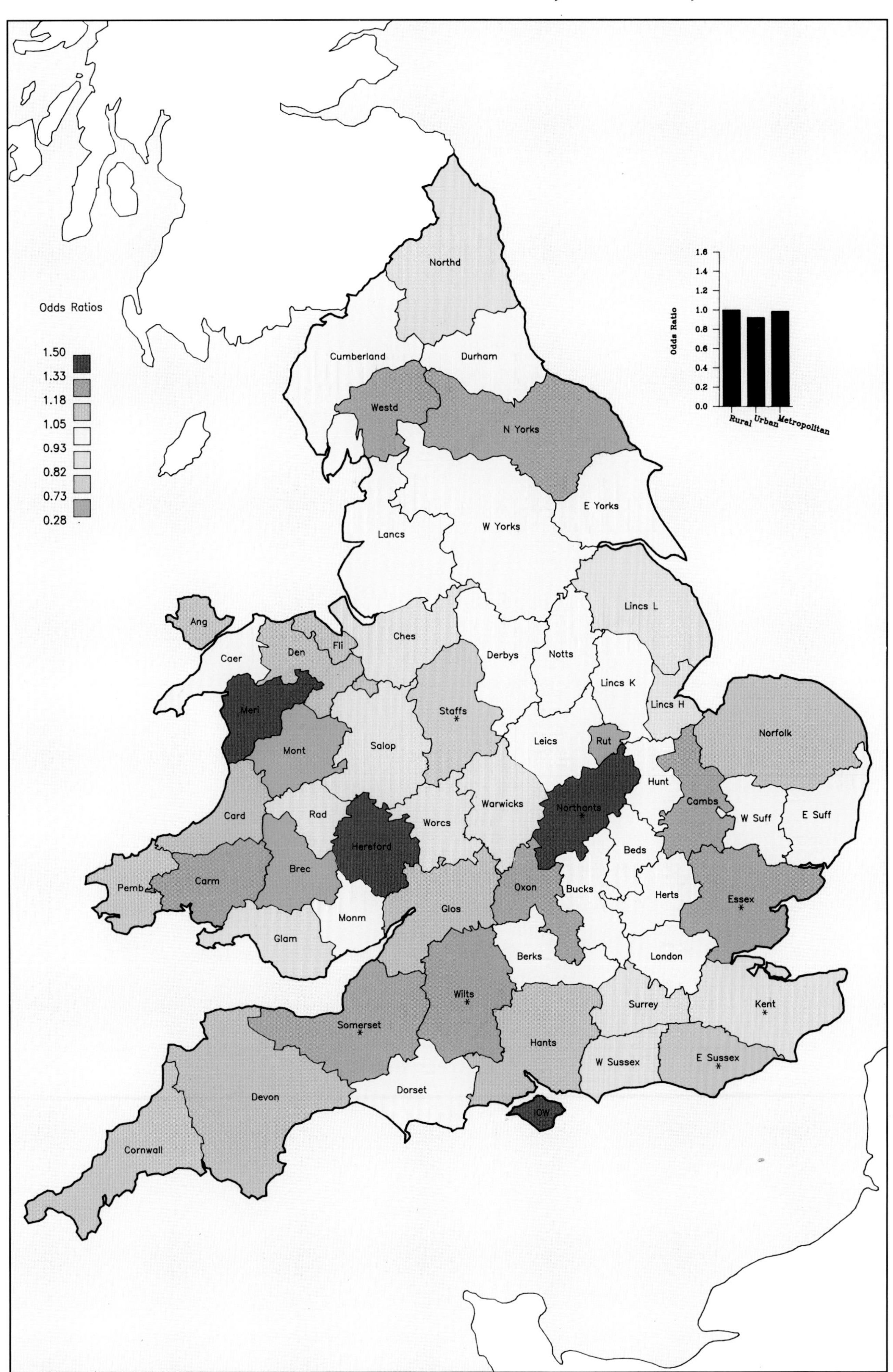

*p<0.05

MAP 39 MALIGNANT MELANOMA OF SKIN, MALES, 1968–85

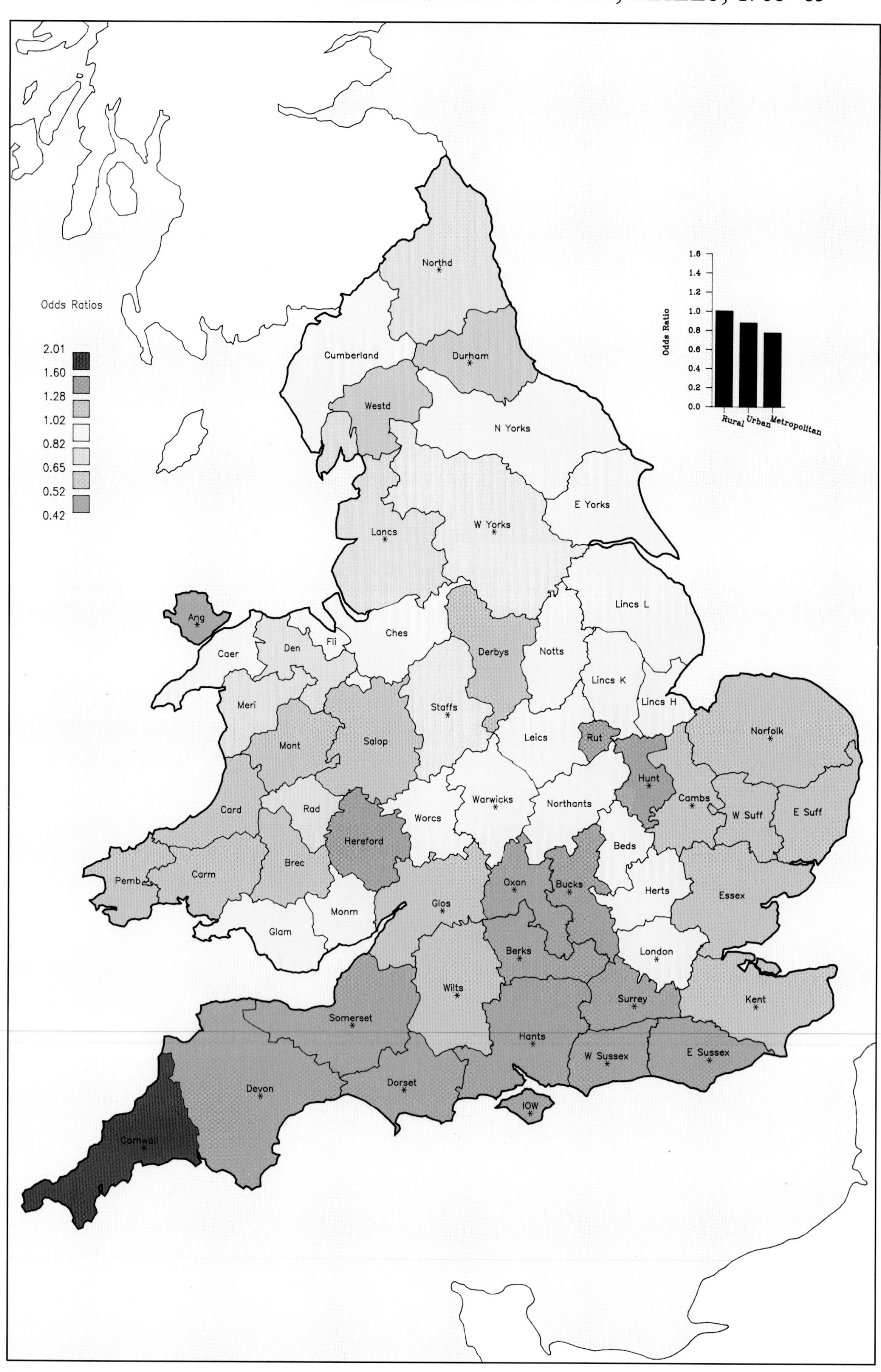

*p<0.05

MAP 40 MALIGNANT MELANOMA OF SKIN, FEMALES, 1968–85

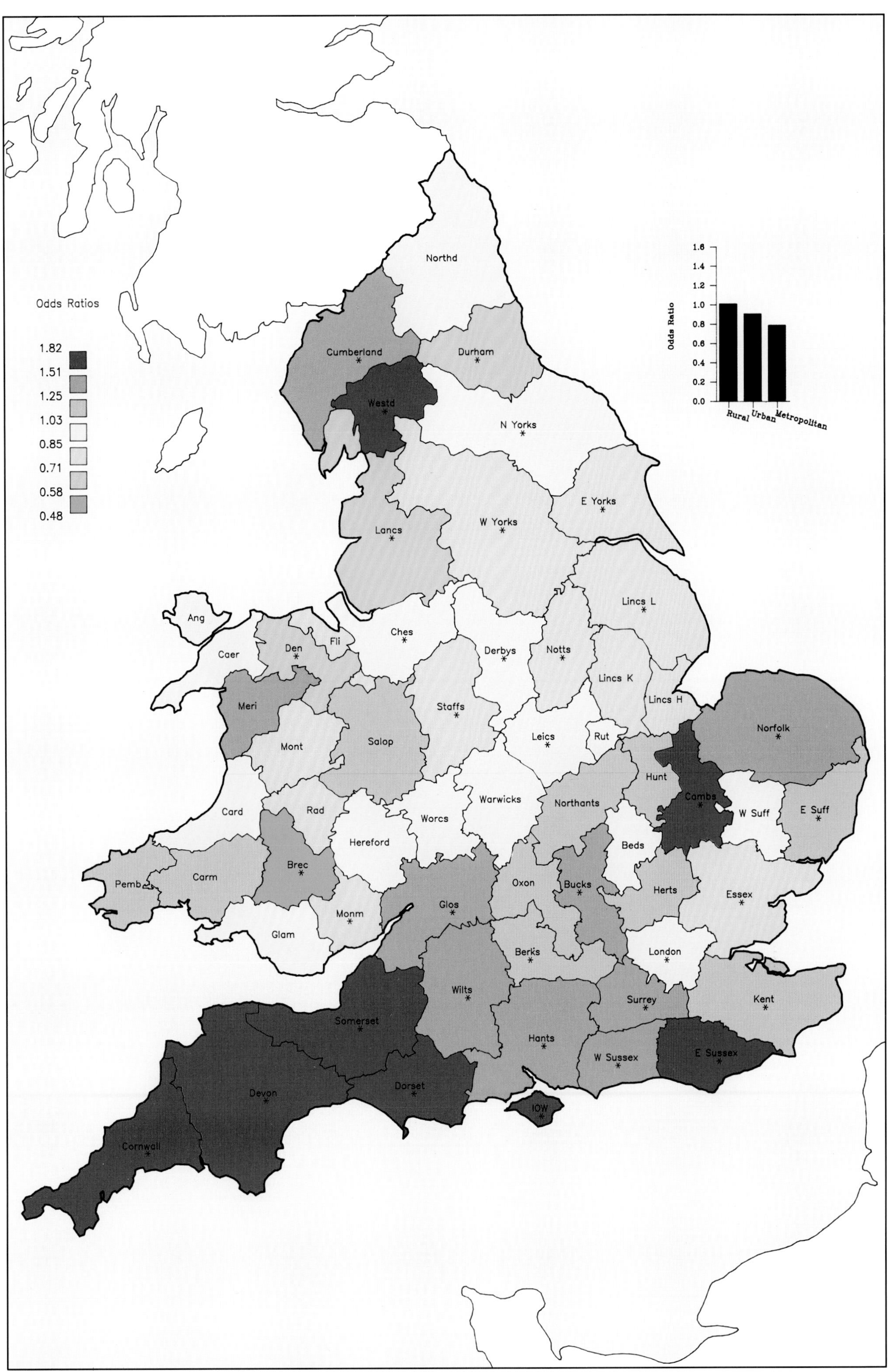

*p<0.05

MAP 41 CANCER OF BREAST, FEMALES, AGES 0–44, 1968–85

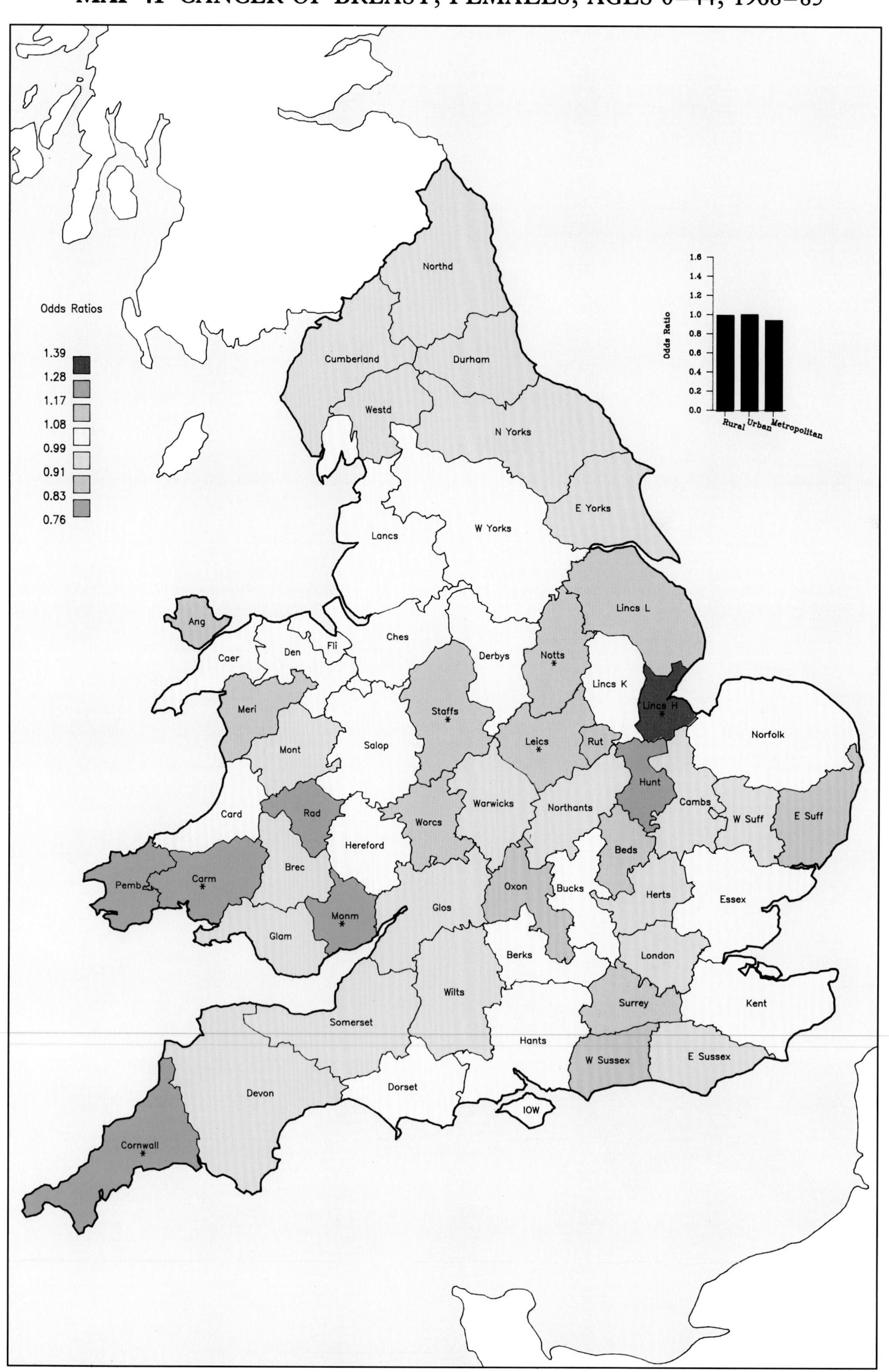

*p<0.05

MAP 42 CANCER OF BREAST, FEMALES, AGES 45+, 1968–85

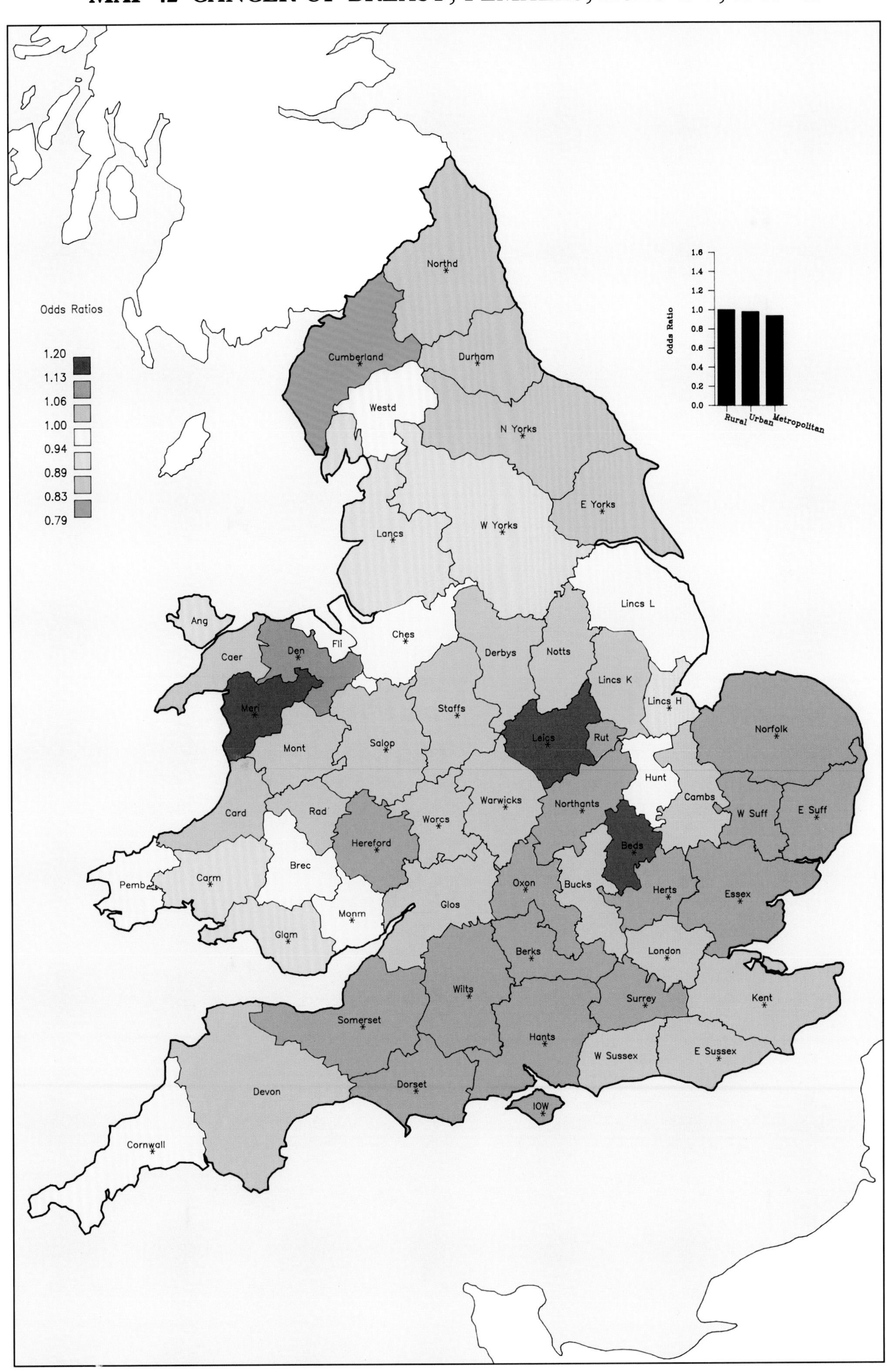

*p<0.05

MAP 43 CANCER OF BREAST, MALES, 1968–85

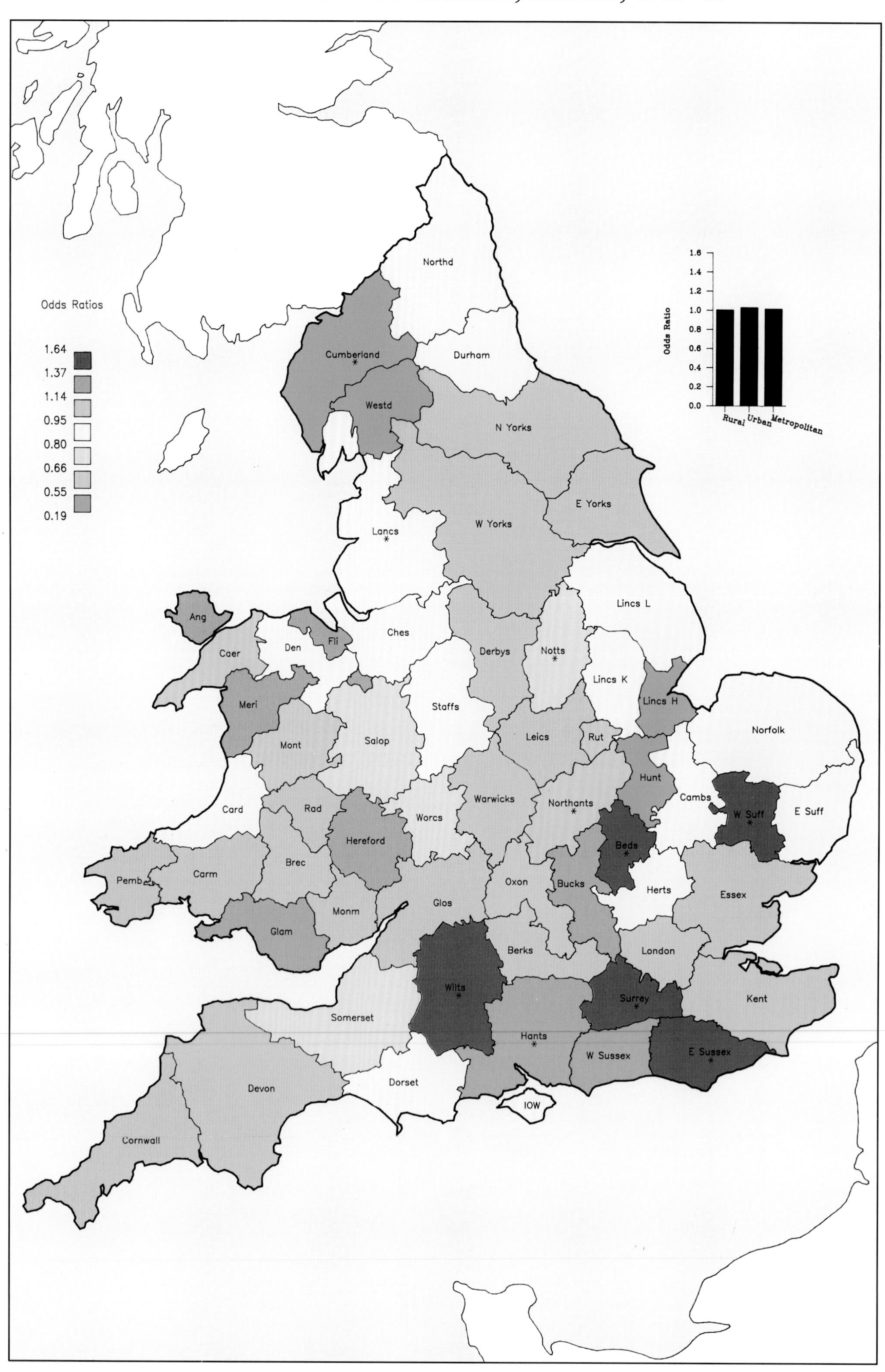

*p<0.05

MAP 44 CANCER OF CERVIX UTERI, 1968–85

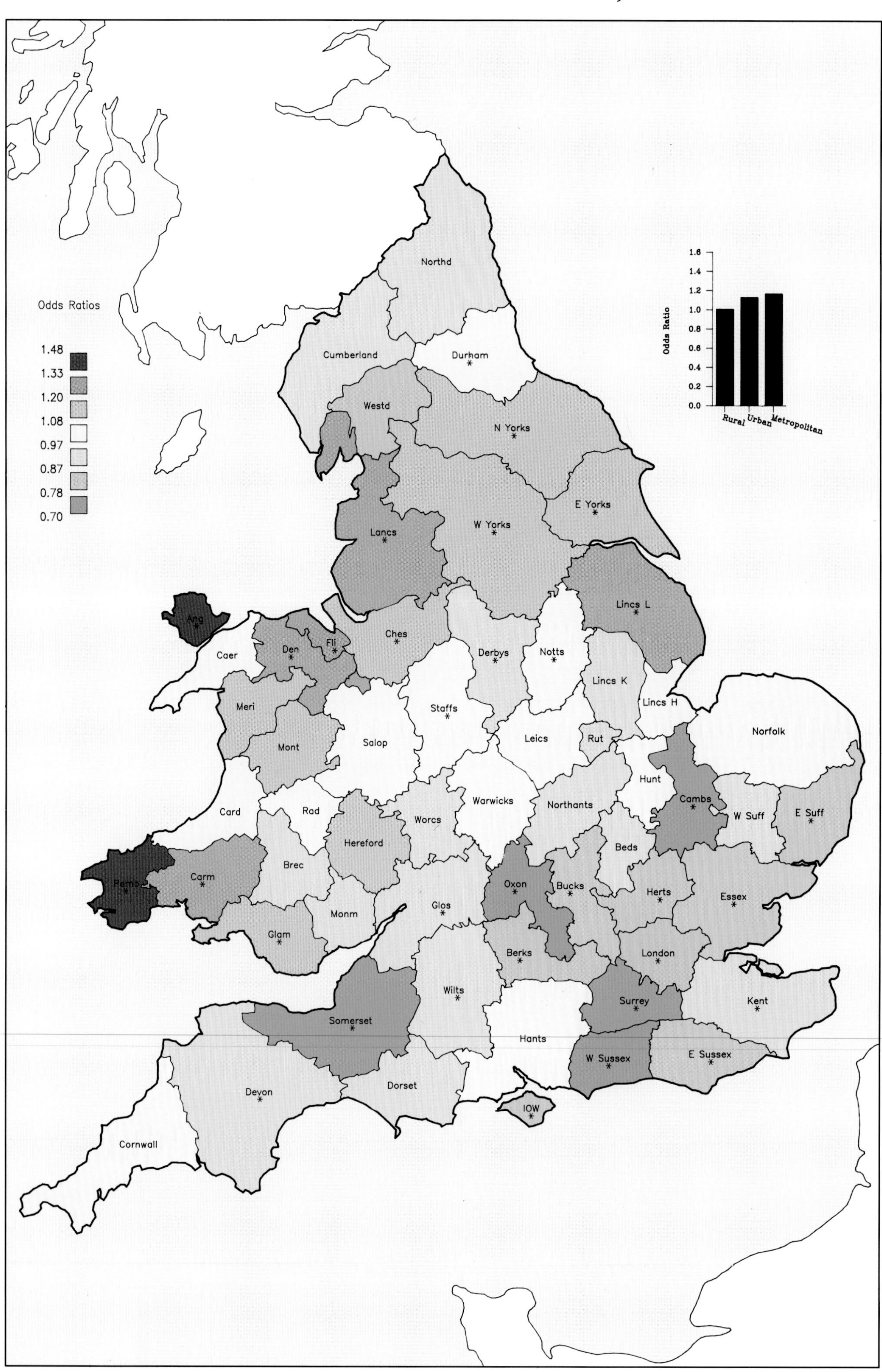

*p<0.05

MAP 45 CANCER OF PLACENTA, 1968–85

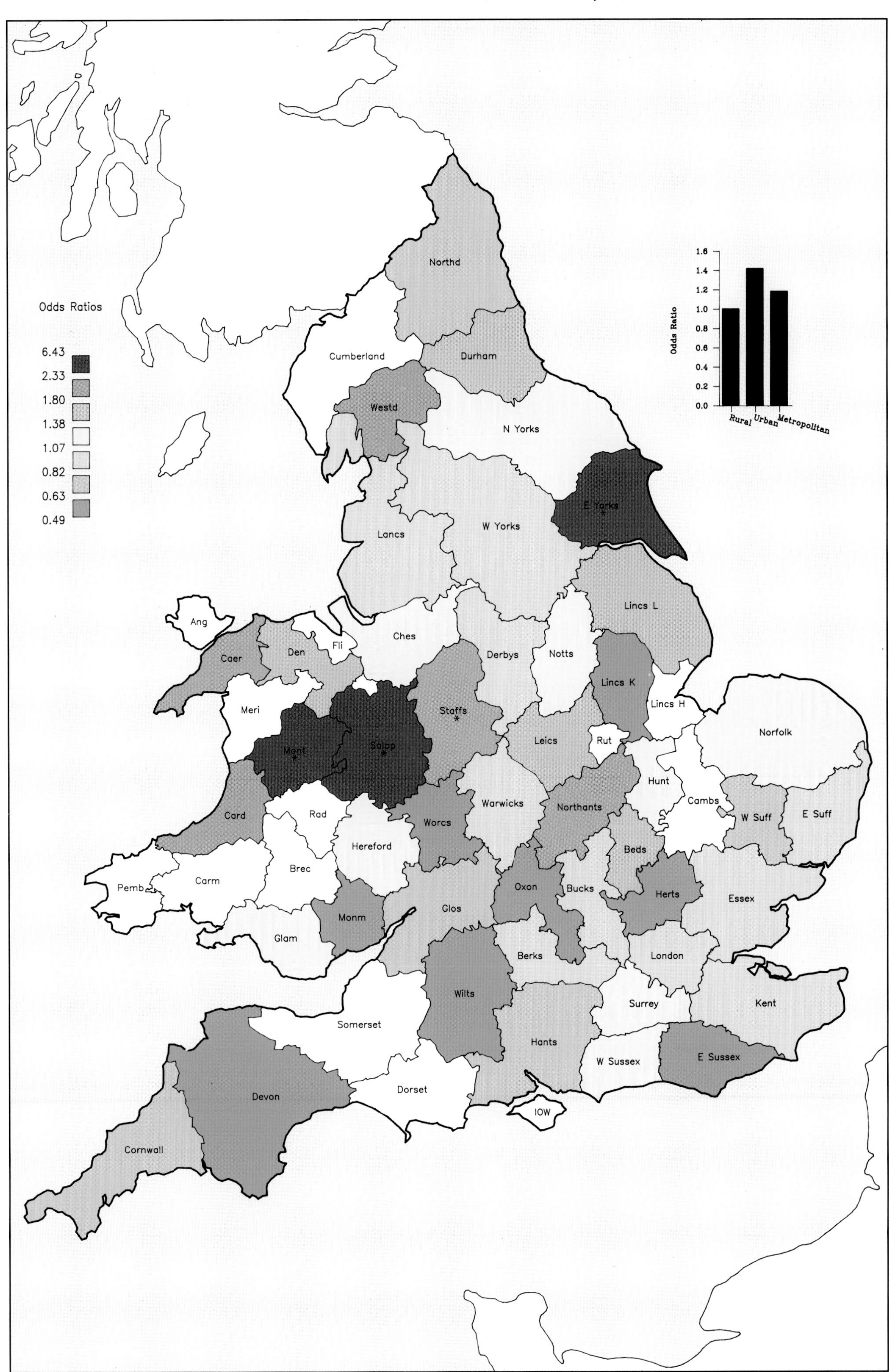

*p<0.05

In counties coloured white, no cases occurred during the period

MAP 46 CANCER OF CORPUS UTERI, 1968–85

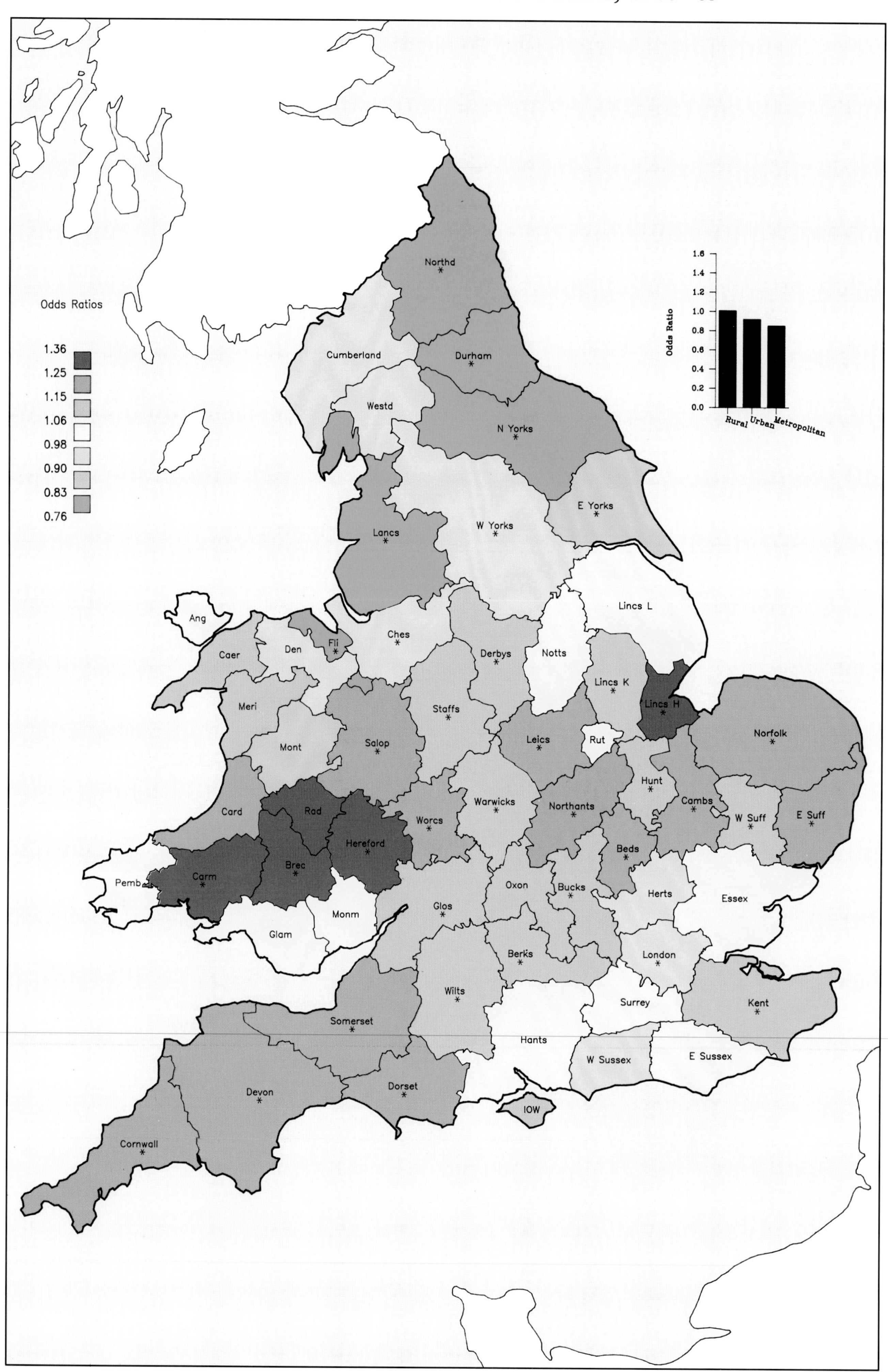

*p<0.05

MAP 47 CANCER OF OVARY, 1968–85

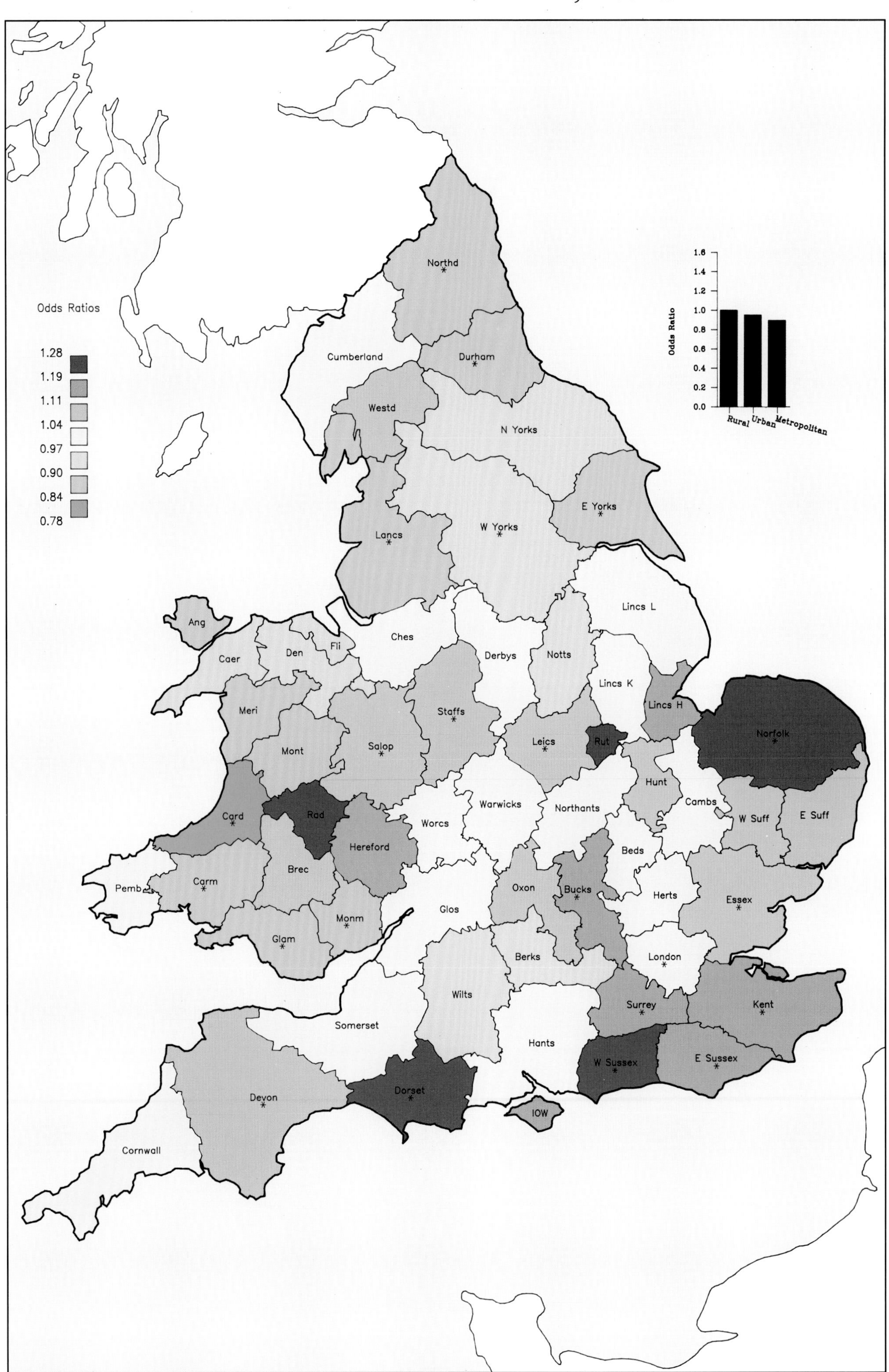

*p<0.05

MAP 48 CANCERS OF VAGINA AND VULVA, 1968–85

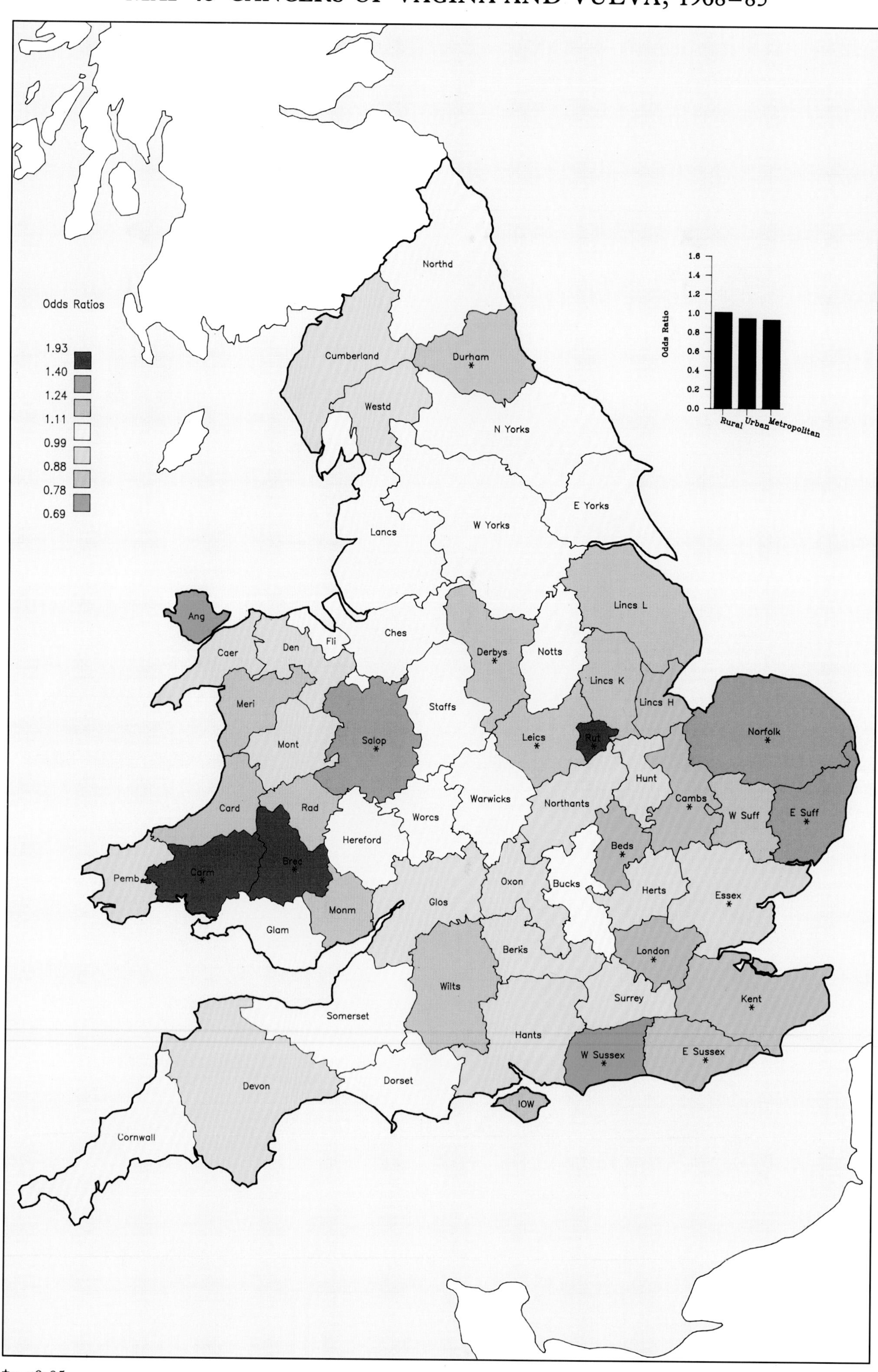

*p<0.05

MAP 49 CANCER OF PROSTATE, 1968–85

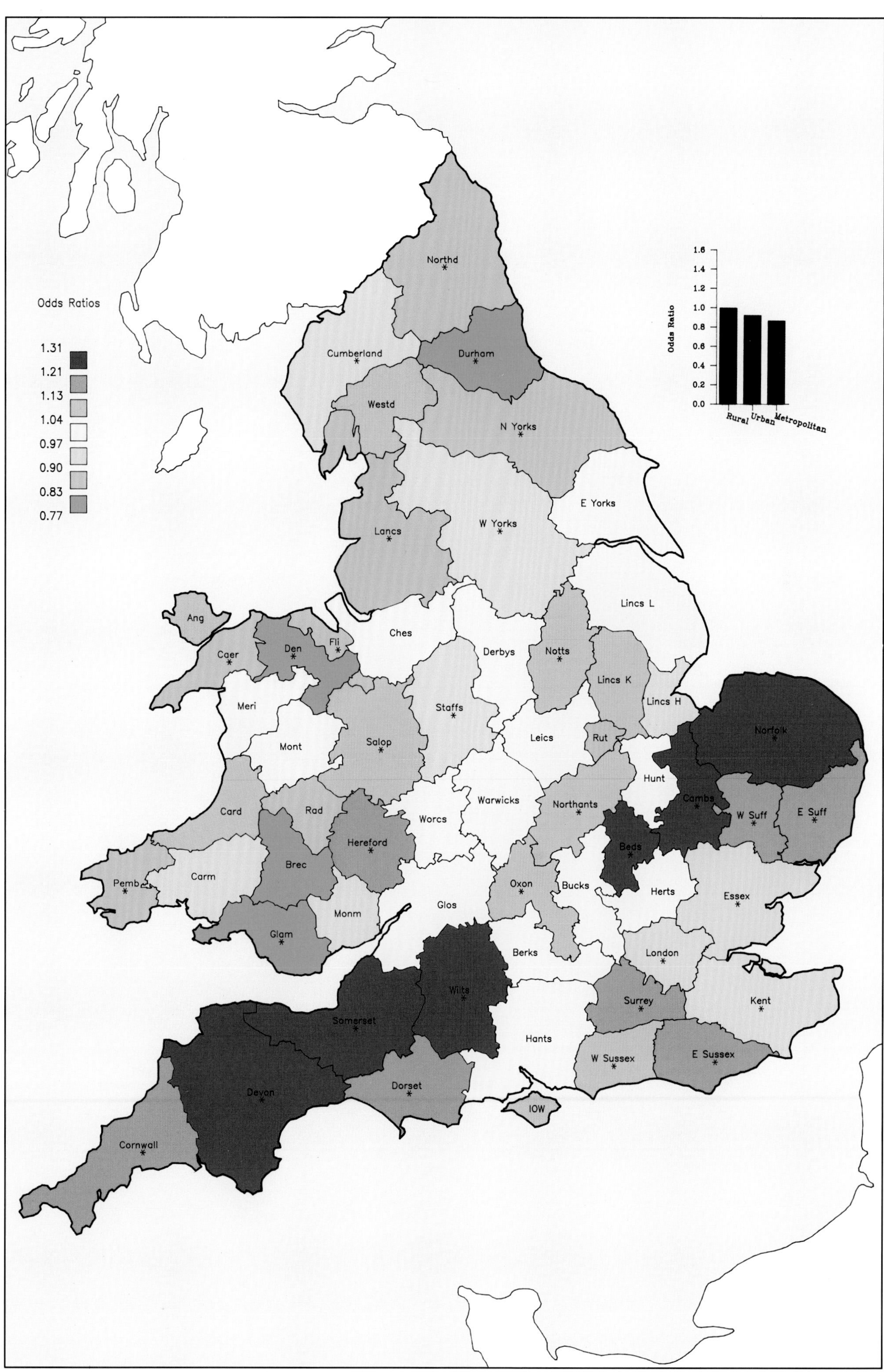

*p<0.05

MAP 50 CANCER OF TESTIS, AGES 0–49, 1968–85

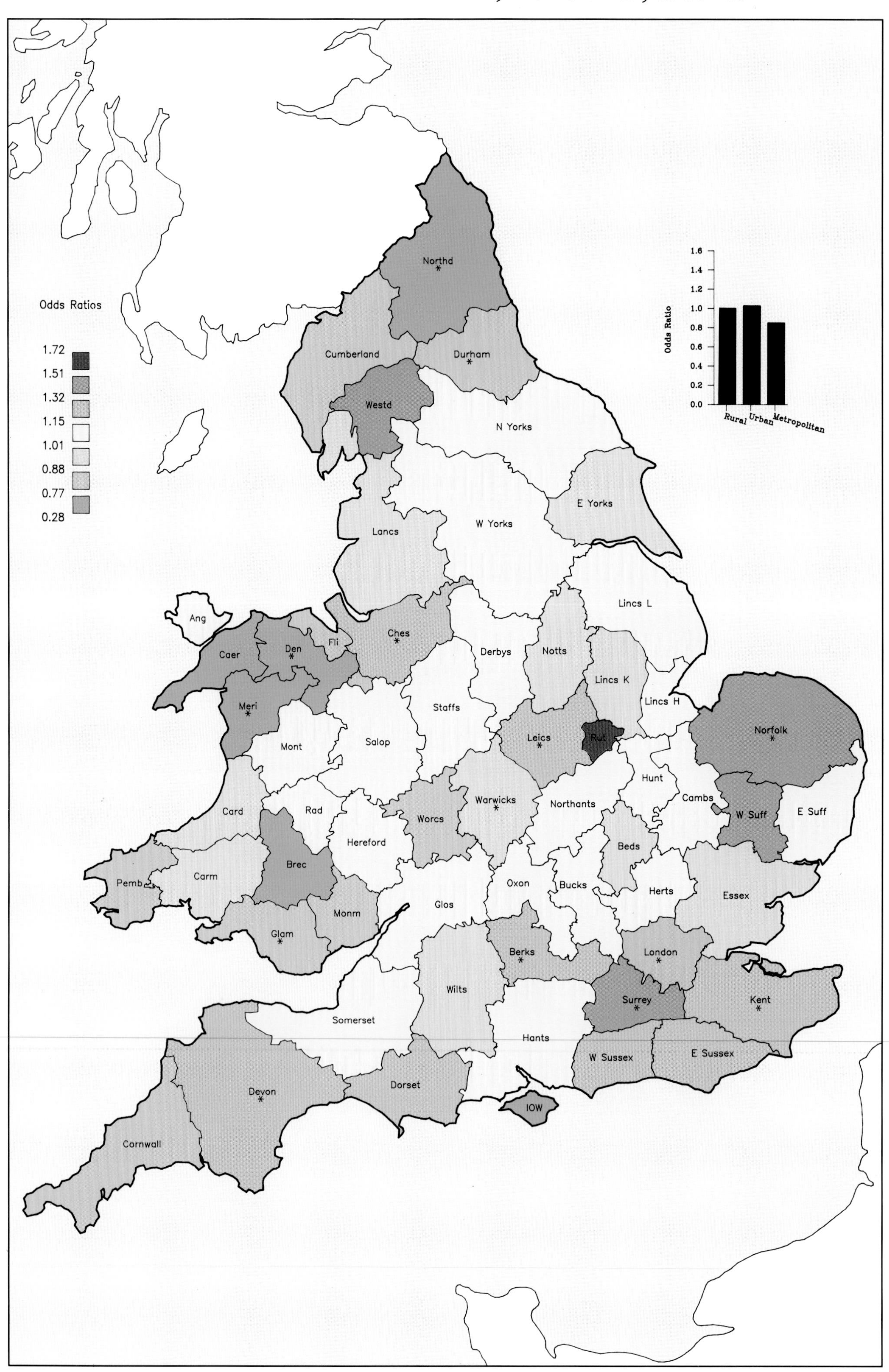

*p<0.05

MAP 51 CANCER OF TESTIS, AGES 50+, 1968–85

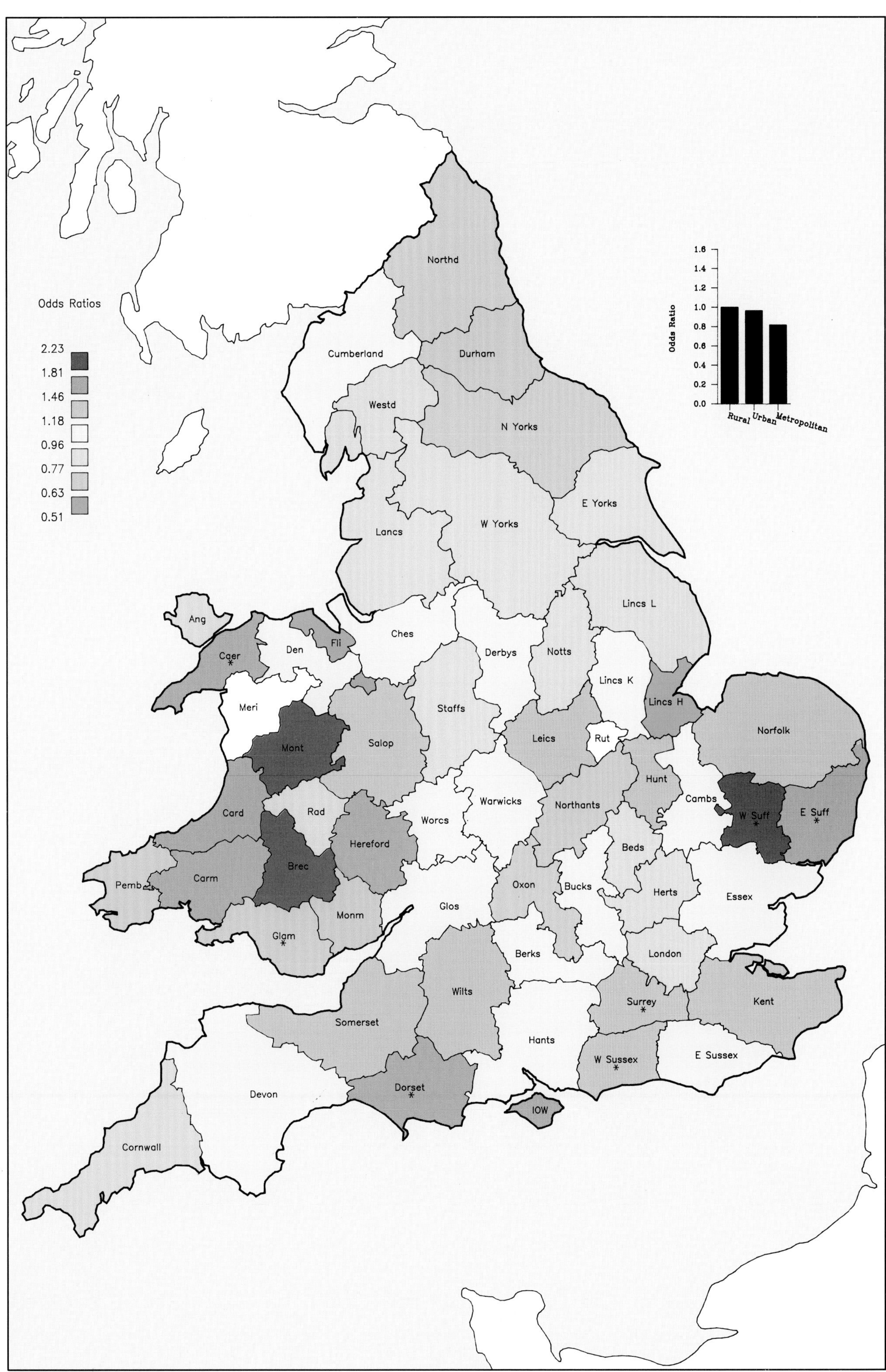

*p<0.05

In counties coloured white, no cases occurred during the period

MAP 52 CANCER OF PENIS, 1968–85

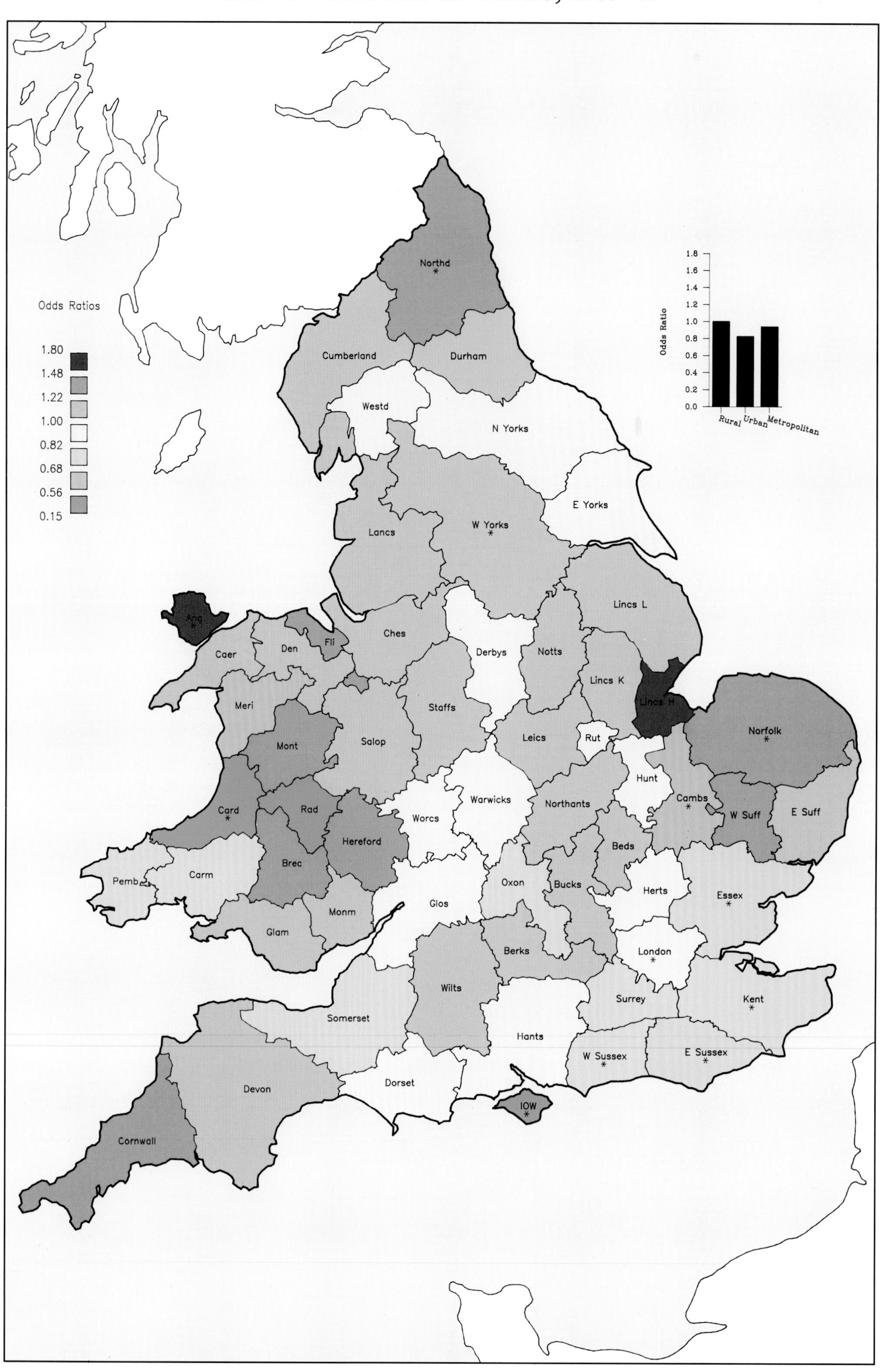

*p<0.05

MAP 53 CANCER OF SCROTUM, 1968–85

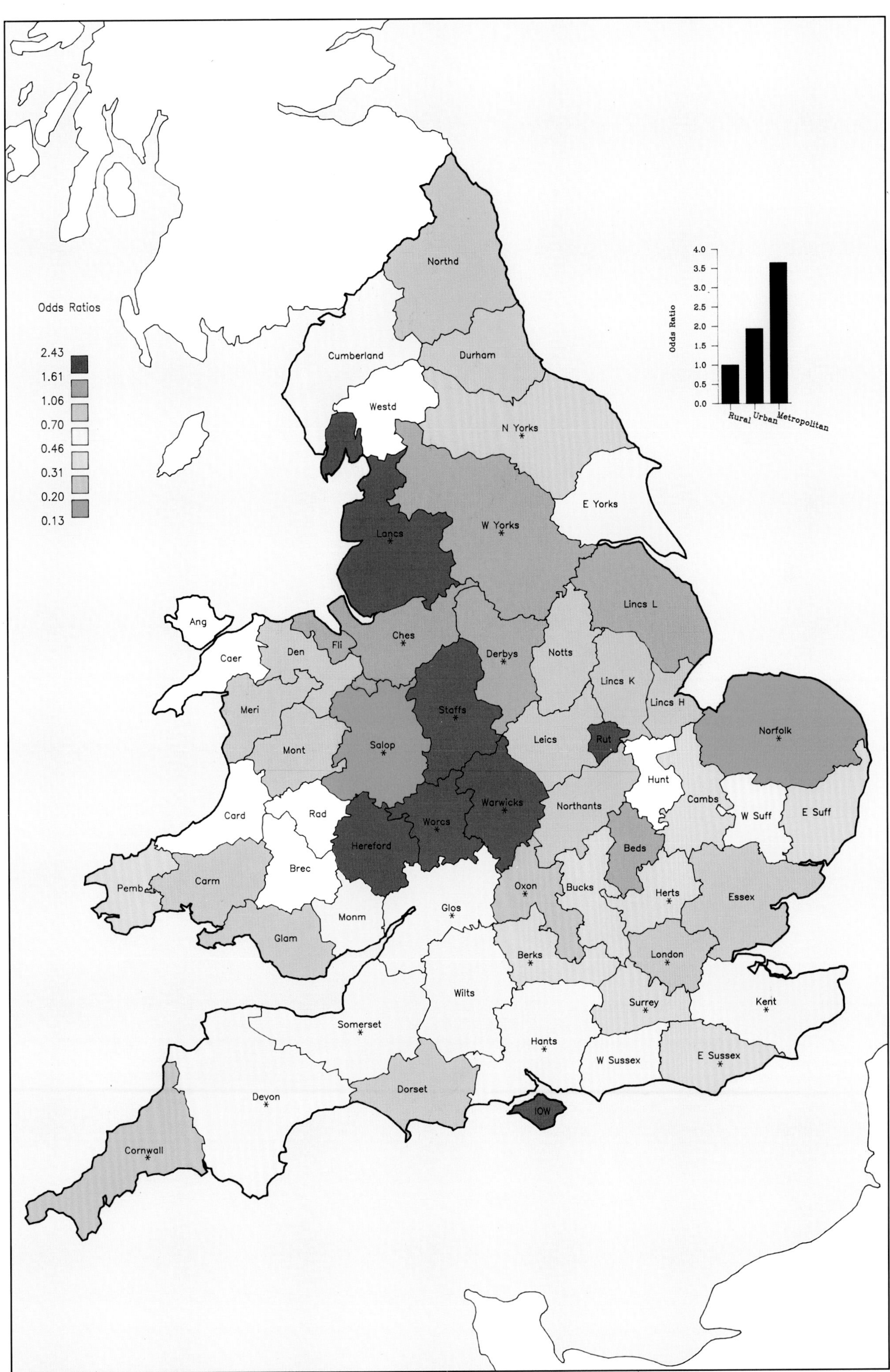

*p<0.05

In counties coloured white, no cases occurred during the period

MAP 54 CANCER OF BLADDER, MALES, 1968–85

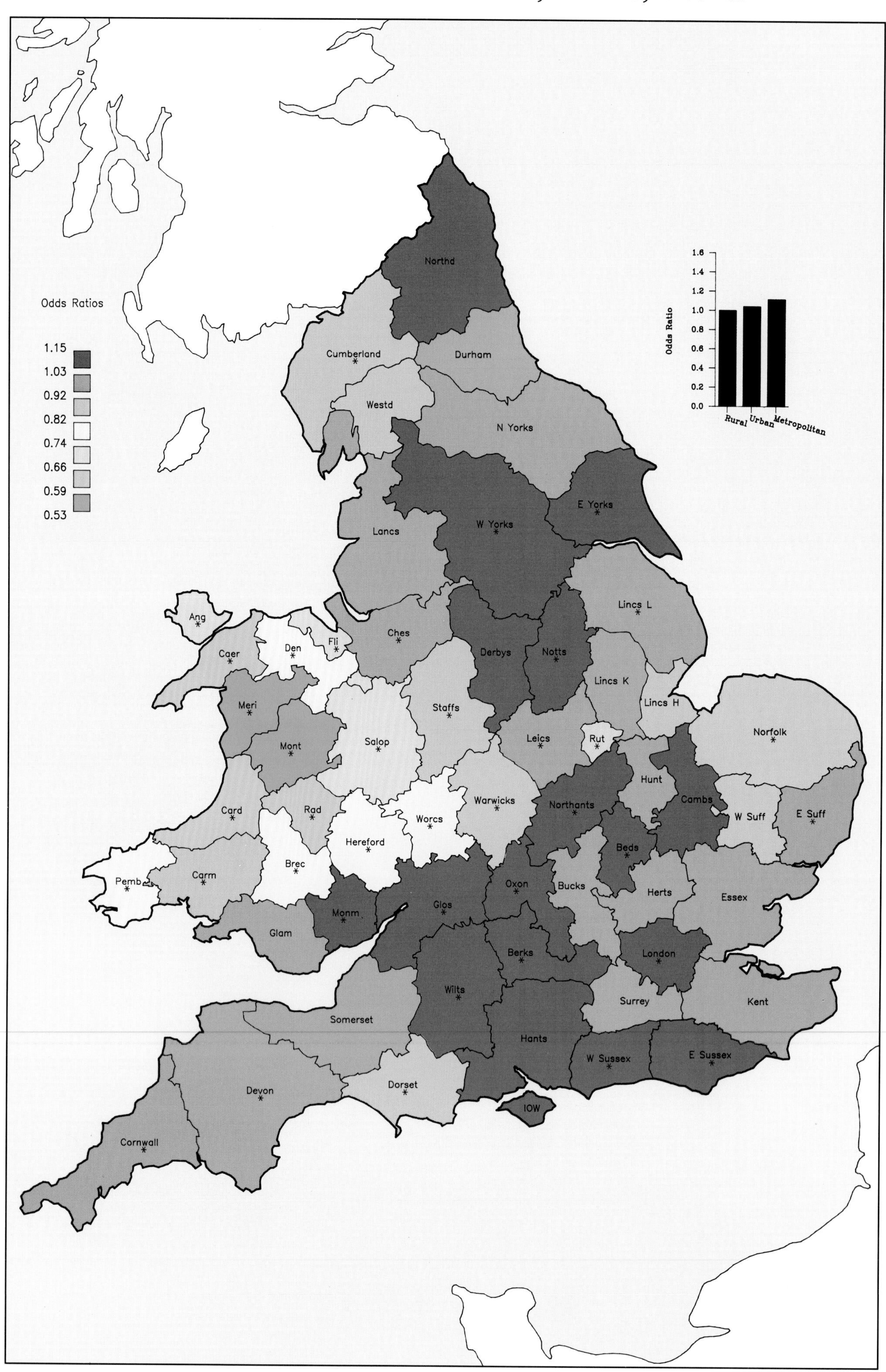

*p<0.05

MAP 55 CANCER OF BLADDER, FEMALES, 1968–85

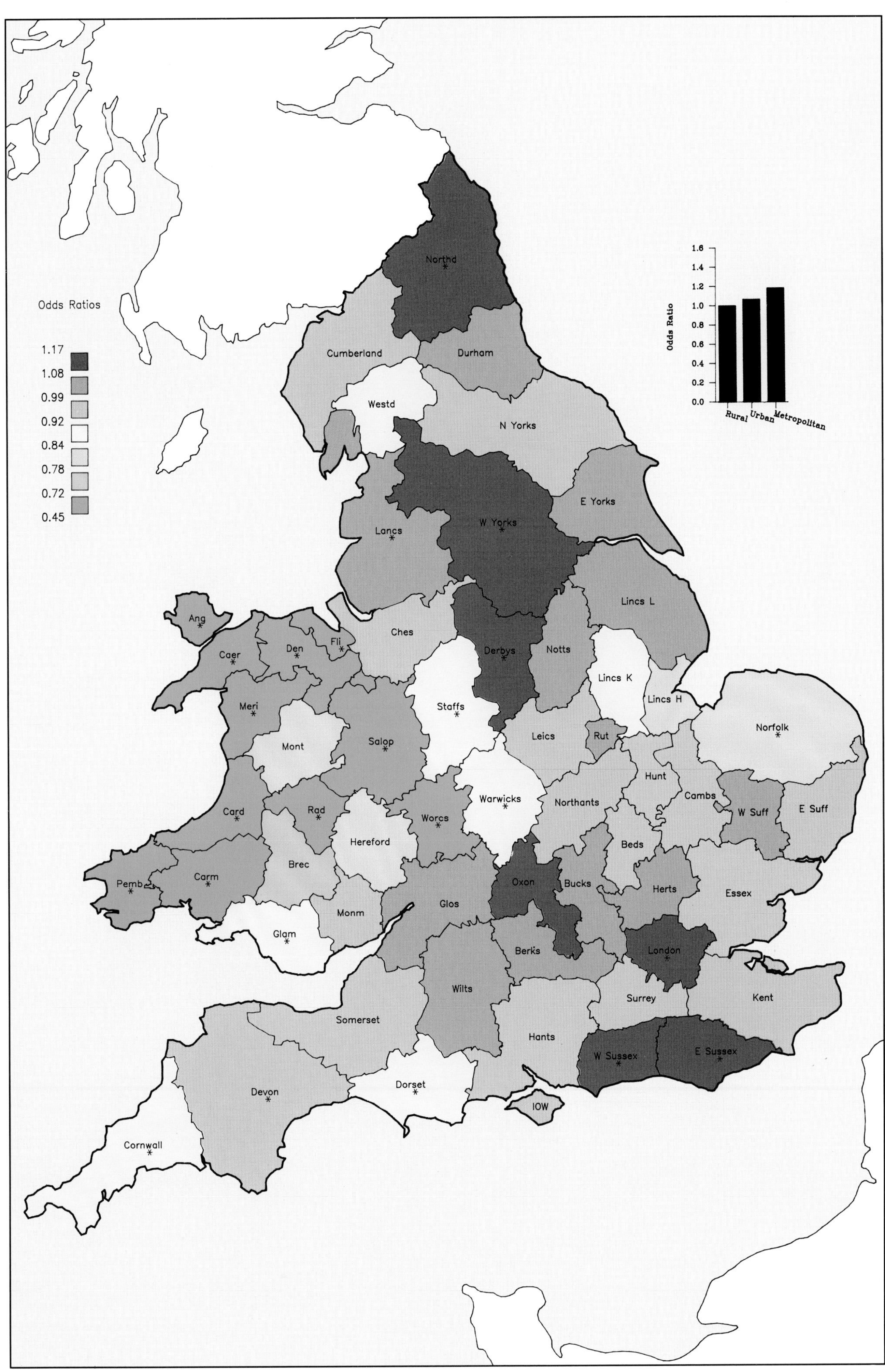

*p<0.05

MAP 56 CANCER OF KIDNEY, MALES, 1968–85

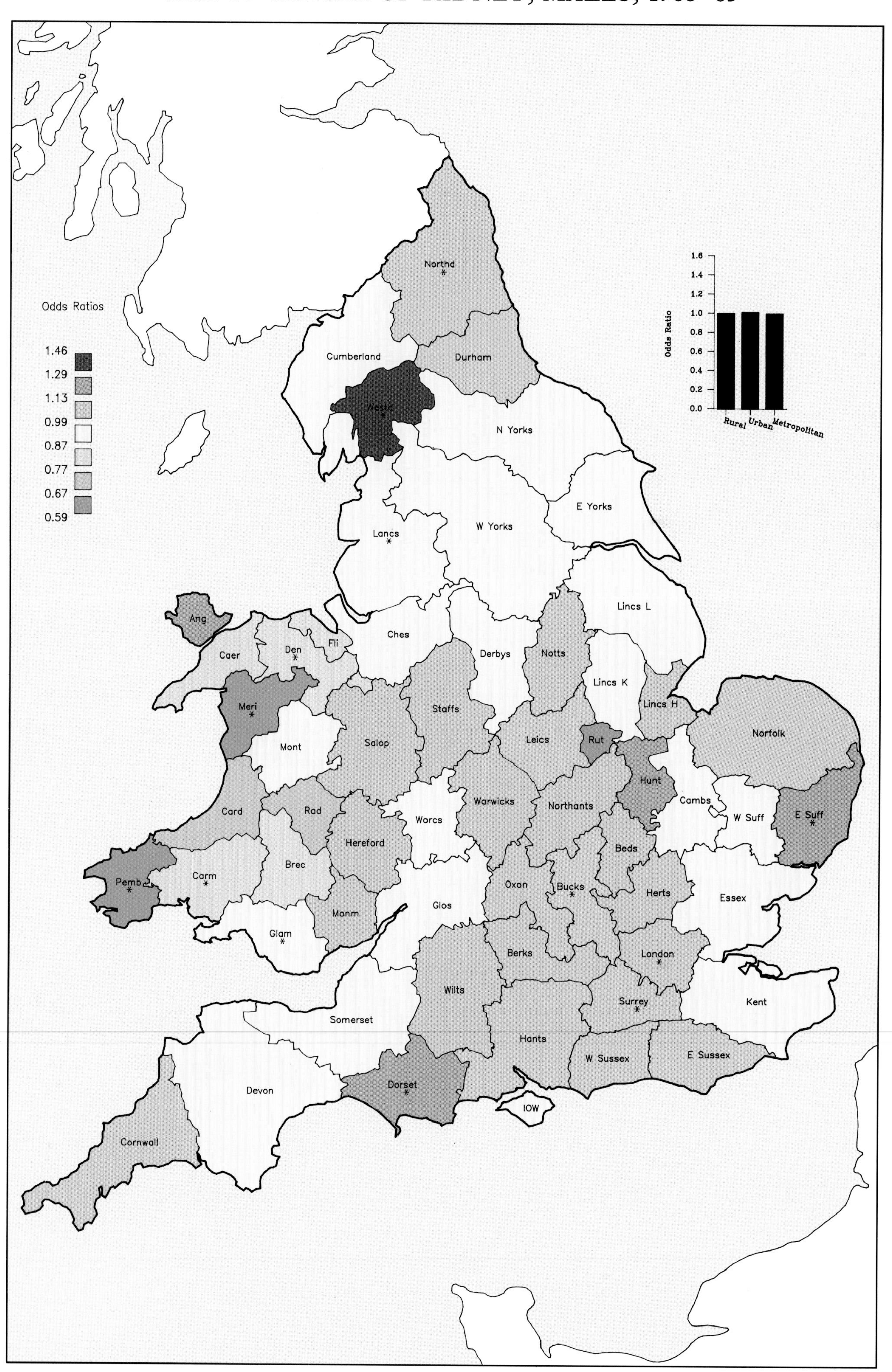

*p<0.05

MAP 57 CANCER OF KIDNEY, FEMALES, 1968–85

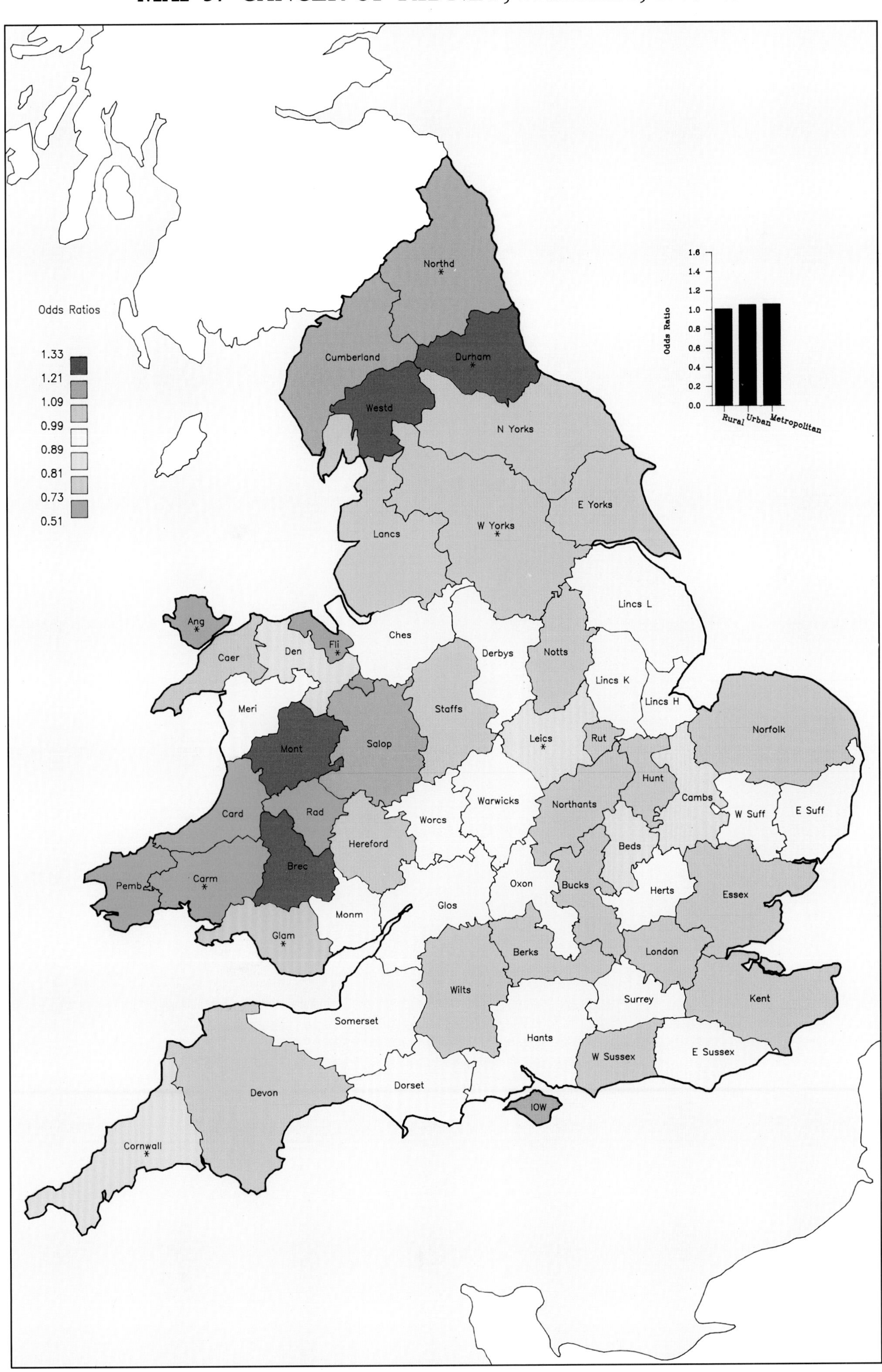

*p<0.05

MAP 58 CANCER OF EYE, MALES, AGES 15+, 1968–85

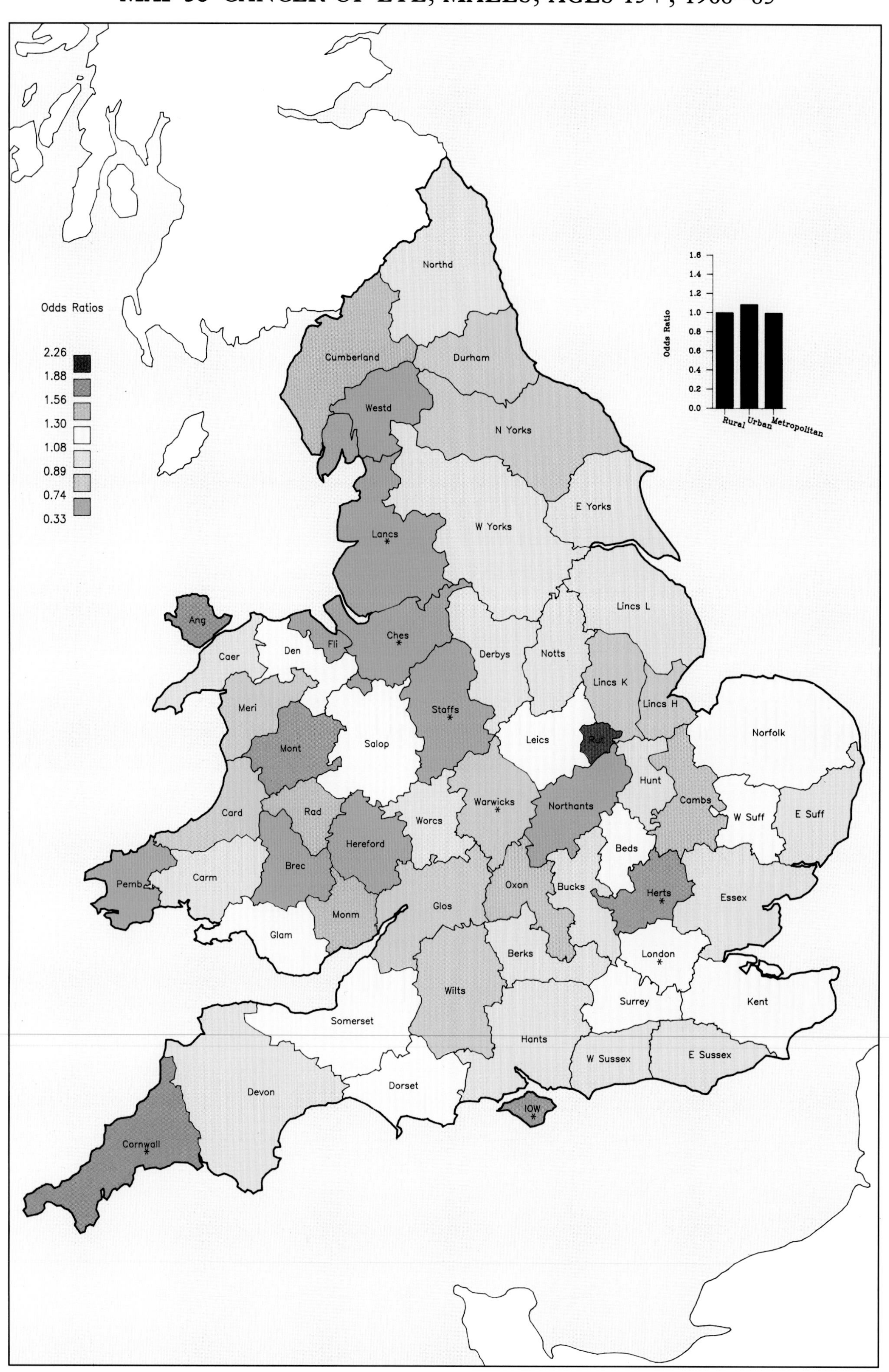

*p<0.05

MAP 59 CANCER OF EYE, FEMALES, AGES 15+, 1968–85

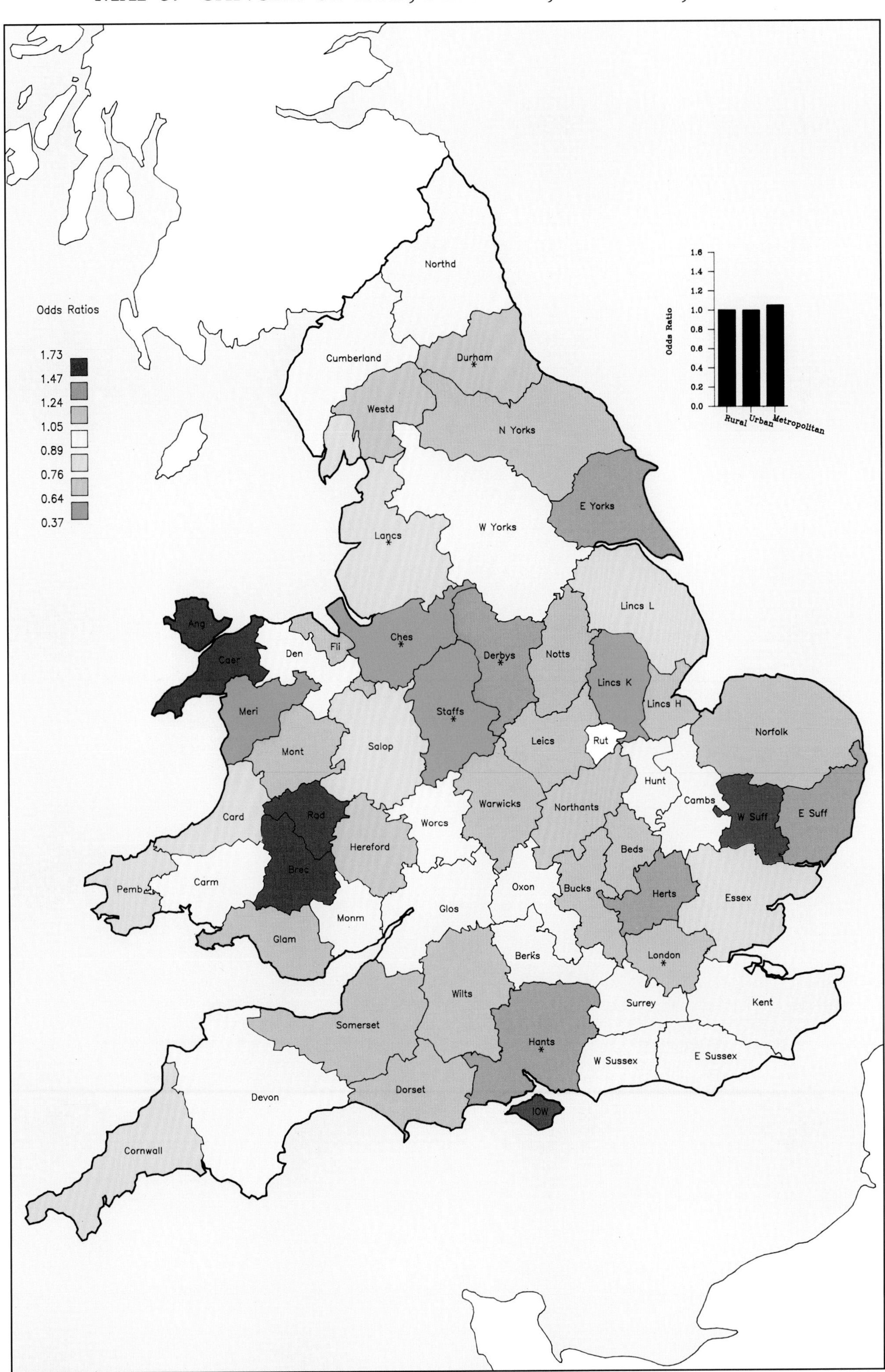

*p<0.05

In counties coloured white, no cases occurred during the period

MAP 60 CANCER OF NERVOUS SYSTEM, MALES, 1968–85

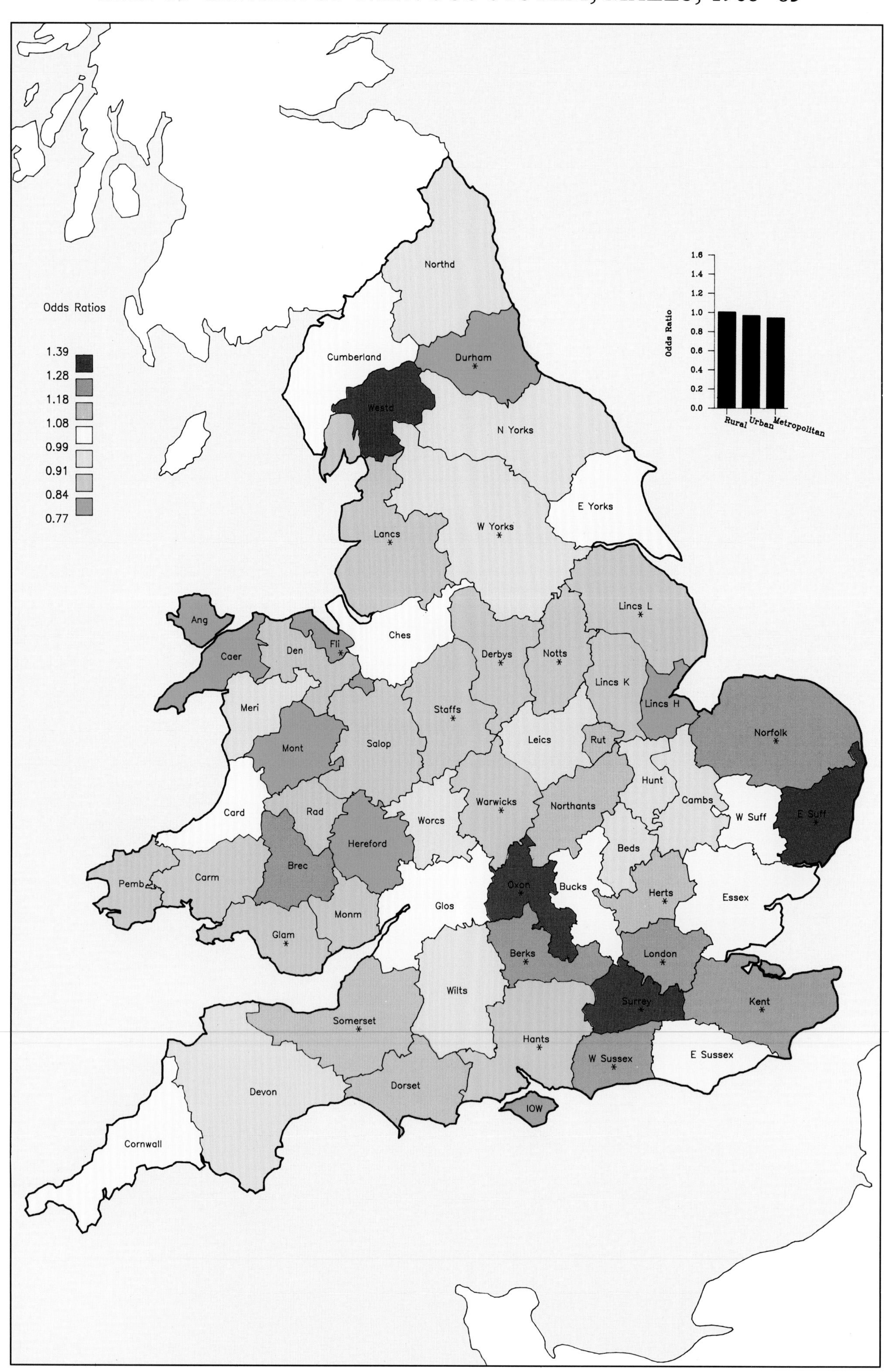

*p<0.05

MAP 61 CANCER OF NERVOUS SYSTEM, FEMALES, 1968–85

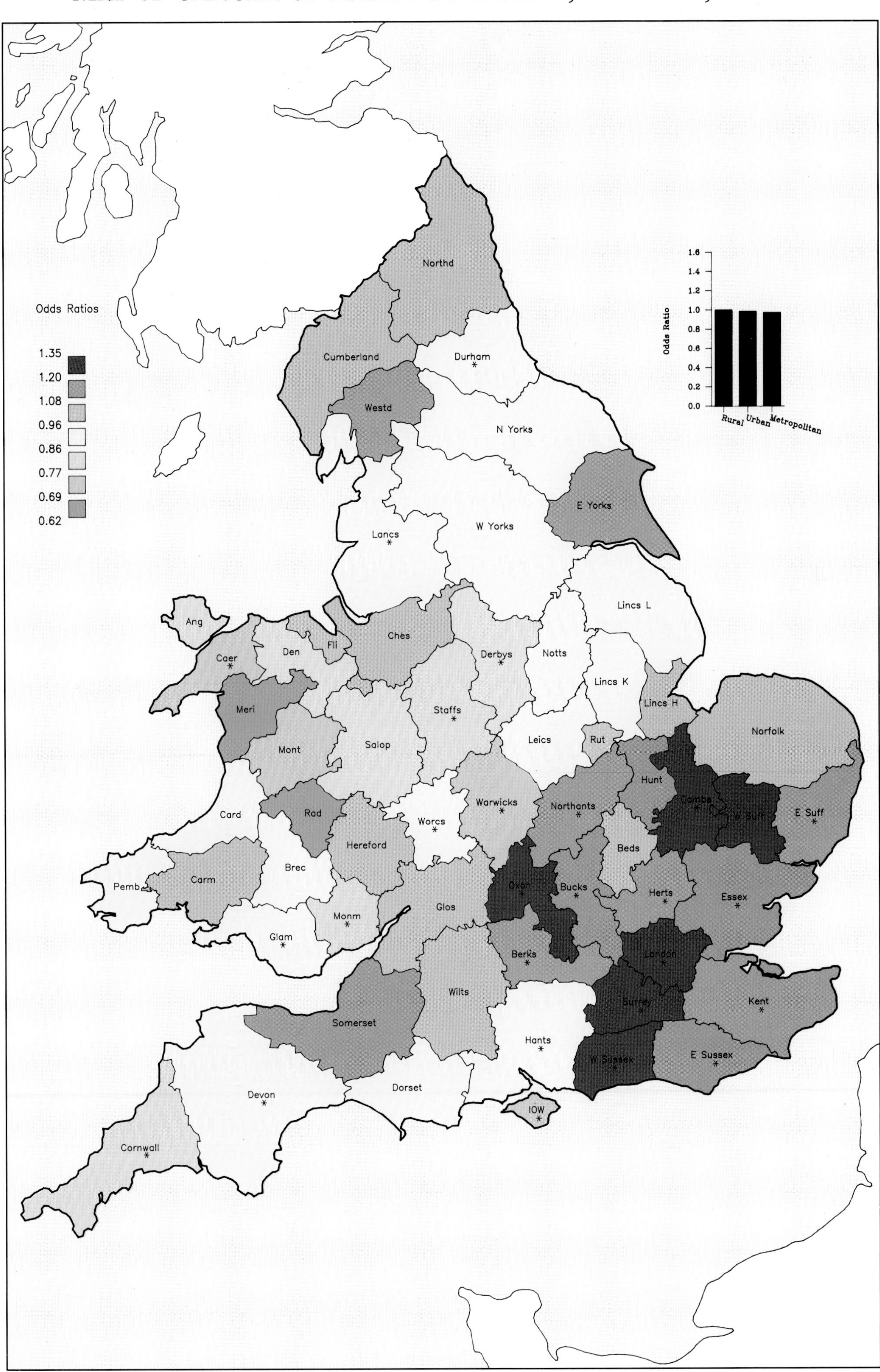

*p<0.05

MAP 62 CANCER OF THYROID, MALES, 1968–85

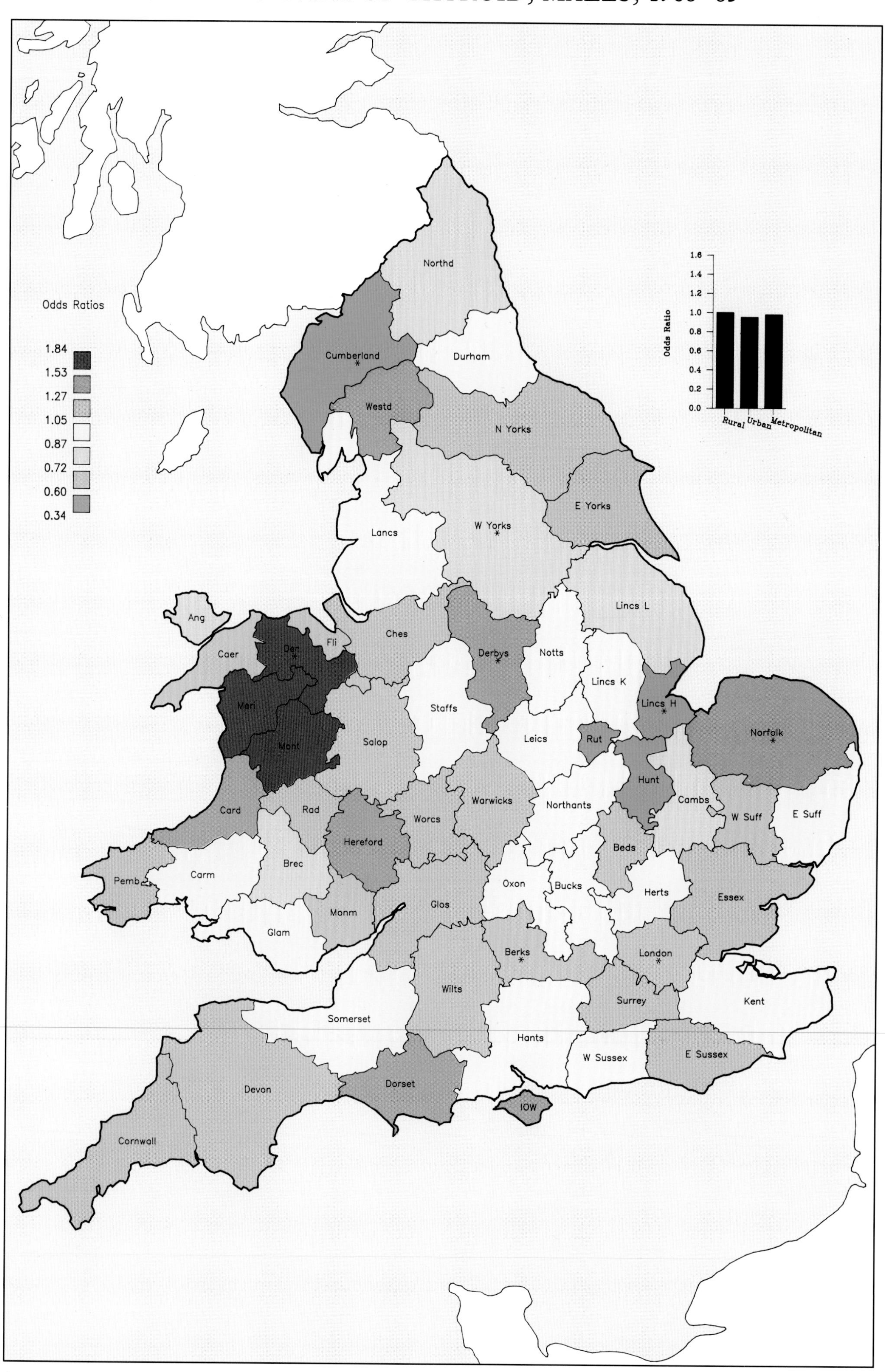

*$p<0.05$

MAP 63 CANCER OF THYROID, FEMALES, 1968–85

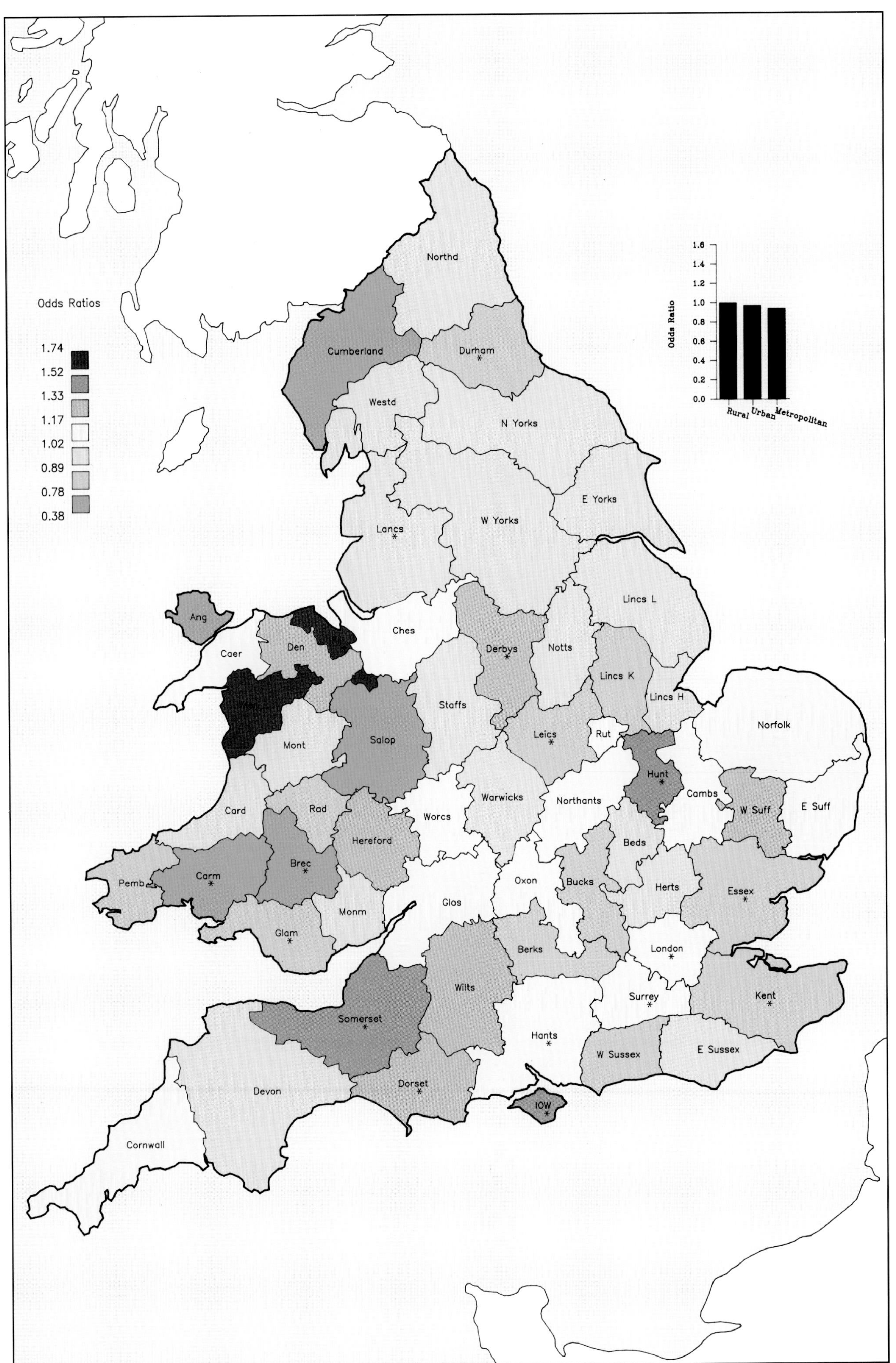

*p<0.05

MAP 64 HODGKIN'S DISEASE, MALES, AGES 0–44, 1968–85

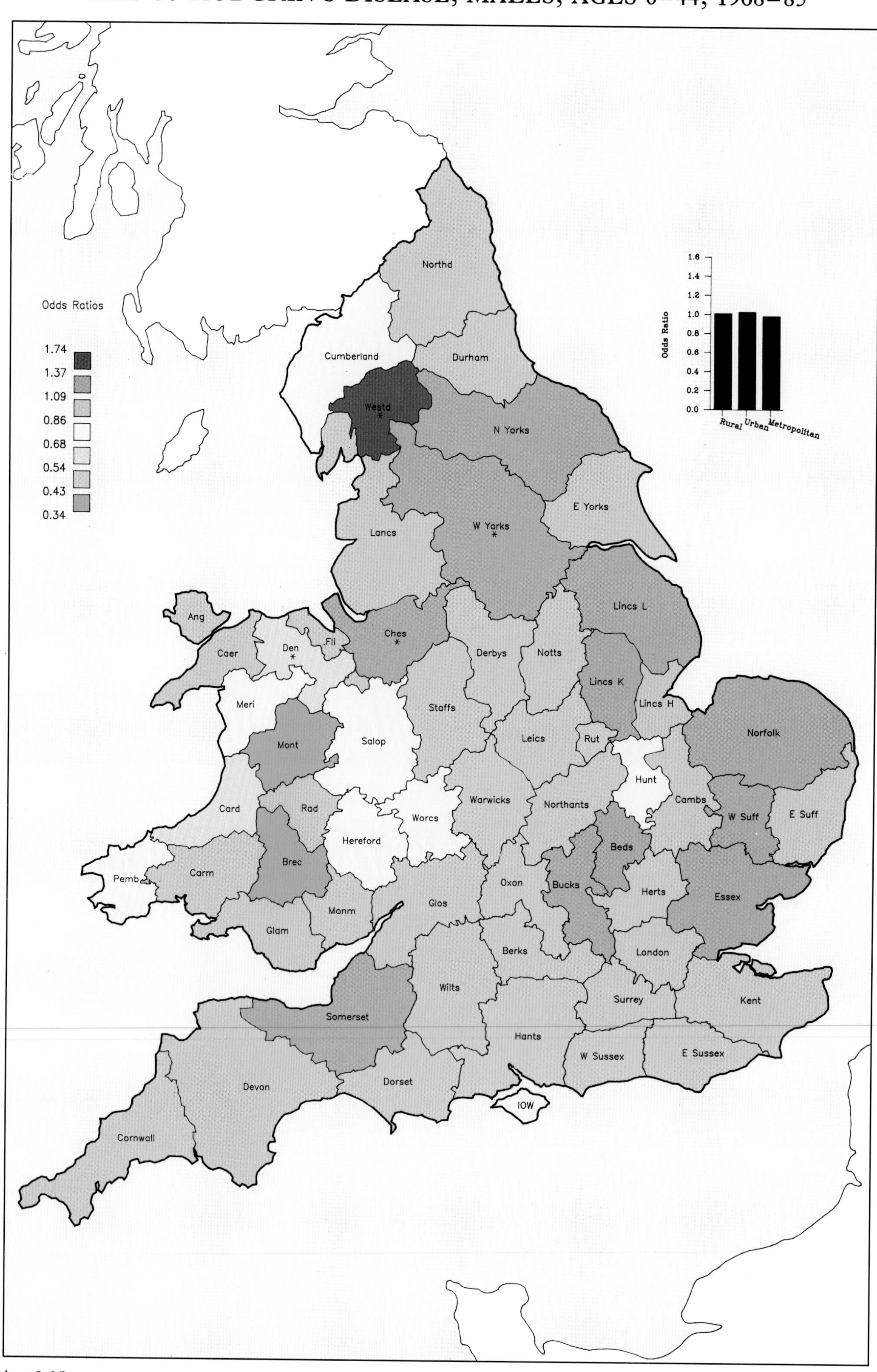

*p<0.05

MAP 65 HODGKIN'S DISEASE, FEMALES, AGES 0–44, 1968–85

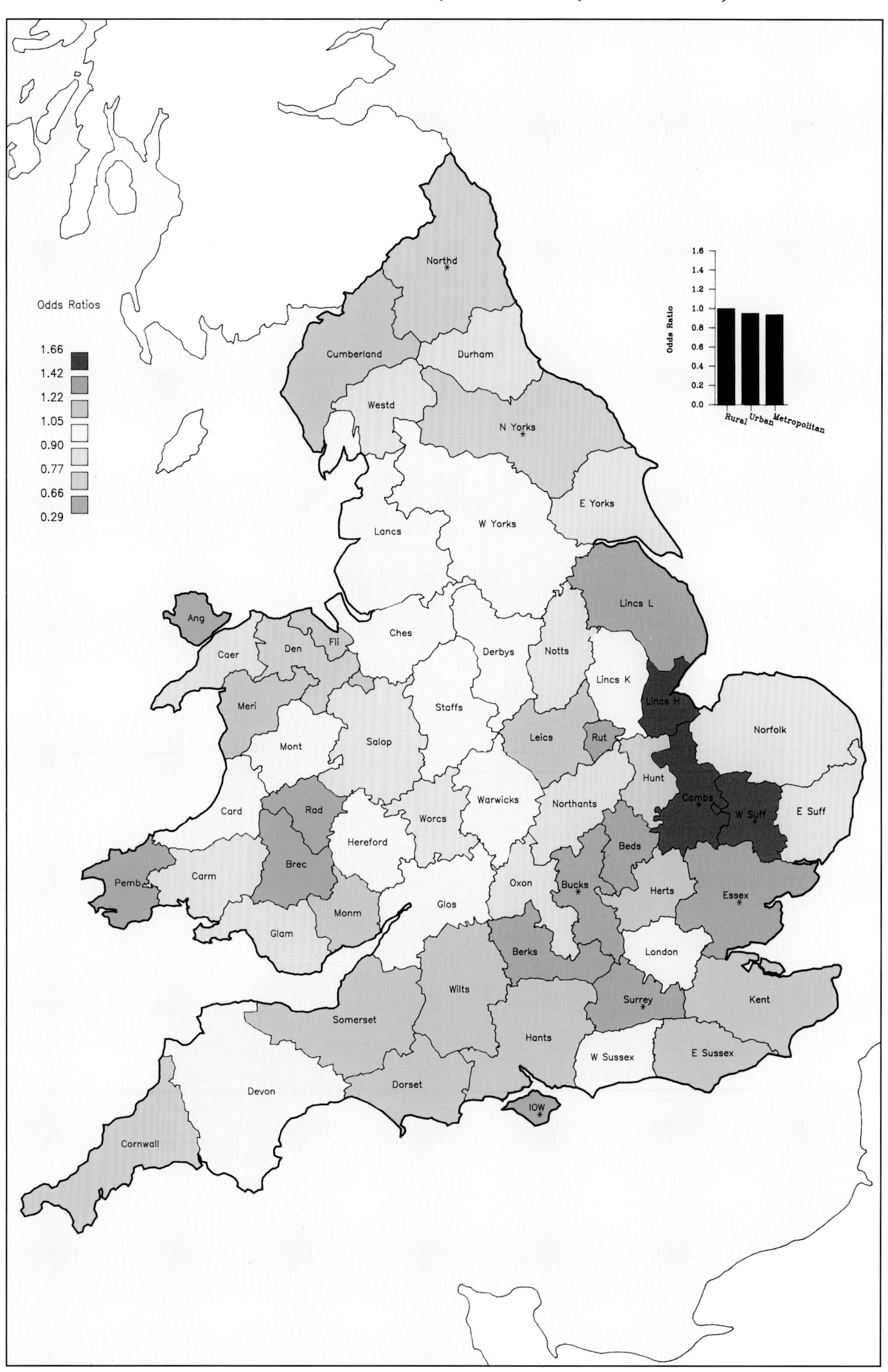

*p<0.05

MAP 66 HODGKIN'S DISEASE, MALES, AGES 45+, 1968–85

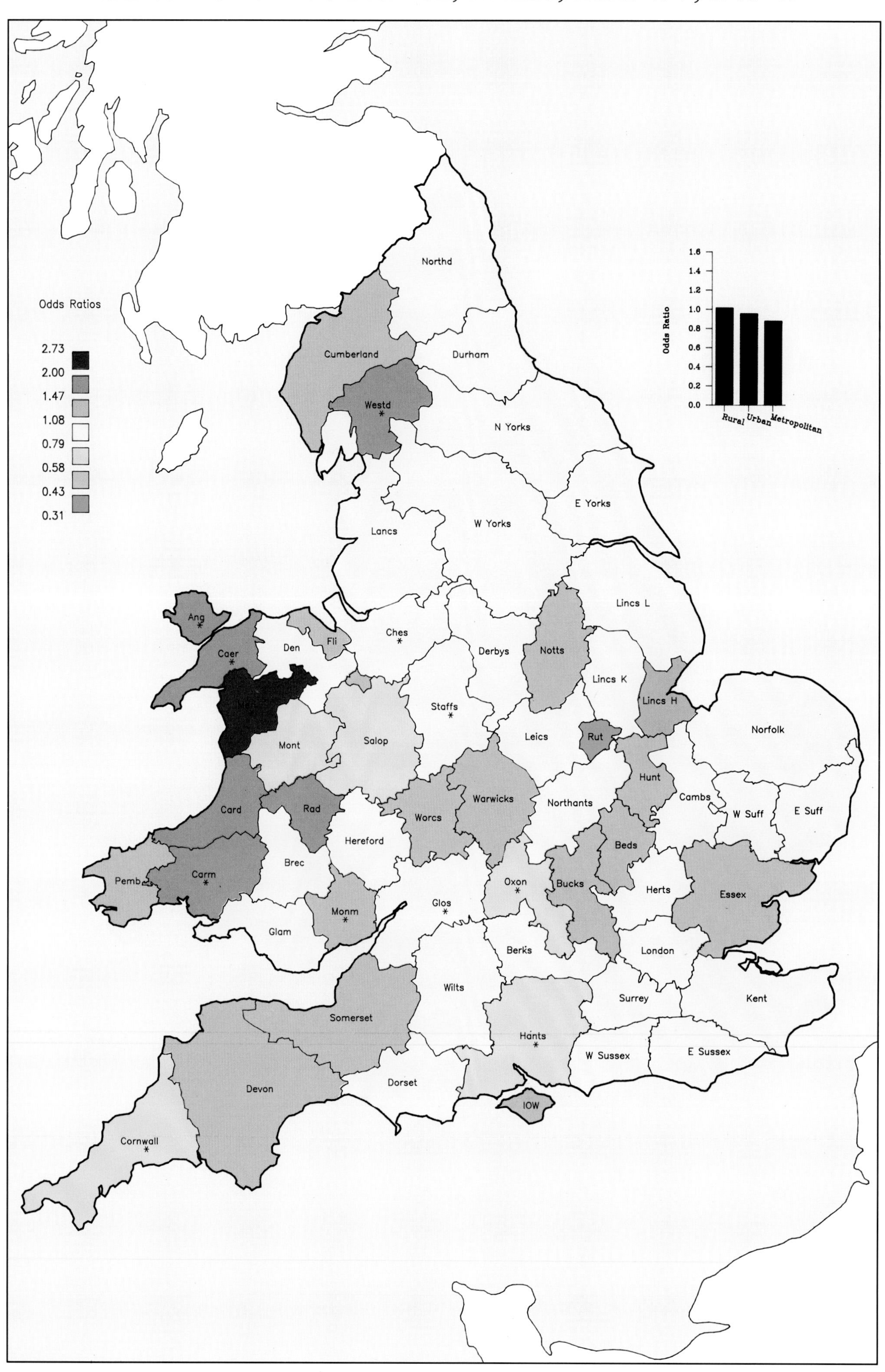

*p<0.05

MAP 67 HODGKIN'S DISEASE, FEMALES, AGES 45+, 1968–85

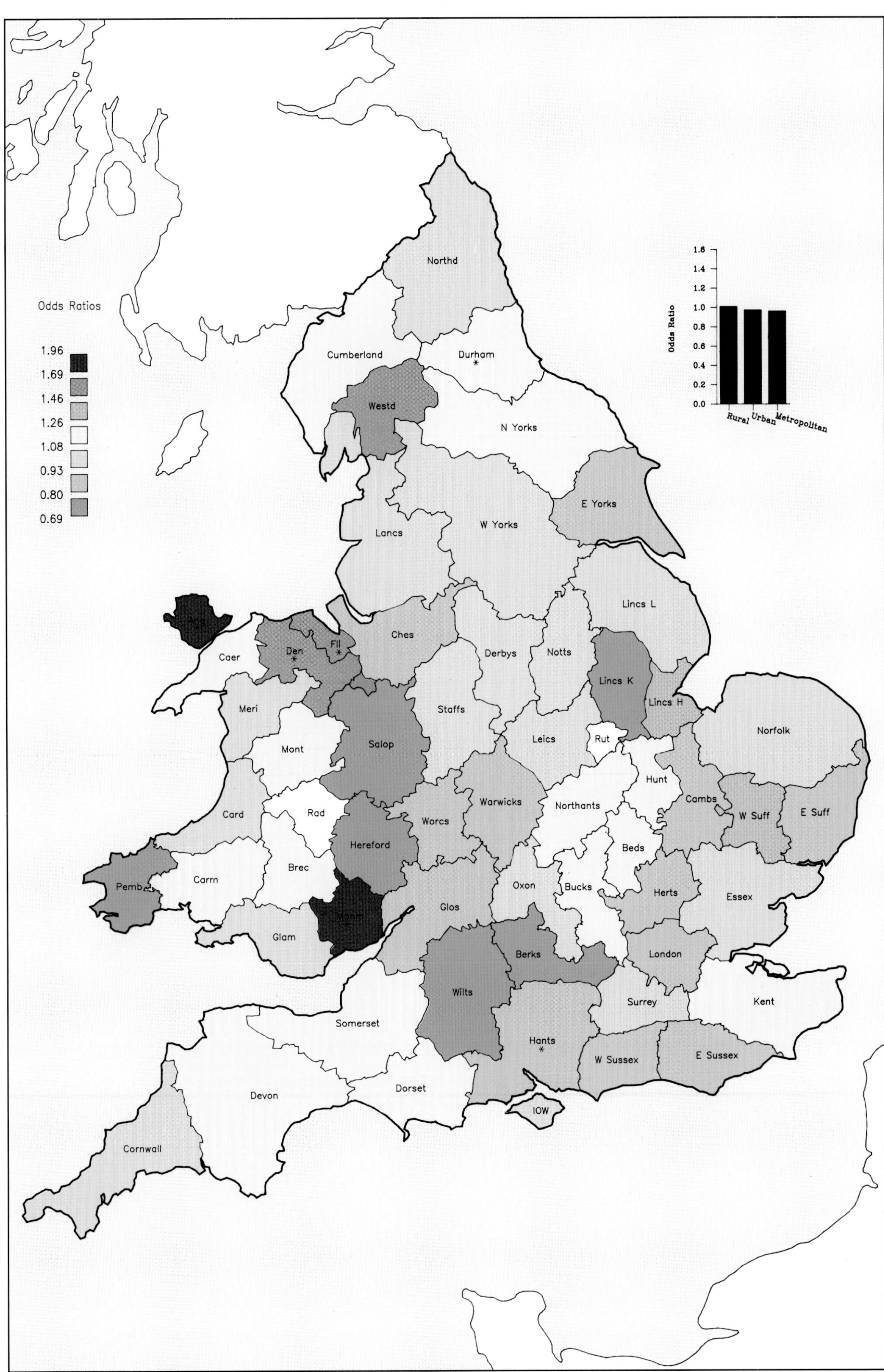

*p<0.05

In counties coloured white, no cases occurred during the period

MAP 68 NON-HODGKIN'S LYMPHOMA, MALES, 1968–85

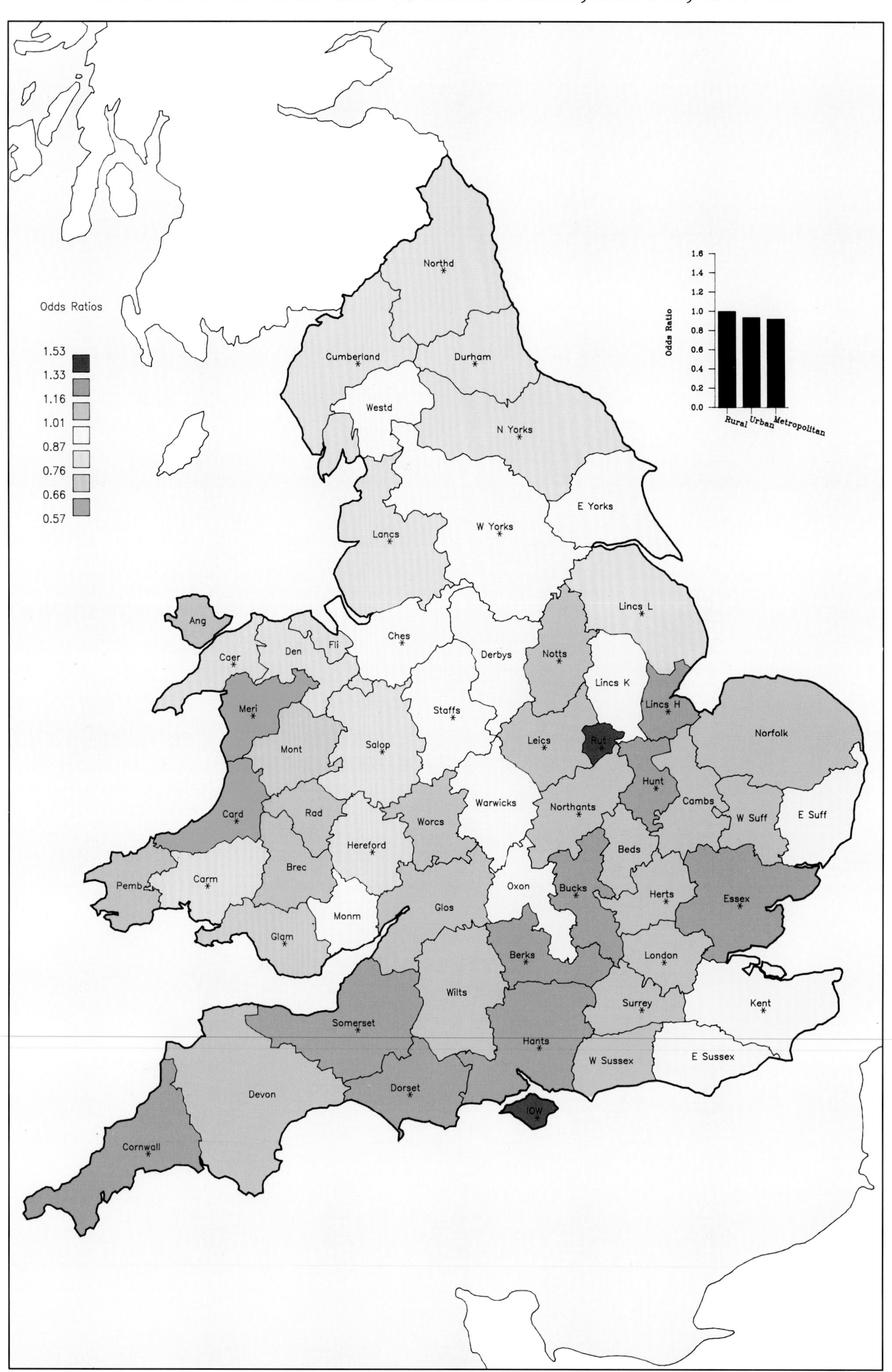

*p<0.05

MAP 69 NON-HODGKIN'S LYMPHOMA, FEMALES, 1968–85

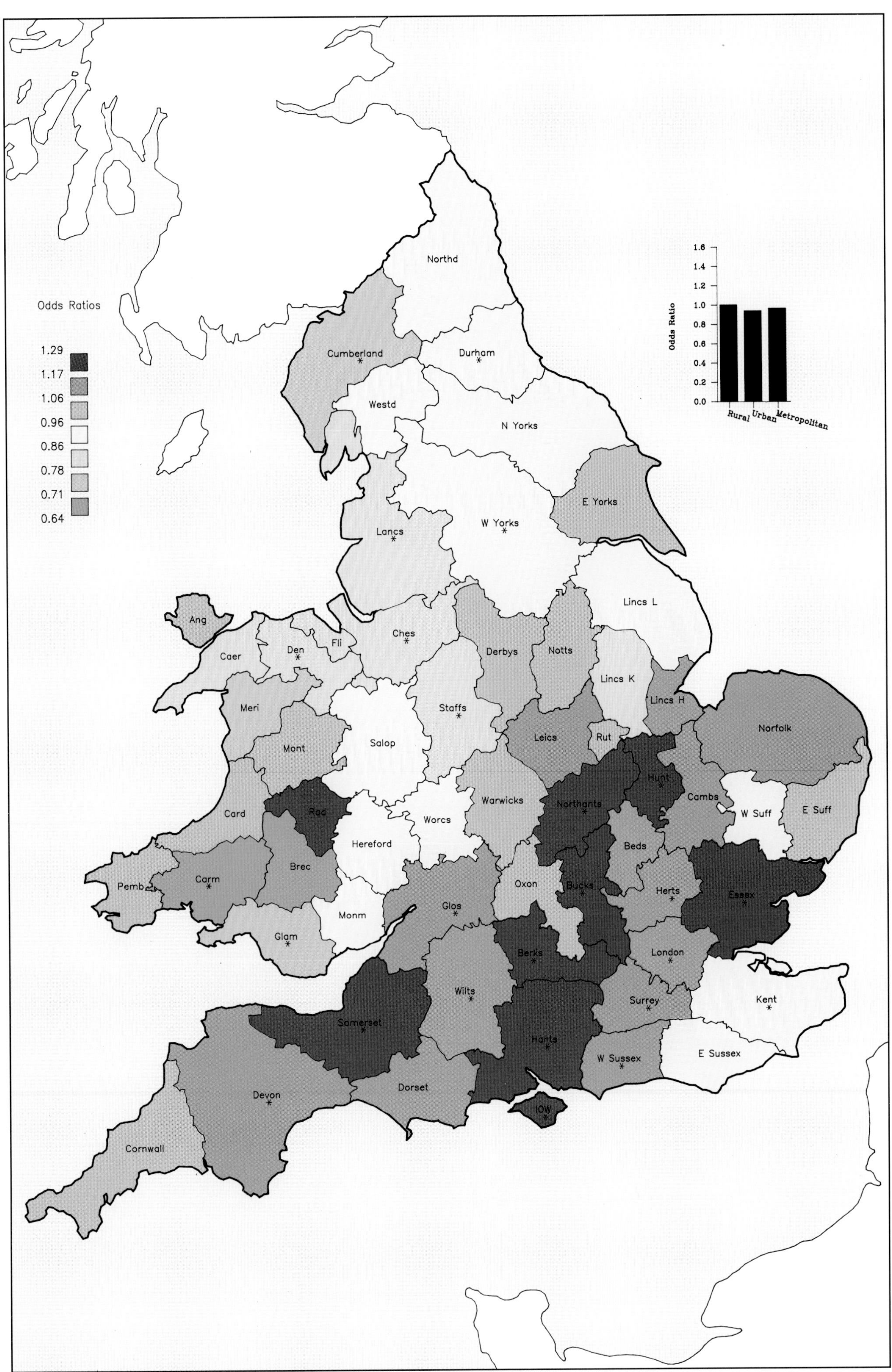

*p<0.05

MAP 70 MULTIPLE MYELOMA, MALES, 1968–85

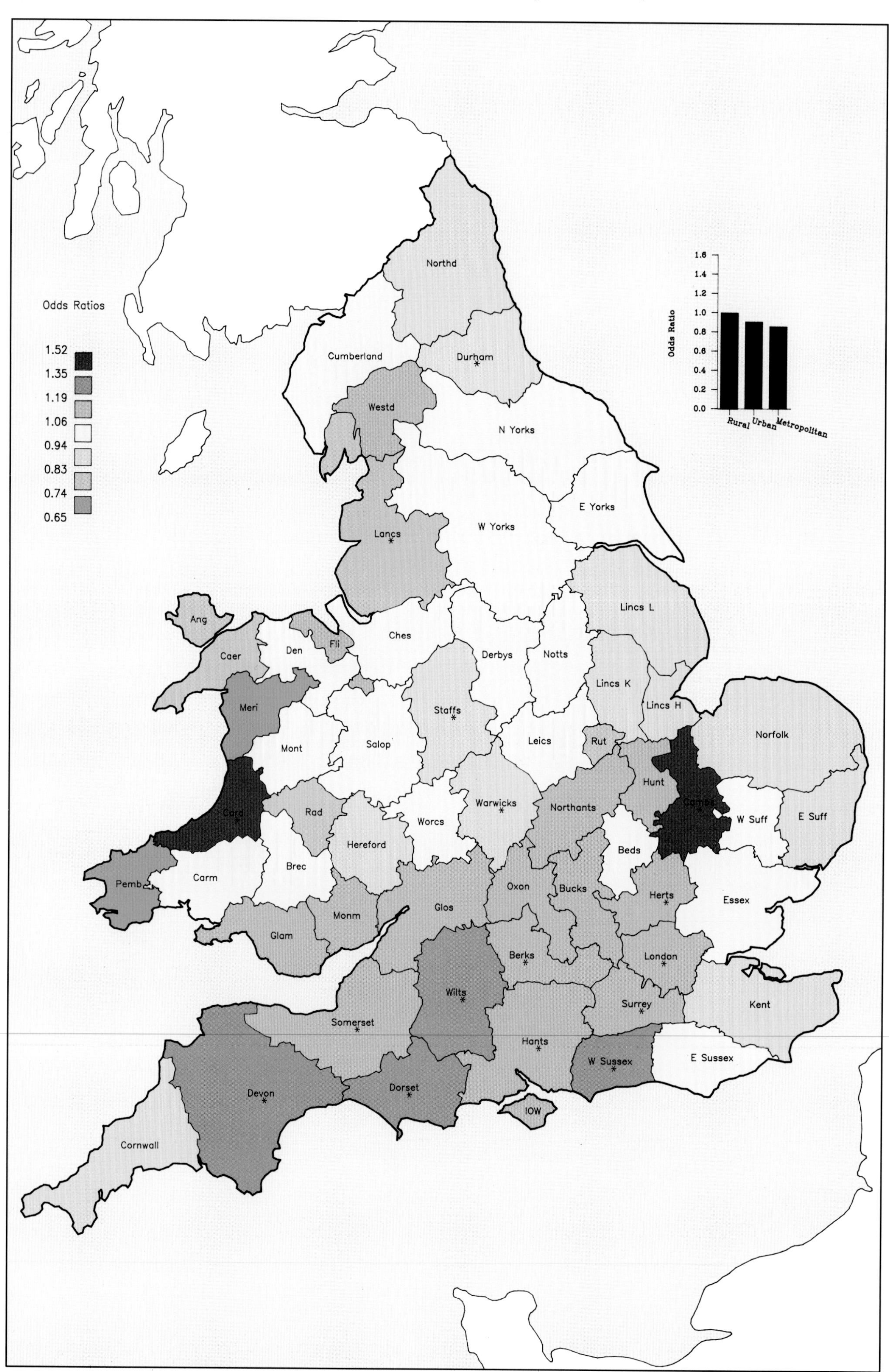

*p<0.05

MAP 71 MULTIPLE MYELOMA, FEMALES, 1968–85

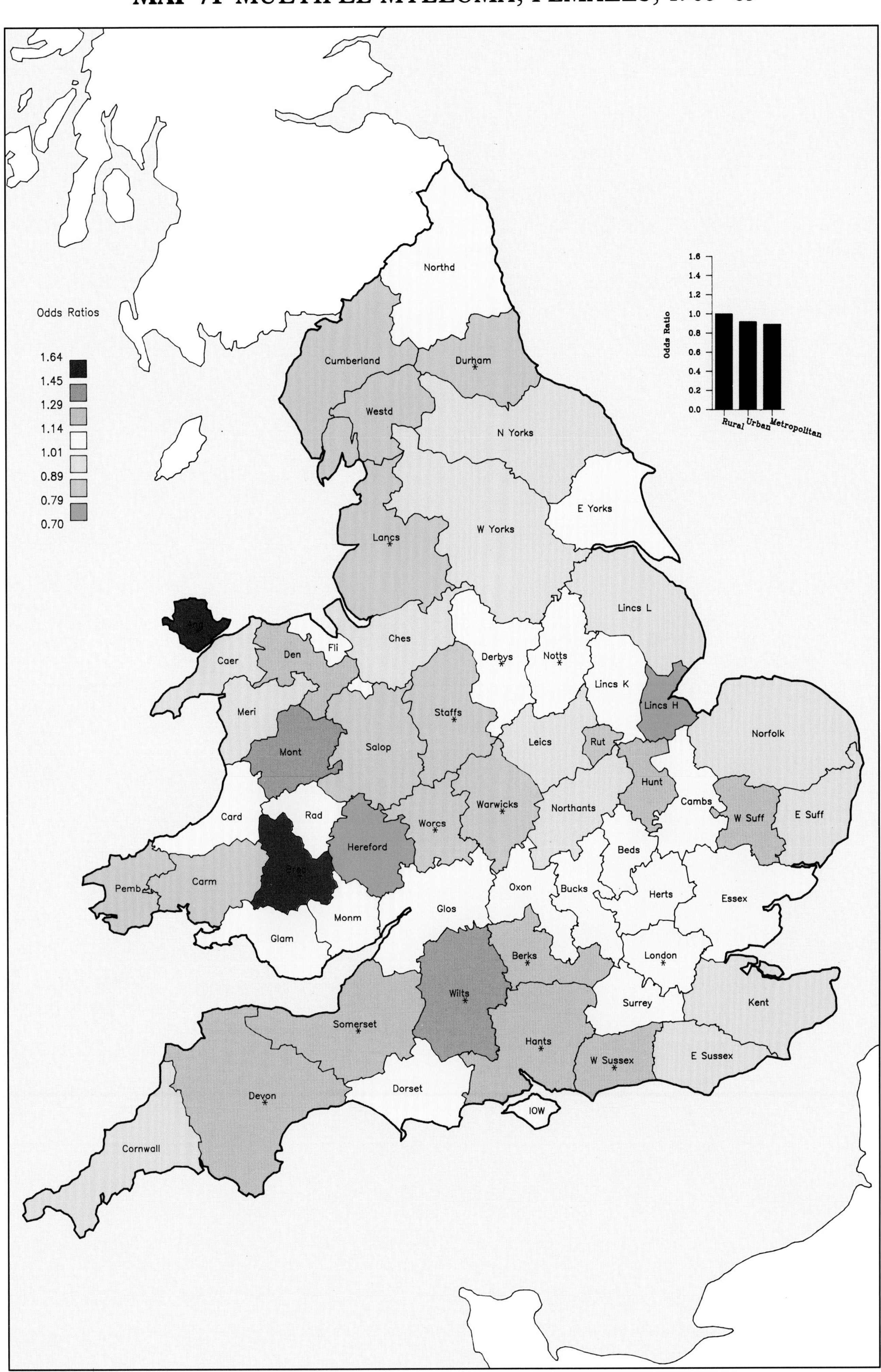

*p<0.05

MAP 72 LEUKAEMIA, MALES, ALL AGES, 1968–85

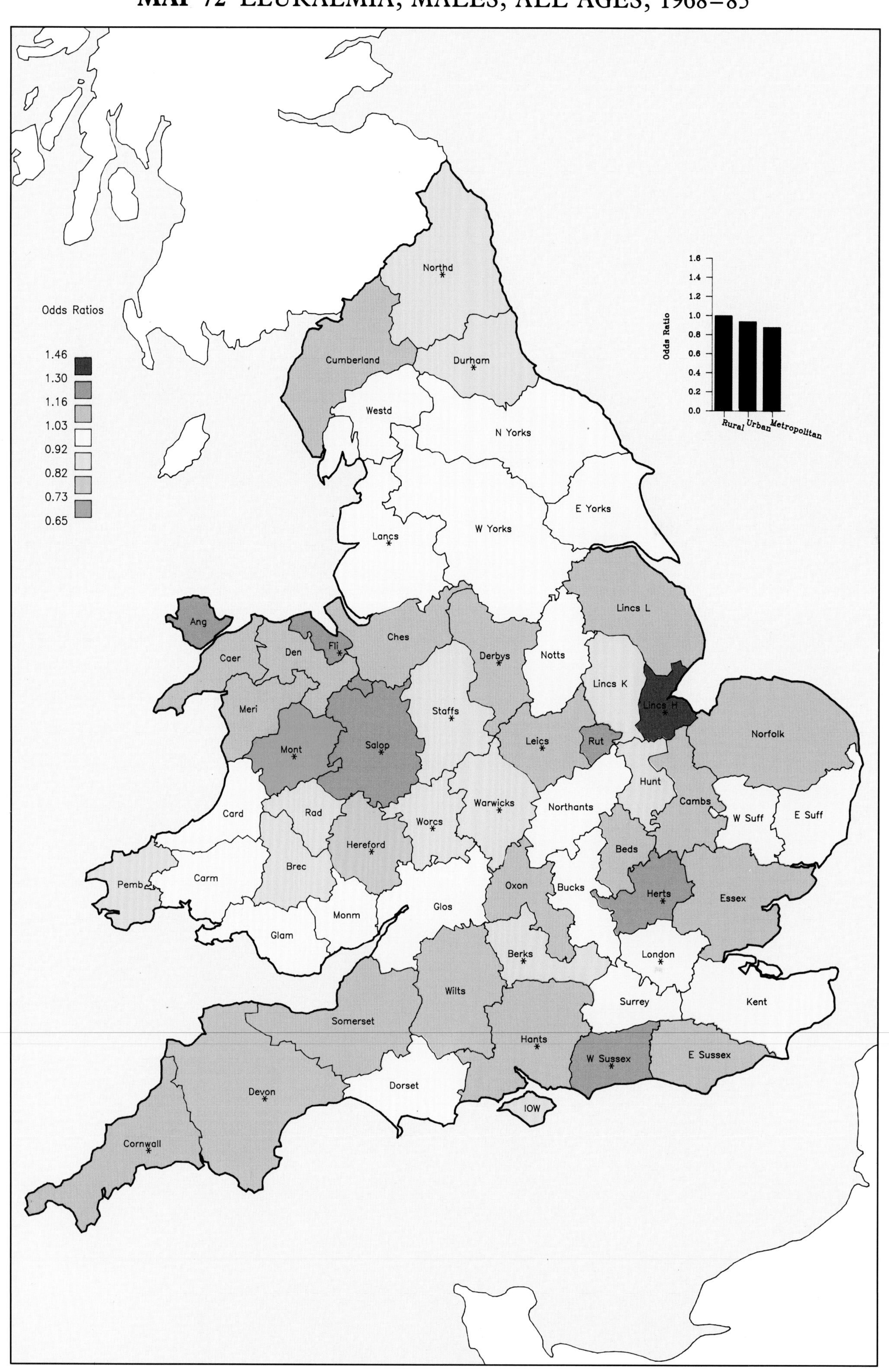

*p<0.05

MAP 73 LEUKAEMIA, FEMALES, ALL AGES, 1968–85

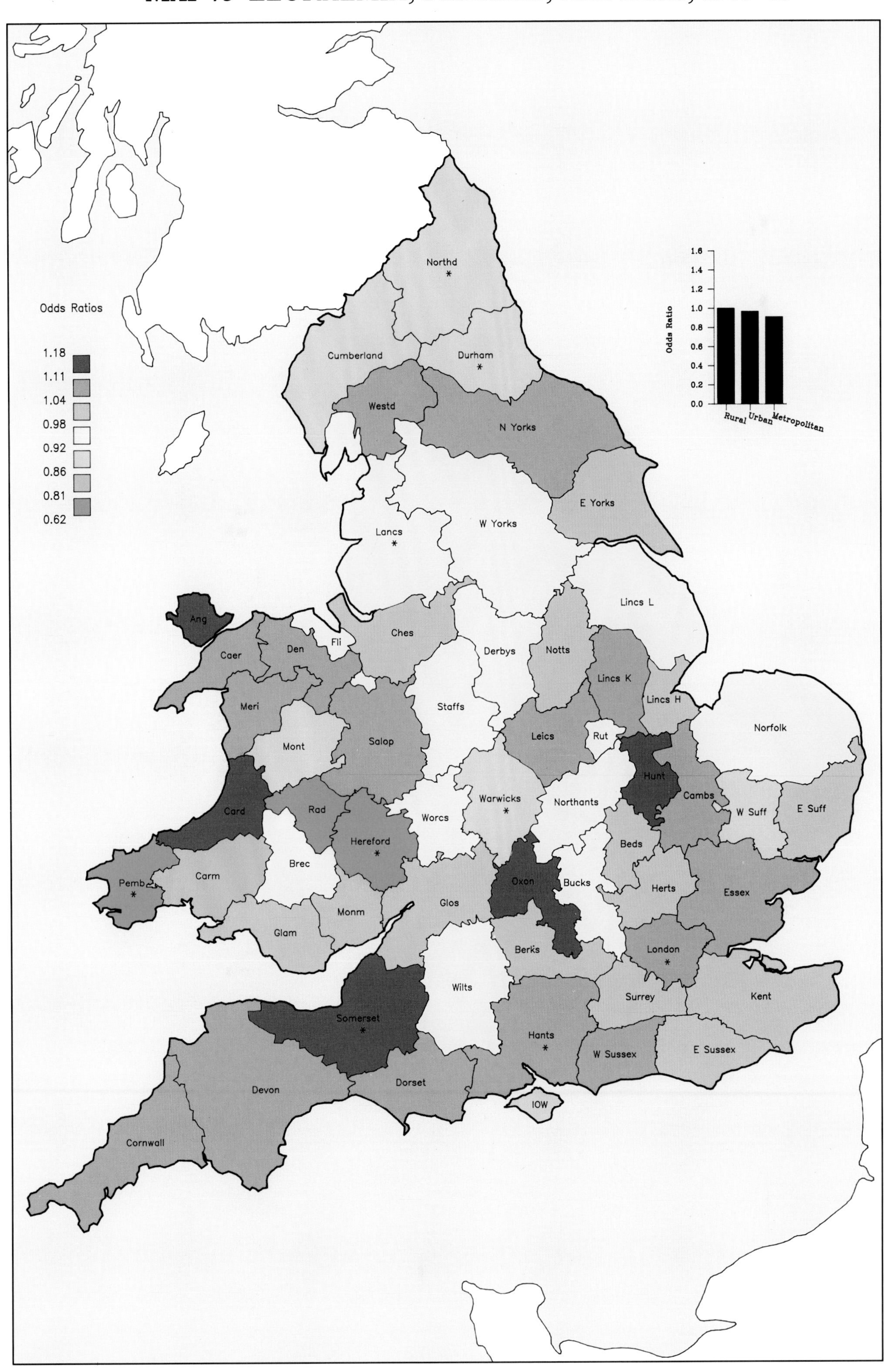

*p<0.05

MAP 74 LEUKAEMIA, MALES, AGES 0–14, 1966–83

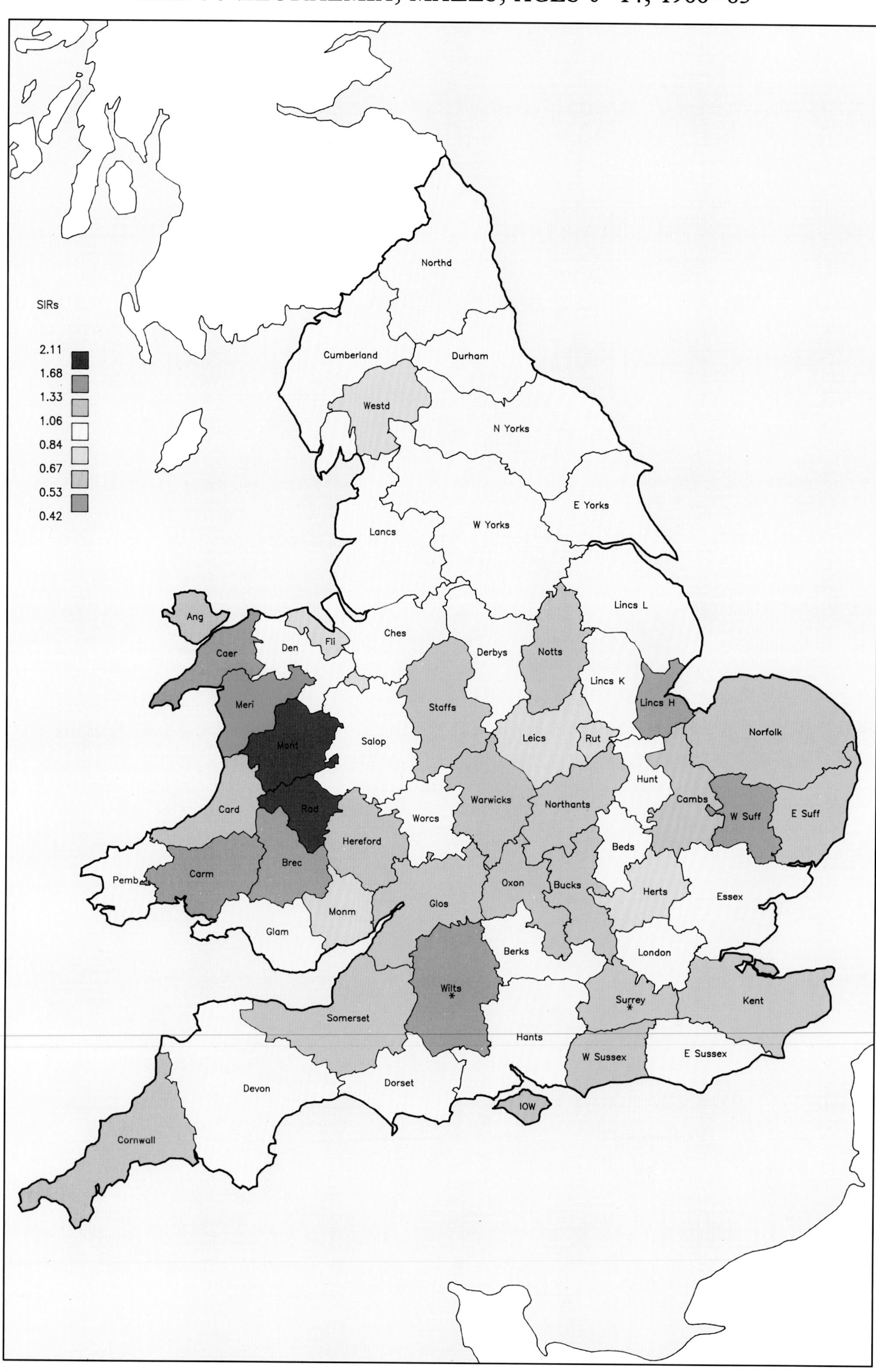

*p<0.05

MAP 75 LEUKAEMIA, FEMALES, AGES 0–14, 1966–83

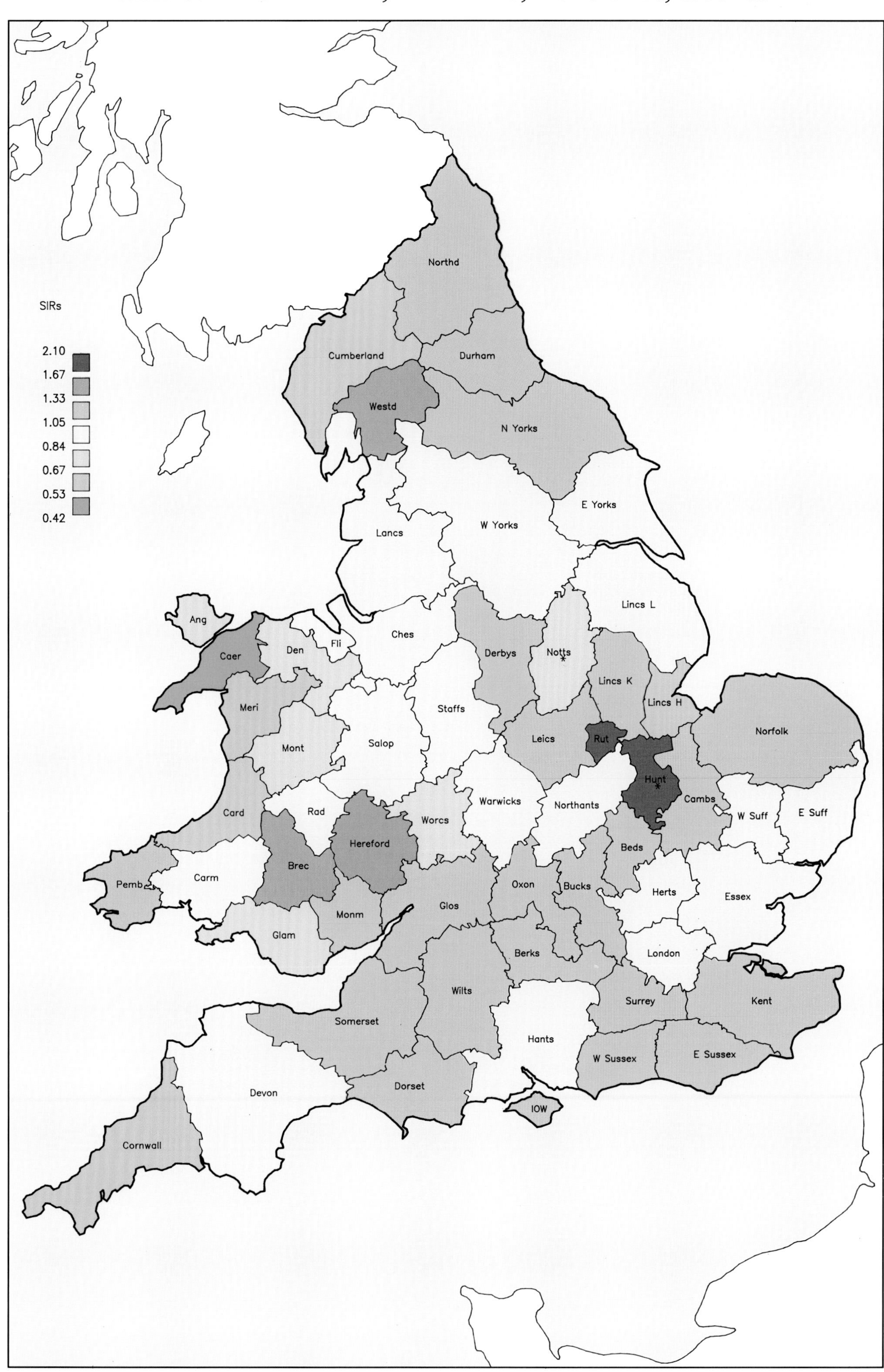

*$p<0.05$

Appendix 1

Counties, regions, and county boroughs of England and Wales

The *counties* of England and Wales for which cancers are mapped in this Atlas (Map E1) are those which had existed with little change for several hundred years until the 1974 reorganization of local government[1]. The distribution of some 'exposures', for instance radon, were available only for the post-1974 reorganized counties, which we have designated 'new counties'. The boundaries of the two are compared in Map A1.1.

The counties presented in the current cancer maps are in general the same as those in the maps by Stocks (1936, 1937, 1939) reproduced in this volume (Maps S1–S9), except that he presented separate data for the Soke of Peterborough and for the Isle of Ely, which were combined with Huntingdonshire and Cambridgeshire respectively in our data, and he showed data separately for Middlesex and London, whereas by the time of the current maps Middlesex had been abolished as an administrative entity, and Greater London covered a larger area (including much of what had been Middlesex) than that included in London in Stocks's time.[2]

Two types of region have commonly been used in analysing 'exposure' data — 'standard' and 'health' regions:-

The boundaries of the *standard regions* in 1971, and their relationship to county boundaries, are shown in Map A1.2. Only in Derbyshire and Dorset did the regional boundaries not follow county boundaries. The definitions of standard regions have changed slightly over time; differences between the 1971 definitions and those in 1951 and 1961 can be found in OPCS (1981). The basis of the standard regions was altered considerably in 1974, and the new standard region boundaries in relation to county boundaries are shown in Map A1.2.

Health regions before April 1974 were the geographical areas covered by the Regional Hospital Boards (RHBs). Their boundaries are shown in Map A1.3. Exact definitions of their composition can be found in OPCS (1973*b*). The boundaries of the health regions were altered on 1 April 1974 when the Regional Health Authorities (RHAs) replaced the RHBs. RHA boundaries are shown in Map A1.3.

Cancer registration regions have followed health region boundaries with certain exceptions. The Mersey registry — not the Welsh registry — covered Anglesey, Caernarvonshire, Denbighshire, Flintshire, Merionethshire, and Montgomeryshire until the end of 1978 (the Welsh registry was responsible for registrations from these counties thereafter). Cancers in the Wessex region were registered by the South Thames registry until the end of 1972. Registration for the North Thames regions was amalgamated with that for the South Thames regions at the start of 1985.

Three regions had registration 'bureaux' in different towns within their region. In Trent there were five bureaux: in Nottingham, Derby, Leicester, Lincoln, and Sheffield, which until early 1990 were responsible for data collection in their areas,

1 It should be noted that Flintshire and Lancashire each consist of two physically separated parts, as shown in Map E2. In the cancer maps and the 'exposure' maps except E2, only the larger part is labelled with the county name.

2 Also, in tables of results Stocks combined Rutland with Lincolnshire Kesteven, whereas we have presented these separately, but in the maps by Stocks they are demarcated separately and sometimes shown with different risks of cancer.

but all coding was conducted at one centre (Sheffield). In the South-western region there were two bureaux, in Plymouth and Bristol, which conducted their own coding and were amalgamated during 1978. The Plymouth bureau covered Devon and Cornwall and the Bristol bureau covered the remainder of the region. In East Anglia there were bureaux in Ipswich, Norwich, and Cambridge, each registering patients treated in their locality, and conducting their own coding. They were amalgamated at the beginning of 1986.

The *county boroughs* in each county are shown in Table A1.1.

Table A1.1 Metropolitan areas (county boroughs) in each county

Bedfordshire
Luton

Berkshire
Reading

Cheshire
Birkenhead, Chester, Stockport, Wallasey

Cumberland
Carlisle

Derbyshire
Derby

Devon
Exeter, Plymouth, Torbay

Durham
Darlington, Gateshead, Hartlepool, South Shields, Sunderland

Essex
Southend-on-Sea

Gloucestershire
Bristol, Gloucester

Hampshire
Bournemouth, Portsmouth, Southampton

Kent
Canterbury

Lancashire
Barrow-in-Furness, Blackburn, Blackpool, Bolton, Bootle, Burnley, Bury, Liverpool, Manchester, Oldham, Preston, Rochdale, St Helens, Salford, Southport, Warrington, Wigan

Leicestershire
Leicester

Lincolnshire (Parts of Kesteven)
Lincoln

Lincolnshire (Parts of Lindsey)
Grimsby

London (Greater)*
City of London, all London boroughs

Norfolk
Great Yarmouth, Norwich

Northamptonshire
Northampton

Northumberland
Newcastle upon Tyne, Tynemouth

Nottinghamshire
Nottingham

Oxfordshire
Oxford

Somerset
Bath

Staffordshire
Burton-upon-Trent, Dudley, Stoke-on-Trent, Walsall, West Bromwich, Wolverhampton

Suffolk (East)
Ipswich

Sussex (East)
Brighton, Eastbourne, Hastings

Warwickshire
Birmingham, Coventry, Solihull

Worcestershire
Warley, Worcester

Yorkshire (East Riding)
Kingston upon Hull

Yorkshire (North Riding)
Teeside

Yorkshire (West Riding)
Barnsley, Bradford, Dewsbury, Doncaster, Halifax, Huddersfield, Leeds, Rotherham, Sheffield, Wakefield, York

Glamorgan
Cardiff, Merthyr Tydfil, Swansea

Monmouthshire
Newport

---

* Referred to in the text and maps simply as 'London'

MAP A1.1 COUNTY BOUNDARIES BEFORE AND AT 1 APRIL 1974

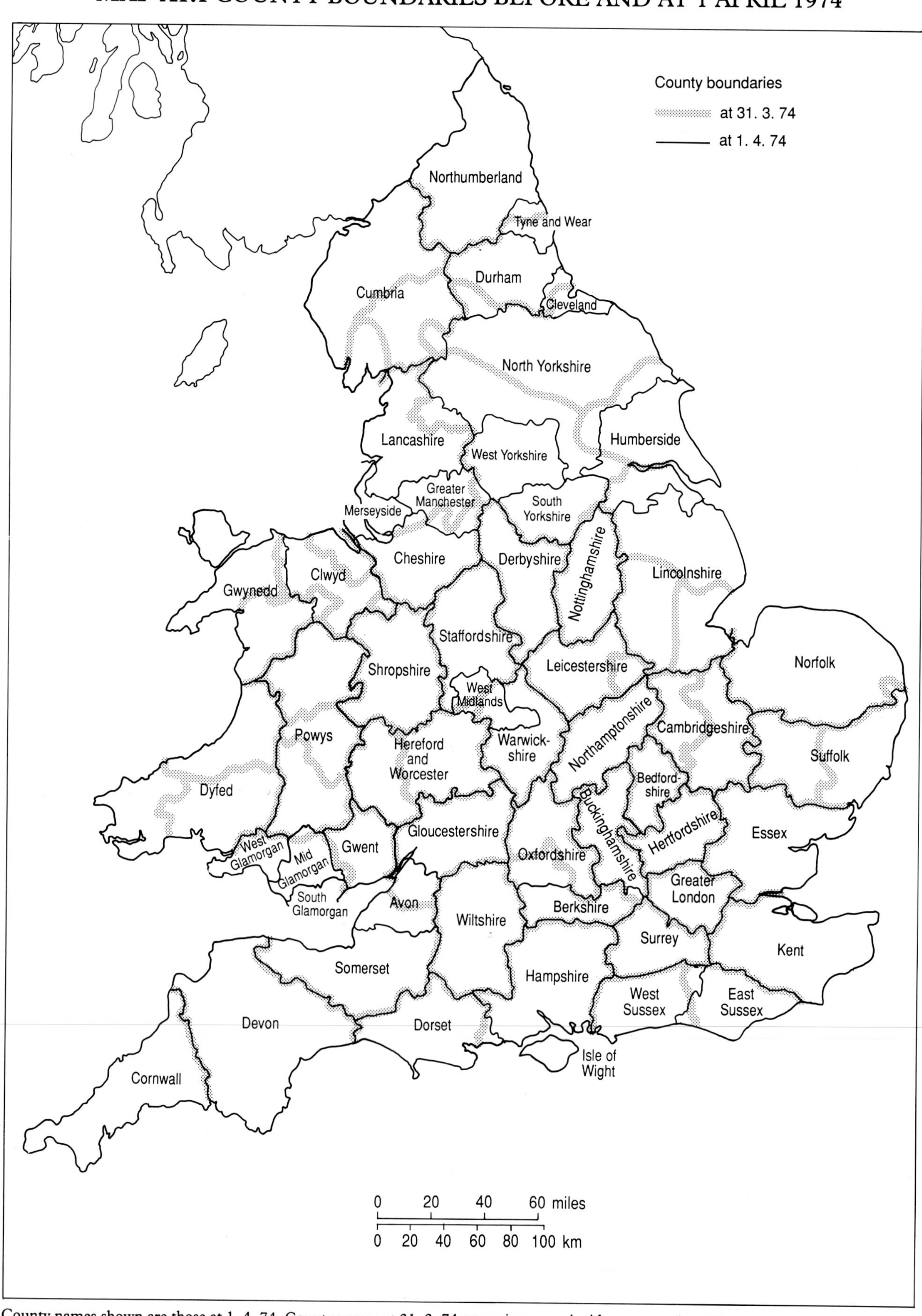

County names shown are those at 1. 4. 74. County names at 31. 3. 74 are as in cancer incidence maps 1 to 75.

MAP A1.2 STANDARD REGION BOUNDARIES BEFORE AND AT 1 APRIL 1974

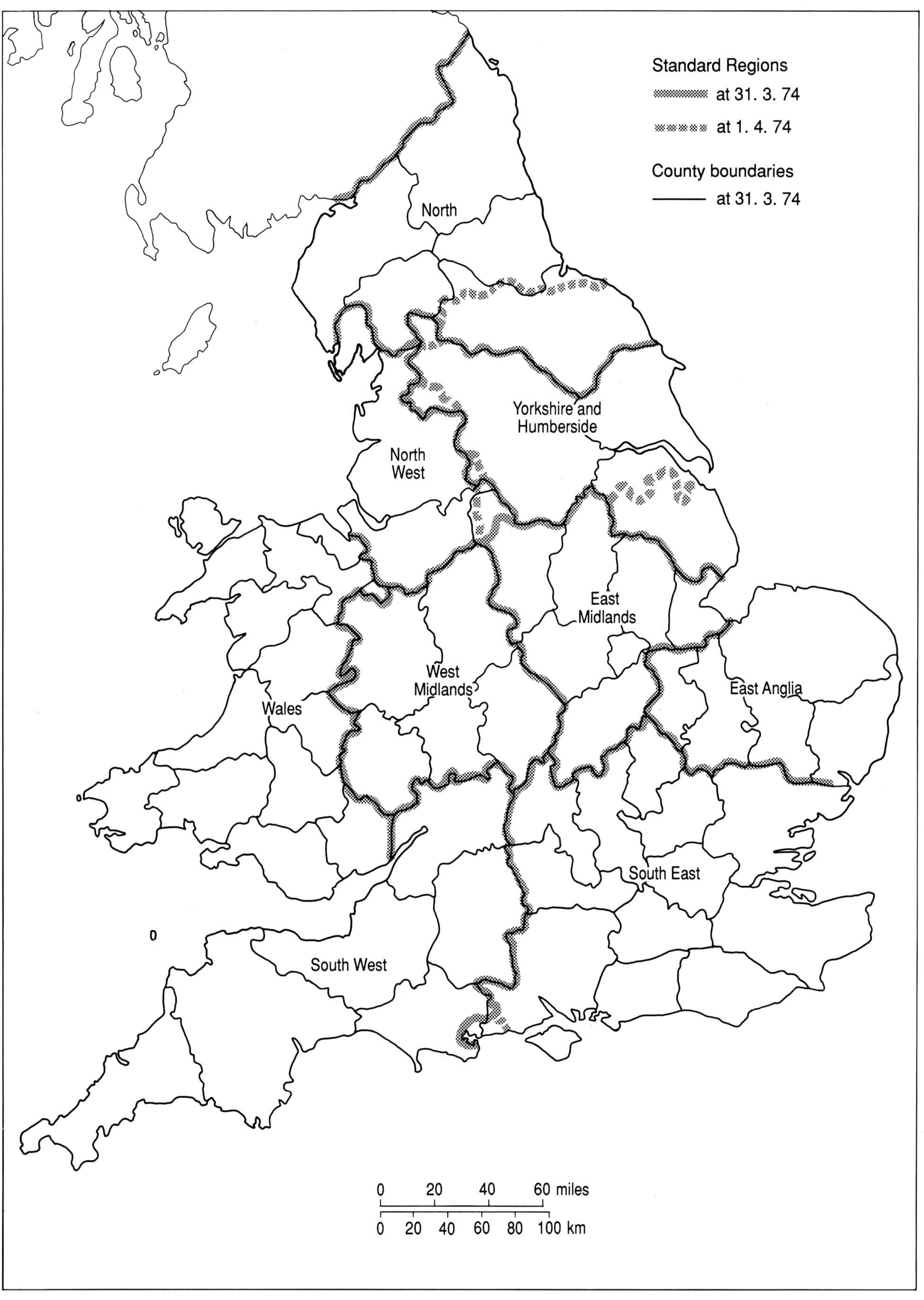

MAP A1.3 HEALTH REGION BOUNDARIES BEFORE AND AT 1 APRIL 1974

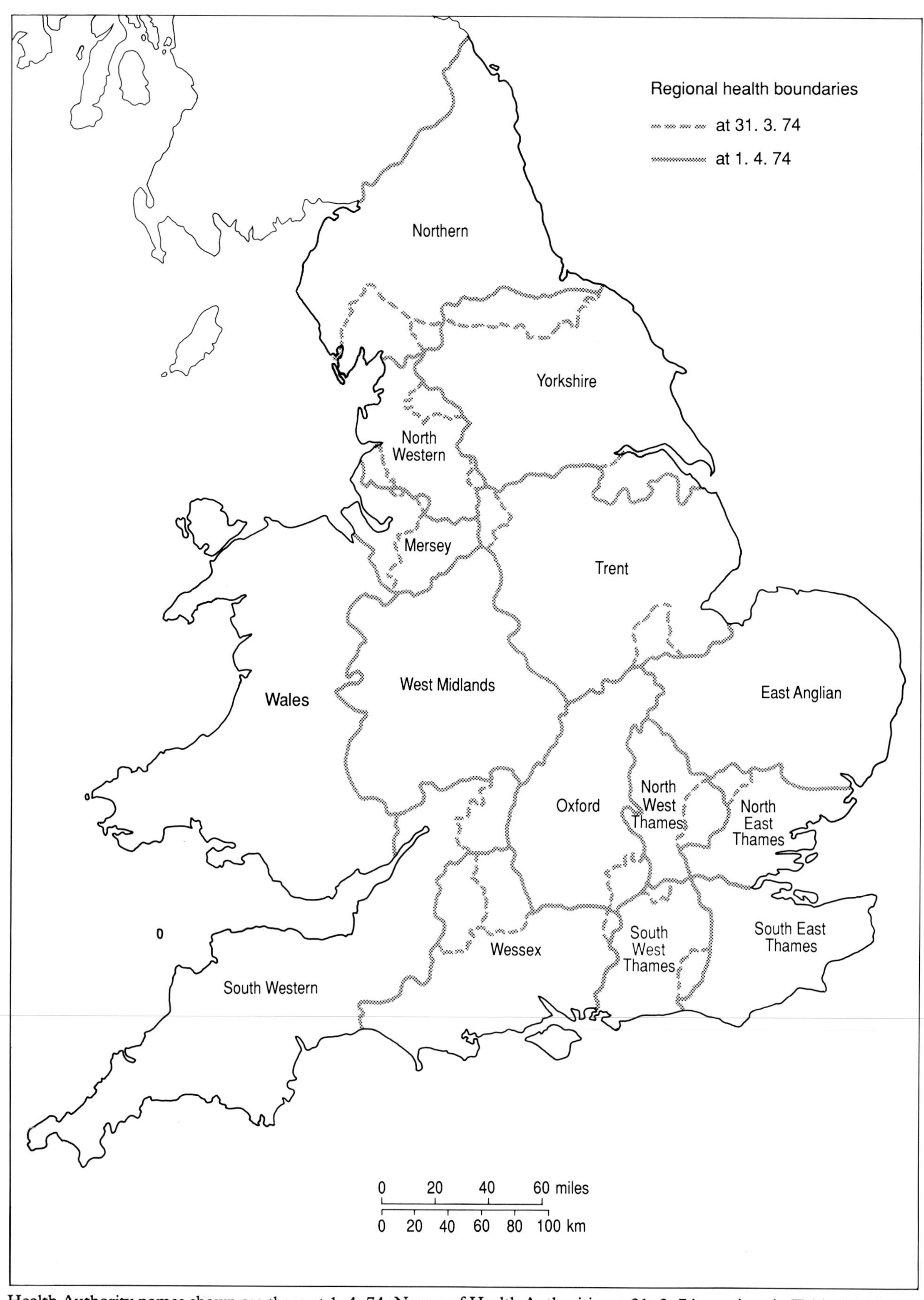

Health Authority names shown are those at 1. 4. 74. Names of Health Authorities at 31. 3. 74 are given in Table A4.18

Appendix 2

County populations, and cancers incident in each county

In the study period, England and Wales had a population of 50 million, of whom (in 1971) 38·2 per cent were aged under 25 years, 48·5 per cent aged 25–64 years, and 13·3 per cent aged 65 years and over. The populations of each county are shown in Table A2.1. The smallest, Radnorshire, had a population of 18 279 and the largest — Greater London — had a population of 7 452 346. Most counties, however, had populations between 100 000 and one million.

The numbers of cancers of all sites in each county are presented in Table A2.2. The numbers of cancers in a county are of course approximately proportional to the county population. Because of the large number of years of data included in the analyses, however, even the least-populous counties (Rutland and Radnorshire) have very substantial numbers of cancers included in the analyses — 767 and 808 respectively for males, and 704 and 751 for females.

Table A2.1 County populations by sex and urbanization, 1971

County	Total		Metropolitan		Urban		Rural	
	Males	Females	Males	Females	Males	Females	Males	Females
Bedfordshire	232 414	231 863	81 358	80 047	78 452	80 243	72 604	71 573
Berkshire	315 528	321 329	65 193	67 746	74 520	78 411	175 815	175 172
Buckinghamshire	291 132	296 427	—	—	144 954	145 915	146 178	150 512
Cambridgeshire*	150 830	152 214	—	—	78 159	77 982	72 671	74 232
Cheshire	745 897	800 490	209 198	228 424	415 272	445 465	121 427	126 601
Cornwall	181 735	199 937	—	—	100 299	113 558	81 436	86 379
Cumberland	142 661	149 526	34 198	37 384	43 573	46 047	64 890	66 095
Derbyshire	436 361	448 770	108 139	111 443	190 068	198 543	138 154	138 784
Devon	426 783	471 621	211 140	233 298	91 195	108 345	124 448	129 978
Dorset	173 293	188 626	—	—	103 140	115 023	70 153	73 603
Durham	689 947	719 690	288 582	306 657	257 662	266 303	143 703	146 730
Essex	661 065	696 963	75 205	87 565	424 103	442 304	161 757	167 094
Gloucestershire	524 373	552 335	250 329	266 560	87 808	95 101	186 236	190 674
Hampshire	758 032	807 451	270 123	296 295	298 945	317 026	188 964	194 130
Herefordshire	68 160	70 479	—	—	29 746	32 156	38 414	38 323
Hertfordshire	453 870	470 762	—	—	319 002	333 551	134 868	137 211
Huntingdonshire†	101 602	101 021	—	—	63 393	64 922	38 209	36 099
Kent	673 458	726 005	15 811	17 365	438 051	479 143	219 596	229 497
Lancashire	2 472 610	2 645 813	1 257 477	1 351 661	996 846	1 067 495	218 287	226 657
Leicestershire	380 500	391 602	138 497	145 711	112 153	114 048	129 850	131 843
Lincoln. (Holland)	52 078	53 612	—	—	20 756	22 220	31 322	31 392
Lincoln. (Kesteven)	114 660	117 889	35 866	38 403	27 647	29 398	51 147	50 088
Lincoln. (Lindsey)	233 012	237 897	46 828	48 712	87 360	91 707	98 824	97 478
London (Greater)	3 578 238	3 874 108	3 578 238	3 874 108	—	—	—	—
Norfolk	300 595	317 021	82 222	90 097	46 131	50 542	172 242	176 382
Northamptonshire	230 254	238 369	61 194	65 448	98 622	101 301	70 438	71 620
Northumberland	384 124	411 628	139 798	151 749	187 529	200 876	56 797	59 003
Nottinghamshire	481 101	495 312	146 766	153 864	219 971	227 024	114 364	114 424
Oxfordshire	191 833	189 757	55 085	53 720	38 216	40 185	98 532	95 852
Rutland	14 153	13 316	—	—	3 061	3 353	11 092	9 963
Shropshire	167 043	170 059	—	—	60 398	62 572	106 645	107 487
Somerset	327 631	355 033	39 578	45 092	136 815	152 228	151 238	157 713
Staffordshire	921 276	937 079	554 721	566 758	218 853	222 003	147 702	148 318
Suffolk (East)	187 571	193 889	60 176	63 136	55 226	60 171	72 169	70 582
Suffolk (West)	81 864	82 870	—	—	31 105	33 201	50 759	49 669
Surrey	483 294	519 595	—	—	385 910	415 602	97 384	103 993
Sussex (East)	339 323	408 651	136 740	167 942	103 961	128 979	98 622	111 730
Sussex (West)	227 130	265 365	—	—	131 380	158 085	95 750	107 280
Warwickshire	1 030 690	1 051 539	721 850	735 153	173 704	179 465	135 136	136 921
Westmorland	34 798	38 038	—	—	17 314	20 111	17 484	17 927
Wight (Isle of)	51 377	58 135	—	—	40 906	46 338	10 471	11 797
Wiltshire	240 162	246 585	—	—	114 484	120 049	125 678	126 536
Worcestershire	340 645	352 608	116 420	120 599	155 738	162 259	68 487	69 750
Yorks. (East)	262 962	280 354	138 765	147 205	61 014	69 466	63 183	63 683
Yorks. (North)	357 475	368 183	195 321	200 909	69 890	76 926	92 264	90 348
Yorks. (West)	1 841 933	1 943 082	966 392	1 025 145	617 056	655 650	258 485	262 287
Anglesey	29 411	30 350	—	—	11 060	11 907	18 351	18 443
Breconshire	26 606	26 771	—	—	7 525	7 920	19 081	18 851
Caernarvonshire	57 274	65 790	—	—	34 925	41 512	22 349	24 278
Cardiganshire	26 528	28 354	—	—	8 847	9 918	17 681	18 436
Carmarthenshire	78 582	83 980	—	—	29 523	33 107	49 059	50 873
Denbighshire	88 471	96 721	—	—	44 150	51 080	44 321	45 641
Flintshire	84 704	91 065	—	—	43 830	48 171	40 874	42 894
Glamorgan	612 047	646 683	244 999	262 842	250 137	264 448	116 911	119 393
Merionethshire	16 764	18 566	—	—	7 237	8 584	9 527	9 982
Monmouthshire	228 009	234 162	54 859	57 427	138 228	141 457	34 922	35 278
Montgomeryshire	21 469	21 650	—	—	9 350	9 984	12 119	11 666
Pembrokeshire	48 569	50 399	—	—	24 352	26 205	24 217	24 194
Radnorshire	9 073	9 206	—	—	3 094	3 508	5 979	5 698
England and Wales	23 682 980	25 066 595	10 381 068	11 098 465	8 062 646	8 609 093	5 239 266	5 359 037

* Includes Isle of Ely
† Includes Soke of Peterborough

Table A2.2 Numbers of cancers incident 1968–85, by sex and county

County	Number of cancers	
	Male	Female
Bedfordshire	12 548	11 675
Berkshire	19 061	18 774
Buckinghamshire	18 121	17 105
Cambridgeshire*	11 637	10 967
Cheshire	49 976	49 917
Cornwall	16 694	16 288
Cumberland	9 152	8 575
Derbyshire	30 582	28 974
Devon	38 720	38 514
Dorset	13 523	13 823
Durham	48 052	43 077
Essex	36 237	34 310
Gloucestershire	36 833	35 791
Hampshire	52 228	51 115
Herefordshire	5 091	4 883
Hertfordshire	23 939	22 848
Huntingdonshire†	6 701	6 113
Kent	45 220	44 042
Lancashire	177 503	171 408
Leicestershire	22 196	22 833
Lincoln. (Holland)	4 119	3 690
Lincoln. (Kesteven)	7 987	7 694
Lincoln. (Lindsey)	15 370	13 910
London (Greater)	228 029	218 518
Norfolk	24 307	23 014
Northamptonshire	17 059	16 144
Northumberland	30 634	27 776
Nottinghamshire	33 261	31 189
Oxfordshire	12 921	12 348
Rutland	767	704
Shropshire	10 648	10 011
Somerset	27 016	26 781
Staffordshire	52 128	47 931
Suffolk (East)	15 013	14 261
Suffolk (West)	6 205	5 610
Surrey	31 353	32 131
Sussex (East)	30 238	32 348
Sussex (West)	19 901	20 434
Warwickshire	66 475	62 444
Westmorland	2 696	2 766
Wight (Isle of)	4 428	4 457
Wiltshire	15 717	14 991
Worcestershire	22 441	21 322
Yorks. (East)	19 295	17 416
Yorks. (North)	22 966	20 884
Yorks. (West)	126 286	121 310
Anglesey	2 487	2 399
Breconshire	1 698	1 620
Caernarvonshire	5 784	6 070
Cardiganshire	2 118	2 256
Carmarthenshire	5 957	6 439
Denbighshire	8 005	8 766
Flintshire	7 132	7 324
Glamorgan	43 469	42 191
Merionethshire	1 526	1 624
Monmouthshire	15 260	13 845
Montgomeryshire	1 657	1 600
Pembrokeshire	3 557	3 663
Radnorshire	808	751
England and Wales	1 620 732	1 559 664

* Includes Isle of Ely
† Includes Soke of Peterborough

Appendix 3

STATISTICAL METHODS

Method of weighting the odds ratios

In a case-control analysis using persons with disease as the controls, it is of concern that for any specific control diagnosis, the aetiological factors for the condition may make persons with it seriously unrepresentative of the catchment population, and hence bias may occur. It is therefore generally held to be desirable that the comparison group should be formed of persons with a wide variety of conditions, so that any bias introduced by specific diseases should be minimized (Cole 1980). If all cancers incident in 1968–85, except those of the site under study, were used as the controls, however, they would be dominated by a few sites (Table 1). Three tumours (lung, non-melanoma skin, and prostate cancers in males, and breast, non-melanoma skin, and colon cancers in females) represented almost 50 per cent of the total cancers in each sex, and at some ages the domination by a small number of sites was greater than this.

As an alternative to using all non-case cancers as the controls in the analysis, we have therefore taken as the controls a weighted sample of other cancers, such that no single site contributed more than a small proportion of the total controls. In each sex and five-year age-group, for all counties combined, the numbers of cancers in the commonest sites were iteratively reduced so that no single site contributed more than 7 per cent of the total number of cancers in that category. (The exact percentage was arbitrary, but we have tried other percentages within the range 5 to 10 per cent and these gave similar results.) For each cancer site, an age- and sex-specific weight was then obtained by dividing the number of cancers of the site in this amended (reduced) file by the corresponding number of cancers of the site in the original file. This set of site-and age-specific weights was then applied to the original site-specific data in each county, to create a weighted control file.

In this weighted control file, consisting of the contributions from each sex- and age-group, no tumour contributed more than 5·6 per cent[1] of the total for all ages in each sex (Table A3.1). The numbers of controls contributed by common sites had been reduced, but the numbers from less-common sites remained unchanged, while their relative contribution was increased because of the reduction in the total. The control group for the case-control analysis for each individual cancer site then consisted of all cancers in this weighted file except the ones from the site under study. The composition of the control group before and after weighting is illustrated in Table A3.1.

Calculation of cancer risks in relation to urbanization

Cancer site risks by degree of urbanization were calculated for England and Wales. Since information on degree of urbanization was not available in the OPCS files for 1982 onwards, the urbanization risks refer only to 1968–81. Risks in metropolitan and in urban areas of England and Wales overall were compared with those in

1 This percentage is less than the 7 per cent mentioned above, mainly because it is the outcome of an iterative computer calculation, and in part because it is produced by summation of results for different age-groups.

Table A3.1 Composition of the control group: numbers and percentages of cancers of the most common sites and of selected less common sites, before and after weighting

Site of cancer	ICD9	Males				Females			
		Unweighted controls		Weighted controls*		Unweighted controls		Weighted controls*	
		No.	(%)	No.	(%)	No.	(%)	No.	(%)
Stomach	151	126 226	(7·8)	32 952	(5·5)	86 291	(5·5)	38 698	(5·4)
Colon	153	103 279	(6·4)	33 442	(5·6)	136 888	(8·8)	40 158	(5·6)
Lung	162	471 433	(29·1)	33 398	(5·6)	133 581	(8·6)	39 649	(5·5)
Non-melanoma skin	173	178 968	(11·0)	33 597	(5·6)	157 661	(10·1)	40 330	(5·6)
Breast (female)	174	—		—		369 254	(23·7)	40 174	(5·6)
Prostate	185	133 840	(8·3)	29 062	(4·9)	—		—	
Lip	140	5 628	(0·3)	5 628	(0·9)	999	(0·1)	999	(0·1)
Thyroid	193	3 441	(0·2)	3 441	(0·6)	9 585	(0·6)	9 398†	(1·3)
Multiple myeloma	203	15 258	(0·9)	15 258	(2·5)	15 293	(1·0)	15 293	(2·1)
All primary malignant neoplasms	140–195; 199–208	1 620 732	(100·0)	594 843	(100·0)	1 559 664	(100·0)	719 211	(100·0)

* Subjects in weighted control file: for each cancer site, the controls consisted of all cancers in this file except the cancers of the site under study

† Weighted file contains fewer cancers than unweighted because at young ages thyroid cancer was sufficiently common for numbers to be reduced by the weighting procedure

rural areas overall by calculating age-adjusted odds ratios. The controls in each of these analyses were a weighted sample of all cancers except the site under study, such that in each five-year age-group and urbanization stratum no single site represented more than seven per cent of the total controls for that category (see above). For the analyses of geographical risks within urbanization strata, weighted odds ratios were calculated to compare the risk of the cancer under analysis in the urbanization stratum analysed (e.g. the rural part) of a county, with the risk in the same urbanization stratum of all other counties combined in England and Wales.

Histograms in the maps display the site-specific England and Wales cancer risks by degree of urbanization. The data underlying these are given in Table A5.45. The results of the analyses of geographical risks within urbanization strata are presented in the text for each cancer site.

Appendix 4

Geographical distribution of 'exposures'

Tables A4.1–A4.24.

Table A4.1 Legally induced abortion rates in women aged 10–49 years by county of residence, England and Wales, 1968–73

County	Abortion rate per 1 000	County	Abortion rate per 1 000
Bedfordshire	6·27	Shropshire	4·97
Berkshire	5·39	Somerset	4·26
Buckinghamshire	5·63	Staffordshire	4·61
Cambridgeshire	9·52	Suffolk (East)	3·98
Cheshire	3·95	Suffolk (West)	5·95
Cornwall	3·64	Surrey	5·56
Cumberland	2·83	Sussex (East)	5·82
Derbyshire	4·21	Sussex (West)	5·60
Devon	4·30	Warwickshire	7·27
Dorset	5·57	Westmorland	—
Durham	3·81	Wight (Isle of)	4·65
Essex	6·40	Wiltshire	4·07
Gloucestershire	6·30	Worcestershire	4·68
Hampshire	5·16	Yorks. (East)	4·42
Herefordshire	5·93	Yorks. (North)	4·89
Hertfordshire	5·47	Yorks. (West)	3·75
Huntingdonshire	5·66	Anglesey	—
Kent	5·48	Breconshire	—
Lancashire	4·11	Caernarvonshire	4·73
Leicestershire	4·87	Cardiganshire	—
Lincolnshire (Holland)	3·22	Carmarthenshire	5·88
Lincolnshire (Kesteven)	2·62	Denbighshire	3·78
Lincolnshire (Lindsey)	3·51	Flintshire	3·92
London (Greater)	11·13	Glamorgan	5·60
Norfolk	3·73	Merionethshire	—
Northamptonshire	4·57	Monmouthshire	5·63
Northumberland	5·53	Montgomeryshire	—
Nottinghamshire	4·35	Pembrokeshire	1·15
Oxfordshire	6·83	Radnorshire	—
Rutland	—		

Calculated from abortions notification data (OPCS 1970–74)
— no data in published tables

Table A4.2 Air pollution by region of England and Wales, 1968–9

Standard region	Smoke (micrograms/ metre^3)	Sulphur dioxide (micrograms/ metre^3)
North	108	97
Yorkshire and Humberside	97	140
North-west	109	147
East Midlands	77	102
West Midlands	63	119
East Anglia	51	87
South-east		
Greater London	46	151
Rest of South-east	39	78
South-west	33	68
Wales	39	62

Data from National Survey of Air Pollution (Central Statistical Office 1972)

Table A4.3 Percentages of population in various alcohol consumption categories, by sex and region. Persons aged 18 and over, England and Wales, 1978.

Standard region	General Household Survey					Survey by Wilson			
	%* of moderate† drinkers		%* of heavy‡ drinkers			% of heavy¶ drinkers		% who have drunk >8 units (♂) or >6 units (♀) any day last week	
	Males	Females	Males	Females		Males	Females	Males	Females
North	18	5	43	1		18	2	45	15
Yorkshire and Humberside	15	5	28	2		11	3	27	14
North-west	16	6	33	2		20	2	31	19
East Midlands	18	3	20	1		12	0	19	2
West Midlands	15	3	30	2		12	7	25	13
East Anglia	14	2	16	1		10	0	23	13
South-east	13	3	17	1	Inner London	19	2	22	9
					Outer London	15	2	31	17
					Other SE	12	6	23	11
South-west	14	2	14	1		16	1	29	2
Wales	17	4	33	3		18	4	34	20

Data from General Household Survey (OPCS 1980) and Wilson (1980)
* Age-standardized
† Defined as five to six alcohol units at least once a week or more than six units once or twice a month (1 unit = 9 grams of alcohol)
‡ Defined as more than six units once a week
¶ Defined as >50 units last week for men, or >35 units last week for women, or was drunk at least three times in the previous three months, or is a problem drinker, based on various physical dependence and psychological criteria

Table A4.4 Liquor-licensed premises ('on'-plus 'off'-licenses) by county of England and Wales, 1968

County	No. of liquor licensed premises per 1 000 persons	County	No. of liquor licensed premises per 1 000 persons
Bedfordshire	2·07	Shropshire	3·25
Berkshire	2·19	Somerset	2·95
Buckinghamshire	1·91	Staffordshire	2·18
Cambridgeshire	2·84	Suffolk (East)	2·51
Cheshire	1·78	Suffolk (West)	3·08
Cornwall	4·12	Surrey	1·56
Cumberland	2·84	Sussex (East)	2·64
Derbyshire	2·62	Sussex (West)	2·20
Devon	3·18	Warwickshire	1·55
Dorset	2·97	Westmorland	3·95
Durham	1·78	Wight (Isle of)	6·25
Essex	1·67	Wiltshire	2·05
Gloucestershire	2·30	Worcestershire	2·43
Hampshire	2·13	Yorks. (East)	2·05
Herefordshire	3·63	Yorks. (North)	2·31
Hertfordshire	1·58	Yorks. (West)	2·11
Huntingdonshire	2·42	Anglesey	2·70
Kent	2·61	Breconshire	4·75
Lancashire	2·13	Caernarvonshire	3·75
Leicestershire	2·35	Cardiganshire	3·76
Lincolnshire (Holland)	3·21	Carmarthenshire	3·45
Lincolnshire (Kesteven)	2·46	Denbighshire	2·51
Lincolnshire (Lindsey)	2·17	Flintshire	2·64
London (Greater)	1·53	Glamorgan	1·72
Norfolk	3·31	Merionethshire	3·44
Northamptonshire	2·48	Monmouthshire	2·02
Northumberland	1·85	Montgomeryshire	4·16
Nottinghamshire	2·06	Pembrokeshire	4·68
Oxfordshire	2·90	Radnorshire	4·94
Rutland	3·34		

Calculated from Liquor Licensing Statistics (Home Office 1969)

Table A4.5 Household food consumption by region of England and Wales, 1970–75 (oz. per person per week)

Standard region	Meat products	Fish	Fats	Sugar	Fresh green vegetables	Fresh fruit
North	39·12	5·81	11·89	16·64	9·97	14·97
Yorkshire and Humberside	37·73	6·16	12·34	17·93	12·61	16·20
North-west	38·31	4·65	11·76	17·42	9·39	16·58
East Midlands	34·79	4·62	11·96	18·08	14·99	17·58
West Midlands	38·59	4·46	11·68	18·30	14·18	17·58
East Anglia and South-east	37·94	4·73	10·93	15·93	15·40	21·73
South-west	36·76	4·13	11·39	16·32	15·60	18·87
Wales	39·53	4·48	12·85	17·85	13·47	17·67

Data from National Food Survey (MAFF 1977)

Table A4.6 Regional means (standard deviations) of daily nutrient intakes, England and Wales, 1982

Nutrient	Sex	North, Yorks., and Humberside	Midlands and East Anglia	South-east and London	South-west	Wales
Energy (MJ)	Male	10·4	10·2	9·6	10·4	10·1
		(2·6)	(2·4)	(2·2)	(2·6)	(2·7)
	Female	7·0	6·8	7·1	7·0	6·4
		(1·9)	(1·9)	(1·9)	(1·7)	(2·1)
Protein (g)	Male	84·5	83·8	80·0	81·8	83·3
		(19·6)	(19·9)	(16·6)	(18·3)	(18·8)
	Female	62·6	61·5	63·3	61·6	56·7
		(14·6)	(13·9)	(14·7)	(12·2)	(14·4)
Fat (g)	Male	105·6	102·5	100·0	108·4	103·0
		(30·9)	(26·4)	(25·2)	(30·9)	(29·3)
	Female	75·3	72·5	76·9	75·8	67·8
		(23·2)	(23·4)	(23·6)	(20·1)	(25·1)
Carbohydrate (g)	Male	269	272	246	275	261
		(32·5)	(75·9)	(66·2)	(78·5)	(76·4)
	Female	185	182	187	184	173
		(61·6)	(59·5)	(60·1)	(58·9)	(67·4)
Total fibre (g)	Male	19·0	19·5	18·5	20·8	18·6
		(6·8)	(7·0)	(6·3)	(7·2)	(5·5)
	Female	14·0	14·9	15·9	15·6	13·8
		(5·0)	(5·2)	(6·2)	(6·0)	(5·6)
Total sugars (g)	Male	97·2	99·8	92·6	102·2	93·7
		(44·6)	(41·1)	(36·3)	(41·1)	(39·2)
	Female	66·2	66·4	69·4	65·1	58·6
		(32·2)	(30·2)	(31·0)	(28·8)	(31·7)
Iron (mg)	Male	12·9	12·6	12·8	13·1	12·3
		(4·0)	(3·8)	(3·6)	(3·5)	(3·0)
	Female	9·9	9·8	10·5	10·1	9·2
		(4·8)	(3·2)	(3·9)	(3·2)	(3·5)
Calcium (mg)	Male	941	981	892	965	848
		(314·7)	(328·6)	(259·3)	(297·8)	(262·3)
	Female	722	738	781	731	599
		(230·4)	(272·6)	(253·1)	(228·8)	(255·7)
Vitamin C (mg)	Male	57·0	61·3	63·1	63·4	59·1
		(31·1)	(32·5)	(40·4)	(27·4)	(29·8)
	Female	47·6	56·8	66·8	58·4	50·6
		(24·7)	(31·0)	(87·6)	(31·6)	(27·8)

Adapted from Braddon *et al.* (1988)

Table A4.7 Height and Body Mass Index of adults aged 16–64 years by region of England and Wales, 1980

Standard region	Height (cm)		Body Mass Index*	
	Males	Females	Males	Females
North	173·3	160·0	24·5	24·0
Yorks. and Humberside	174·1	160·9	24·5	24·0
North-west	173·1	160·2	24·4	23·9
East Midlands	174·4	161·0	24·6	24·3
West Midlands	173·5	160·6	24·3	24·1
East Anglia	174·8	160·9	24·7	24·3
South-east				
Greater London	173·7	161·0	24·3	23·9
Rest of South-east	174·7	161·9	24·0	23·7
South-west	175·1	161·9	24·3	24·4
Wales	171·9	159·4	24·7	24·1

Data from a survey by Knight (1984)
* Weight/Height^2

Table A4.8 Acute hepatitis B: rates of new laboratory reports by hospital region of reporting, England and Wales, 1980–84

Hospital region	Mean annual rate per 100 000 population
Northern	0·61
Yorkshire	3·04
Trent	1·97
East Anglia	3·36
North-west Thames	5·55
North-east Thames	2·03
South-east Thames	2·72
South-west Thames	2·89
Wessex	2·76
Oxford	2·64
South-western	3·53
West Midlands	2·58
Mersey	2·81
North-western	2·69
Wales	1·40
England and Wales	2·68

Based on laboratory reports sent to the Communicable Disease Surveillance Centre

Table A4.9 Percentage of males born outside United Kingdom and Republic of Ireland by country of birth, in each county of England and Wales, 1971

County of residence	Country of birth						
	Indian Subcontinent*	China and other east Asian countries*	Africa (Commonwealth and Rep. South Africa)*	West Indies (Commonwealth)*	Europe (outside British Isles)*	Other (outside British Isles)*	Total†
Bedfordshire	2·0	0·2	0·4	1·1	2·6	1·6	8·0
Berkshire	1·0	0·4	0·4	0·5	1·7	1·2	5·2
Buckinghamshire	2·4	0·3	0·5	0·8	2·2	1·3	7·4
Cambridgeshire	0·5	0·3	0·4	0·1	1·6	1·6	4·6
Cheshire	0·3	0·1	0·1	0·1	0·7	0·6	1·9
Cornwall	0·2	0·2	0·3	0·1	0·7	0·8	2·4
Cumberland	0·1	0·1	0·1	0·0	0·6	0·4	1·4
Derbyshire	0·8	0·1	0·1	0·3	0·9	0·4	2·6
Devon	0·3	0·3	0·3	0·1	0·9	0·7	2·6
Dorset	0·4	0·3	0·3	0·1	1·1	0·7	2·9
Durham	0·2	0·1	0·1	0·0	0·4	0·2	1·0
Essex	0·5	0·2	0·3	0·1	1·0	0·7	2·8
Gloucestershire	0·5	0·2	0·3	0·6	1·1	0·7	3·4
Hampshire	0·6	0·4	0·4	0·2	1·4	0·9	3·9
Herefordshire	0·2	0·1	0·2	0·0	0·9	0·5	1·9
Hertfordshire	0·9	0·2	0·3	0·3	1·7	0·9	4·5
Huntingdonshire	1·2	0·3	0·2	0·3	2·6	3·6	8·3
Kent	0·9	0·3	0·4	0·1	1·0	0·7	3·3
Lancashire	1·1	0·1	0·3	0·3	0·7	0·6	3·1
Leicestershire	2·1	0·2	1·2	0·4	1·2	0·7	5·8
Lincoln. (Holland)	0·1	0·1	0·1	0·0	0·6	0·4	1·3
Lincoln. (Kesteven)	0·3	0·3	0·2	0·1	1·2	0·7	2·8
Lincoln. (Lindsey)	0·3	0·2	0·1	0·1	0·9	0·5	2·1
London (Greater)	2·3	0·4	1·4	2·3	2·5	2·4	11·4
Norfolk	0·2	0·2	0·2	0·1	0·7	1·0	2·3
Northamptonshire	0·5	0·1	0·2	0·5	1·3	1·2	3·9
Northumberland	0·4	0·2	0·2	0·0	0·5	0·4	1·6
Nottinghamshire	0·7	0·1	0·2	0·7	1·2	0·6	3·4

Oxfordshire	0·9	0·4	0·5	0·5	1·7	3·7	7·6
Rutland	0·3	0·5	0·3	0·2	1·3	1·0	3·6
Shropshire	0·5	0·2	0·1	0·1	0·9	0·5	2·4
Somerset	0·3	0·2	0·3	0·1	0·9	0·7	2·5
Staffordshire	1·8	0·1	0·2	0·7	0·8	0·4	4·0
Suffolk (East)	0·3	0·2	0·2	0·5	0·9	2·9	5·0
Suffolk (West)	0·3	0·2	0·2	0·1	1·0	5·6	7·3
Surrey	0·8	0·4	0·5	0·2	1·9	1·4	5·2
Sussex (East)	0·6	0·3	0·5	0·1	1·3	1·2	4·1
Sussex (West)	0·7	0·3	0·4	0·1	1·3	1·1	3·9
Warwickshire	3·2	0·2	0·5	1·5	0·9	0·7	6·9
Westmorland	0·2	0·1	0·2	0·0	0·7	0·4	1·6
Wight (Isle of)	0·4	0·2	0·3	0·2	0·9	0·7	2·5
Wiltshire	0·7	0·4	0·3	0·3	2·0	0·8	4·4
Worcestershire	1·7	0·1	0·2	0·5	1·0	0·5	3·9
Yorks. (East)	0·2	0·1	0·1	0·0	0·6	0·3	1·4
Yorks. (North)	0·6	0·2	0·2	0·1	0·8	0·4	2·2
Yorks. (West)	1·6	0·1	0·2	0·4	0·9	0·6	3·9
Anglesey	0·1	0·2	0·2	0·0	0·7	0·7	1·9
Breconshire	0·2	0·1	0·2	0·1	0·6	0·2	1·4
Caernarvonshire	0·2	0·1	0·1	0·0	0·8	0·4	1·7
Cardiganshire	0·2	0·2	0·3	0·0	0·8	0·5	2·0
Carmarthenshire	0·1	0·0	0·1	0·0	0·6	0·3	1·1
Denbighshire	0·2	0·1	0·1	0·0	0·6	0·3	1·3
Flintshire	0·1	0·1	0·1	0·0	0·9	0·3	1·6
Glamorgan	0·3	0·1	0·2	0·1	0·9	0·4	2·0
Merionethshire	0·1	0·1	0·1	0·1	0·6	0·3	1·3
Monmouthshire	0·3	0·1	0·1	0·1	0·7	0·3	1·6
Montgomeryshire	0·0	0·0	0·1	0·0	0·4	0·3	0·9
Pembrokeshire	0·1	0·1	0·1	0·1	1·1	0·4	1·9
Radnorshire	0·1	0·1	0·1	0·0	0·6	0·2	1·0
England and Wales	1·2	0·2	0·4	0·6	1·3	1·0	4·7

Calculated from 1971 Census data (OPCS, unpublished)

* Indian subcontinent: Pakistan, India, and Ceylon. China and other east Asian countries: Hong Kong, Malaysia, Singapore, Burma, China, and others. Africa Commonwealth: Ghana, Kenya, Malawi, Nigeria, Rhodesia, Sierra Leone, Tanzania, Uganda, Zambia, and others. West Indies Commonwealth: Barbados, Guyana, Jamaica, Trinidad and Tobago, and others. Europe (outside British Isles): all continental European countries (except USSR), Malta and Gozo. Other: all other countries except British Isles, visitors to the United Kingdom, and birthplace not stated.

† Totals are not exactly equal to the sum of values in the other columns because of rounding

Table A4.10 Percentage of females born outside United Kingdom and Republic of Ireland by country of birth, in each county of England and Wales, 1971

County of residence	Country of birth						
	Indian Subcontinent*	China and other east Asian countries*	Africa (Commonwealth and Rep. South Africa)*	West Indies (Commonwealth)*	Europe (outside British Isles)*	Other (outside British Isles)*	Total†
Bedfordshire	1·2	0·2	0·4	1·1	2·5	1·1	6·4
Berkshire	0·7	0·3	0·4	0·5	2·0	1·2	5·2
Buckinghamshire	1·3	0·2	0·4	0·7	2·3	1·1	6·1
Cambridgeshire	0·4	0·3	0·3	0·1	1·8	1·5	4·4
Cheshire	0·2	0·1	0·1	0·1	0·8	0·5	1·8
Cornwall	0·3	0·2	0·3	0·1	0·7	0·8	2·3
Cumberland	0·1	0·1	0·1	0·0	0·5	0·3	1·1
Derbyshire	0·5	0·1	0·1	0·3	0·7	0·3	2·0
Devon	0·4	0·3	0·3	0·1	1·0	0·7	2·7
Dorset	0·4	0·3	0·3	0·1	1·3	0·9	3·2
Durham	0·1	0·1	0·1	0·0	0·4	0·2	0·8
Essex	0·4	0·2	0·2	0·1	1·3	0·6	2·9
Gloucestershire	0·4	0·2	0·3	0·6	1·1	0·7	3·2
Hampshire	0·6	0·4	0·4	0·2	1·8	0·8	4·2
Herefordshire	0·2	0·1	0·2	0·1	0·8	0·5	1·9
Hertfordshire	0·6	0·3	0·3	0·4	2·0	0·9	4·5
Huntingdonshire	0·6	0·3	0·2	0·3	2·5	2·1	6·0
Kent	0·7	0·3	0·3	0·1	1·3	0·8	3·6
Lancashire	0·5	0·1	0·2	0·2	0·7	0·4	2·2
Leicestershire	1·6	0·1	1·0	0·4	1·2	0·5	4·9
Lincoln. (Holland)	0·1	0·1	0·1	0·0	0·7	0·3	1·3
Lincoln. (Kesteven)	0·2	0·3	0·1	0·1	1·1	0·6	2·4
Lincoln. (Lindsey)	0·2	0·1	0·1	0·0	0·8	0·4	1·6
London (Greater)	1·6	0·4	1·1	2·2	3·2	2·3	10·8
Norfolk	0·2	0·2	0·2	0·1	0·9	0·8	2·3
Northamptonshire	0·4	0·1	0·2	0·5	1·3	0·8	3·3
Northumberland	0·2	0·1	0·1	0·0	0·5	0·3	1·4
Nottinghamshire	0·4	0·1	0·1	0·6	1·1	0·4	2·8

Oxfordshire	0·6	0·4	0·5	0·5	2·0	2·7	6·6
Rutland	0·2	0·6	0·3	0·2	1·7	0·9	3·9
Shropshire	0·3	0·2	0·2	0·2	0·9	0·4	2·0
Somerset	0·3	0·2	0·3	0·1	1·0	0·7	2·6
Staffordshire	1·2	0·1	0·2	0·6	0·7	0·2	2·9
Suffolk (East)	0·3	0·2	0·2	0·4	1·1	1·8	3·9
Suffolk (West)	0·3	0·3	0·2	0·1	1·2	3·9	6·1
Surrey	0·7	0·4	0·5	0·2	2·4	1·6	5·8
Sussex (East)	0·6	0·3	0·4	0·2	1·7	1·1	4·3
Sussex (West)	0·7	0·3	0·4	0·1	1·6	0·9	4·0
Warwickshire	1·8	0·1	0·4	1·4	0·9	0·5	5·1
Westmorland	0·2	0·1	0·2	0·1	0·5	0·5	1·6
Wight (Isle of)	0·4	0·2	0·3	0·1	1·1	0·6	2·6
Wiltshire	0·6	0·4	0·3	0·2	2·3	0·6	4·5
Worcestershire	0·9	0·1	0·1	0·4	0·9	0·3	2·8
Yorks. (East)	0·1	0·1	0·1	0·0	0·7	0·3	1·4
Yorks. (North)	0·3	0·2	0·1	0·0	0·8	0·3	1·8
Yorks. (West)	0·8	0·1	0·2	0·4	0·8	0·4	2·6
Anglesey	0·1	0·2	0·1	0·0	0·6	0·5	1·5
Breconshire	0·1	0·1	0·1	0·0	0·5	0·2	1·1
Caernarvonshire	0·1	0·1	0·1	0·0	0·6	0·5	1·4
Cardiganshire	0·2	0·1	0·2	0·0	0·8	0·5	1·8
Carmarthenshire	0·1	0·0	0·1	0·0	0·6	0·1	0·9
Denbighshire	0·1	0·1	0·1	0·0	0·6	0·2	1·2
Flintshire	0·1	0·1	0·1	0·0	0·8	0·3	1·4
Glamorgan	0·2	0·1	0·1	0·1	0·7	0·3	1·5
Merionethshire	0·1	0·1	0·1	0·0	0·5	0·4	1·2
Monmouthshire	0·2	0·1	0·1	0·1	0·6	0·3	1·3
Montgomeryshire	0·1	0·0	0·0	0·0	0·5	0·3	0·9
Pembrokeshire	0·2	0·1	0·1	0·1	1·0	0·3	1·8
Radnorshire	0·1	0·0	0·1	0·0	0·5	0·5	1·1
England and Wales	0·8	0·2	0·4	0·6	1·5	0·8	4·2

Calculated from 1971 Census data (OPCS, unpublished)

* Indian subcontinent: Pakistan, India, and Ceylon. China and other east Asian countries: Hong Kong, Malaysia, Singapore, Burma, China, and others. Africa Commonwealth: Ghana, Kenya, Malawi, Nigeria, Rhodesia, Sierra Leone, Tanzania, Uganda, Zambia, and others. West Indies Commonwealth: Barbados, Guyana, Jamaica, Trinidad and Tobago, and others. Europe (outside British Isles): all continental European countries (except USSR), Malta and Gozo. Other: all other countries except British Isles, visitors to the United Kingdom, and birthplace not stated.

† Totals are not exactly equal to the sum of values in the other columns because of rounding

Table A4.11 Socio-economic and educational status of the population by county, England and Wales (social class 1971, income 1970–71, and education beyond age 16, 1968)

County	% Men in social classes I, II, IIIN*	Total net income[†] (£/case[‡])	Pupils aged 16 as a % of those aged 13 three years earlier
Bedfordshire	34·9	1 642	27·6
Berkshire	43·5	1 648	36·4
Buckinghamshire	42·0	1 774	34·0
Cambridgeshire	39·3	1 601	29·8
Cheshire	40·4	1 642	33·8
Cornwall	37·5	1 350	23·2
Cumberland	30·7	1 502	28·1
Derbyshire	29·4	1 487	25·5
Devon	38·6	1 416	29·9
Dorset	39·1	1 517	30·5
Durham	25·2	1 425	21·3
Essex	42·1	1 678	30·9
Gloucestershire	36·7	1 568	35·7
Hampshire	38·3	1 587[§]	31·9
Herefordshire	36·9	1 584	25·4
Hertfordshire	45·8	1 829	38·0
Huntingdonshire	35·0	1 484	29·6
Kent	38·9	1 555	31·9
Lancashire	29·5	1 423	26·3
Leicestershire	33·3	1 529[¶]	27·3
Lincolnshire (Holland)	32·4		21·7
Lincolnshire (Kesteven)	32·7	1 419	31·6
Lincolnshire (Lindsey)	28·8		25·7
London (Greater)	42·2	1 658	39·2
Norfolk	32·8	1 395	22·1
Northamptonshire	30·0	1 555	23·7
Northumberland	31·2	1 452	25·6
Nottinghamshire	29·8	1 447	22·9
Oxfordshire	38·2	1 722	32·1
Rutland	40·5	1 529[¶]	33·1
Shropshire	33·5	1 485	27·9
Somerset	40·8	1 526	27·9
Staffordshire	27·7	1 502	22·8
Suffolk (East)	32·7	1 545	21·0
Suffolk (West)	32·2		28·5
Surrey	54·0	1 488	42·5
Sussex (East)	45·4	1 566	35·4
Sussex (West)	44·9		41·6
Warwickshire	30·8	1 579	29·1
Westmorland	40·3	1 464	34·0
Wight (Isle of)	38·6	1 587[§]	32·8
Wiltshire	34·0	1 504	30·4
Worcestershire	32·5	1 528	27·2
Yorks. (East)	32·5	1 491	27·6
Yorks. (North)	31·2	1 393	22·6
Yorks. (West)	29·0	1 508	26·6
Anglesey	34·0	1 439	39·7
Breconshire	34·1	1 335	39·6
Caernarvonshire	37·1	1 414	37·7
Cardiganshire	50·9	1 433	48·0
Carmarthenshire	32·7	1 469	40·3
Denbighshire	31·8	1 468	31·3
Flintshire	30·4	1 444	31·8
Glamorgan	29·3	1 420	30·3
Merionethshire	38·7	1 321	50·9
Monmouthshire	25·8	1 463	30·0
Montgomeryshire	44·0	1 305	33·8
Pembrokeshire	36·9	1 406	45·1
Radnorshire	49·3	1 277	34·1

Table A4.11 (*notes cont.*)

Calculated from data on social class at the 1971 Census (OPCS 1975), on income in taxation statistics (Board of Inland Revenue 1973), and on school attendance in education statistics (Department of Education and Science 1969)
* Social Classes I, II, IIIN correspond approximately with non-manual occupations
† Defined as the taxable income (before tax) from all sources after allowable deductions but before reliefs and allowances for tax
‡ 'Cases' are tax-paying units (counting husband and wife as one unit) having incomes in a particular county
¶ Data were combined for Leicestershire and Rutland
§ Data were combined for Hampshire and the Isle of Wight

Table A4.12 Hospital discharge rates per 100 000 population for selected conditions by county of residence, England and Wales, 1959–60

County of residence	Diagnostic group (ICD7) and sex								
	Diseases of thyroid gland* (250–4)		Peptic ulcer* (540–2)		Diseases of gallbladder† (584–6)		Hyperplasia of prostate† (610)	Diseases of breast† (620–1)	Cervicitis* (630·0)
	Males	Females	Males	Females	Males	Females	Males	Females	Females
Bedfordshire	1·1	8·6	15·0	6·4	4·0	11·4	10·3	2·9	12·2
Berkshire	2·3	11·7	14·9	3·6	3·8	10·9	13·2	5·6	13·4
Buckinghamshire	3·3	11·5	18·9	6·7	3·1	14·6	15·2	1·7	14·2
Cambridgeshire	1·8	4·3	19·0	5·4	5·9	10·8	9·5	2·2	8·3
Cheshire	2·3	9·3	20·9	8·2	3·6	14·1	11·3	4·5	18·3
Cornwall	2·8	7·9	14·3	2·5	6·2	19·8	23·4	7·3	6·5
Cumberland	0·4	8·2	28·2	10·5	2·1	9·6	8·4	2·7	14·6
Derbyshire	0·7	5·1	19·7	6·6	4·0	13·2	8·0	3·2	5·4
Devon	1·2	10·3	20·1	7·4	7·7	15·2	20·9	3·5	8·2
Dorset	1·3	6·2	14·7	5·3	5·3	7·0	11·4	3·2	8·4
Durham	1·4	7·7	26·9	10·9	4·4	12·7	10·8	3·5	18·1
Essex	1·9	8·4	21·1	7·7	6·2	12·7	13·0	5·1	11·9
Gloucestershire	1·0	10·3	18·9	7·5	4·2	10·7	13·4	5·9	9·9
Hampshire	1·1	5·8	15·6	5·8	5·0	9·0	9·8	5·1	13·9
Herefordshire	—	9·1	19·5	4·6	3·1	12·3	4·7	—	29·7
Hertfordshire	1·5	11·8	15·7	7·1	3·5	8·1	9·1	4·1	14·0
Huntingdonshire	1·3	4·0	16·2	2·7	3·9	14·6	15·5	2·7	7·3
Kent	1·4	8·6	21·6	7·3	3·9	11·5	12·7	4·4	11·7
Lancashire	1·6	8·3	23·2	7·3	4·9	11·4	11·7	5·6	11·6
Leicestershire	1·2	3·9	18·1	4·2	2·5	12·8	10·9	3·2	5·1
Lincoln. (Holland)	2·0	2·9	18·5	4·8	3·9	23·2	9·8	1·9	15·3
Lincoln. (Kesteven)	1·5	7·4	17·7	3·0	4·3	7·8	11·6	4·7	4·4
Lincoln. (Lindsey)	1·0	5·6	13·6	3·4	2·4	11·3	8·5	4·4	12·6
London and Middx.	2·5	11·0	26·5	10·9	4·3	11·5	12·9	6·7	12·3
Norfolk	1·5	5·4	18·2	5·1	3·9	9·3	10·0	1·8	3·3
Northamptonshire	0·8	11·2	22·1	6·2	3·2	7·0	14·8	7·0	6·9
Northumberland	1·6	9·8	30·3	11·5	6·6	15·7	13·2	3·6	15·9
Nottinghamshire	1·0	4·6	18·2	4·8	3·7	10·8	8·0	3·1	14·0
Oxfordshire	1·6	14·5	20·3	7·5	1·3	7·9	14·4	4·0	14·7
Rutland	—	12·6	15·3	—	—	—	—	—	4·2
Shropshire	1·0	8·6	14·8	4·3	1·3	12·4	12·9	8·3	13·6
Somerset	1·3	7·9	18·8	8·7	3·6	16·3	13·5	3·6	19·7
Staffordshire	1·3	7·1	15·2	5·4	5·1	10·6	6·9	4·9	3·9
Suffolk (East)	3·3	10·5	17·0	5·9	5·4	10·8	14·5	3·4	9·0
Suffolk (West)	0·8	3·8	21·9	10·7	1·5	8·1	13·7	6·5	3·8
Surrey	0·8	8·6	17·6	9·1	3·7	9·9	13·7	5·1	10·3
Sussex (East)	1·1	5·8	19·9	7·3	3·5	7·3	13·5	6·1	4·8
Sussex (West)	1·7	7·8	20·6	5·7	8·0	8·8	20·0	6·1	4·4
Warwickshire	1·3	7·3	20·8	6·5	5·3	8·5	7·4	5·9	7·1
Westmorland	1·6	2·9	17·5	2·9	6·4	11·4	12·7	5·7	10·0
Wight (Isle of)	1·2	4·0	17·3	2·0	2·3	8·0	11·4	8·0	16·1

Table A4.12 *(cont.)*

County of residence	Diagnostic group (ICD7) and sex									
	Diseases of thyroid gland* (250–4)		Peptic ulcer* (540–2)		Diseases of gallbladder† (584–6)		Hyperplasia of prostate† (610)	Diseases of breast† (620–1)	Cervicitis* (630·0)
	Males	Females	Males	Females	Males	Females	Males	Females	Females
Wiltshire	1·4	9·6	29·6	4·6	3·7	12.3	9·2	5·6	9·8
Worcestershire	1·5	10·5	20·2	9·7	2·6	12·9	8·8	4·2	8·5
Yorks. (East)	0·6	4·8	20·5	6·8	4·4	11·5	11·5	6·3	13·2
Yorks. (North)	0·9	6·3	20·1	9·1	4·0	12·6	11·3	7·4	19·0
Yorks. (West)	1·2	6·2	23·7	5·9	4·9	12·2	9·4	3·5	10·6
Anglesey	—	5·7	39·2	7·4	—	3·7	11·8	3·7	18·8
Breconshire	3·6	14·6	17·8	9·1	3·5	7·3	7·1	3·6	11·0
Caernarvonshire	4·5	7·7	34·7	7·7	8·9	6·1	19·6	4·6	6·9
Cardiganshire	1·9	9·1	29·0	3·6	—	17·8	24·0	10·7	—
Carmarthenshire	1·8	16·4	20·5	5·9	1·2	18·7	18·1	5·8	9·9
Denbighshire	1·2	7·9	16·6	6·2	9·8	19·2	20·8	7·9	10·8
Flintshire	1·4	4·7	24·5	9·4	4·2	16·0	11·1	5·3	6·0
Glamorgan	1·5	13·0	24·8	7·7	6·0	15·2	12·3	4·7	19·5
Merionethshire	2·5	15·9	22·3	10·6	5·1	21·1	10·2	—	10·6
Monmouthshire	1·8	6·7	23·4	5·5	5·1	12·4	11·6	2·3	14·7
Montgomeryshire	—	4·5	20·1	11·2	4·5	8·9	8·9	26·8	13·4
Pembrokeshire	—	8·4	17·0	3·1	2·1	23·1	19·1	10·5	3·2
Radnorshire	1·0	21·4	20·4	1·6	10·3	21·2	20·6	52·6	10·7
England and Wales	1·6	8·4	21·3	7·5	4·7	12·1	12·1	5·1	11·1

Recalculated from Hospital In-Patient Enquiry (Ministry of Health and General Register Office 1963*a*, *b*)
* Average rate for the years 1959–60
† Rate for 1959 only. Data not available for 1960.

Table A4.13 Hospital discharge rates per 100 000 population for selected conditions by region of residence, England and Wales, 1970

Hospital region of residence	Diagnostic group (ICD8)				
	Goitre, thyrotoxicosis (240–2)	Cholelithiasis, cholecystitis (574, 575)	Nephritis, nephrosis (580–4)	Urinary calculus (592, 594)	Undescended testis (752·1)
Newcastle	2·1	10·5	2·5	2·4	1·5
Leeds	2·2	11·2	2·1	2·6	2·3
Sheffield	1·8	8·4	1·5	1·5	1·9
East Anglia	3·6	9·4	1·4	2·4	3·1
NW Metropolitan	3·4	7·7	2·4	2·9	2·8
NE Metropolitan	3·3	10·5	1·9	3·0	2·9
SE Metropolitan	2·6	8·4	2·0	2·2	2·4
SW Metropolitan	3·7	9·2	1·7	2·8	2·8
Wessex	2·8	9·5	1·8	2·8	3·6
Oxford	3·3	7·0	1·8	2·7	2·1
South-western	2·6	9·5	2·1	2·8	3·0
Wales	4·6	12·5	1·9	3·0	1·6
Birmingham	2·3	9·0	1·0	2·1	2·0
Manchester	2·0	12·3	1·4	2·4	2·0
Liverpool	2·3	10·2	2·0	2·5	2·7
England and Wales	2·7	9·7	1·8	2·5	2·4

Data from Hospital In-Patient Enquiry (DHSS and OPCS 1972)

Table A4.14 Percentage of male work-force in selected occupations, England and Wales, 1961

County of residence	Occupation*											
	I	I	V	VIII	VIII	IX	IX	X	X	X	X	XIV
	000	001–005	040–045	080–085	081	090–093	091	100–108	100	101	102	140
	Fishermen	Farmers	Furnace, foundry	Wood-workers	Cabinet-makers	Leather-workers	Shoe-makers	Textile-workers	Fibre prep.	Spinners	Warpers	Rubber-workers
Bedfordshire	0·00	5·80	0·84	2·38	0·05	0·38	0·13	0·19	0·00	0·00	0·00	0·22
Berkshire	0·01	5·59	0·35	2·20	0·13	0·22	0·15	0·04	0·01	0·00	0·00	0·03
Buckinghamshire	0·01	5·22	0·77	4·05	0·88	0·20	0·07	0·10	0·01	0·00	0·00	0·31
Cambridgeshire	0·00	11·17	0·17	2·46	0·10	0·29	0·10	0·00	0·00	0·00	0·00	0·09
Cheshire	0·01	3·85	0·75	2·15	0·06	0·30	0·11	0·91	0·08	0·19	0·03	0·13
Cornwall	0·49	14·56	0·39	2·55	0·07	0·22	0·17	0·06	0·00	0·02	0·00	0·00
Cumberland	0·07	9·73	1·50	2·17	0·03	0·88	0·15	0·69	0·08	0·09	0·03	0·13
Derbyshire	0·01	3·48	2·54	2·00	0·09	0·25	0·11	1·66	0·07	0·11	0·09	0·13
Devon	0·11	10·28	0·35	2·33	0·09	0·33	0·14	0·36	0·07	0·01	0·01	0·02
Dorset	0·06	10·33	0·23	2·73	0·05	0·16	0·13	0·14	0·00	0·00	0·01	0·00
Durham	0·03	1·89	1·73	2·51	0·07	0·15	0·12	0·28	0·04	0·02	0·01	0·05
Essex	0·04	2·97	0·60	2·87	0·38	0·46	0·15	0·10	0·01	0·00	0·01	0·11
Gloucestershire	0·01	4·27	0·63	2·48	0·11	0·42	0·12	0·15	0·01	0·01	0·01	0·16
Hampshire	0·02	4·22	0·42	2·53	0·08	0·15	0·12	0·04	0·00	0·00	0·00	0·07
Herefordshire	0·02	21·42	1·36	1·89	0·02	0·20	0·08	0·04	0·00	0·00	0·00	0·10
Hertfordshire	0·00	4·04	0·53	2·22	0·16	0·22	0·15	0·18	0·01	0·00	0·00	0·23
Huntingdonshire	0·00	14·32	0·20	2·37	0·00	0·13	0·10	0·07	0·00	0·00	0·00	0·63
Kent	0·03	4·86	0·37	2·19	0·08	0·21	0·13	0·04	0·00	0·00	0·00	0·05
Lancashire	0·09	1·78	1·15	2·33	0·15	0·53	0·16	2·55	0·35	0·55	0·19	0·51
Leicestershire	0·00	3·99	0·76	2·39	0·12	3·50	0·18	4·01	0·03	0·12	0·03	0·64
Lincoln. (Holland)	0·18	29·81	0·25	2·51	0·03	0·13	0·10	0·00	0·00	0·00	0·00	0·00
Lincoln. (Kesteven)	0·00	16·23	0·68	1·88	0·06	0·25	0·12	0·00	0·00	0·00	0·00	0·21
Lincoln. (Lindsey)	1·55	9·86	2·19	2·18	0·03	0·12	0·07	0·13	0·00	0·02	0·00	0·13
London and Middx.	0·00	0·54	0·35	2·36	0·30	0·40	0·17	0·05	0·01	0·00	0·00	0·18
Norfolk	0·20	16·39	0·29	2·99	0·11	1·93	0·16	0·11	0·01	0·01	0·00	0·01
Northamptonshire	0·01	5·88	1·67	2·25	0·03	10·88	0·14	0·01	0·01	0·00	0·00	0·17
Northumberland	0·24	4·05	0·96	2·54	0·10	0·22	0·15	0·05	0·00	0·01	0·00	0·09
Nottinghamshire	0·00	3·34	0·91	2·13	0·12	0·34	0·12	2·38	0·00	0·09	0·06	0·07
Oxfordshire	0·00	6·85	0·61	2·29	0·21	0·10	0·06	0·45	0·09	0·10	0·03	0·00
Rutland	0·00	16·65	1·01	1·68	0·22	0·11	0·00	0·00	0·00	0·00	0·00	0·00
Shropshire	0·00	15·08	1·39	1·81	0·06	0·09	0·08	0·13	0·00	0·00	0·01	0·08
Somerset	0·01	9·88	0·31	2·42	0·17	1·76	0·13	0·34	0·06	0·05	0·03	0·22
Staffordshire	0·00	2·48	4·35	2·32	0·09	0·43	0·15	0·30	0·00	0·04	0·00	0·85

Table A4.14 *(cont.)*

County of residence	Occupation*											
	I	I	V	VIII	VIII	IX	IX	X	X	X	X	XIV
	000	001–005	040–045	080–085	081	090–093	091	100–108	100	101	102	140
	Fishermen	Farmers	Furnace, foundry	Wood-workers	Cabinet-makers	Leather-workers	Shoe-makers	Textile-workers	Fibre prep.	Spinners	Warpers	Rubber-workers
Suffolk (East)	0·79	11·26	0·79	2·80	0·19	0·43	0·23	0·07	0·00	0·00	0·00	0·02
Suffolk (West)	0·00	18·29	0·34	2·30	0·12	0·18	0·12	0·30	0·10	0·00	0·00	0·00
Surrey	0·00	2·70	0·27	1·83	0·14	0·26	0·16	0·04	0·00	0·00	0·00	0·15
Sussex (East)	0·07	6·34	0·22	2·20	0·17	0·28	0·22	0·02	0·00	0·00	0·00	0·02
Sussex (West)	0·04	7·38	0·34	2·91	0·15	0·18	0·12	0·01	0·00	0·00	0·00	0·04
Warwickshire	0·00	1·78	1·91	2·04	0·09	0·21	0·13	0·15	0·00	0·02	0·01	0·59
Westmorland	0·12	18·39	0·24	2·58	0·04	3·95	0·24	0·60	0·04	0·00	0·00	0·00
Wight (Isle of)	0·03	6·91	0·35	3·44	0·03	0·15	0·15	0·00	0·00	0·00	0·00	0·00
Wiltshire	0·01	9·10	0·51	2·30	0·03	0·39	0·13	0·24	0·05	0·01	0·01	0·89
Worcestershire	0·00	5·68	3·88	2·25	0·13	0·28	0·12	1·61	0·04	0·08	0·06	0·17
Yorks. (East)	2·08	8·23	0·84	2·84	0·11	0·44	0·16	0·07	0·00	0·01	0·00	0·04
Yorks. (North)	0·21	9·04	2·80	2·21	0·05	0·15	0·09	0·15	0·00	0·08	0·00	0·00
Yorks. (West)	0·00	2·32	2·71	2·15	0·11	0·35	0·16	3·88	0·94	0·55	0·22	0·07
Anglesey	0·15	15·00	0·10	2·58	0·10	0·05	0·05	0·00	0·00	0·00	0·00	0·00
Breconshire	0·05	13·44	0·91	1·60	0·05	0·23	0·23	0·18	0·05	0·05	0·00	0·55
Caernarvonshire	0·12	9·18	0·77	1·79	0·00	0·26	0·23	0·02	0·00	0·02	0·00	0·00
Cardiganshire	0·15	26·26	0·20	2·26	0·05	0·30	0·30	0·10	0·00	0·00	0·00	0·00
Carmarthenshire	0·03	11·94	1·75	1·55	0·02	0·14	0·08	0·12	0·00	0·03	0·00	0·02
Denbighshire	0·02	9·23	1·13	1·91	0·10	0·55	0·08	0·31	0·02	0·02	0·03	0·00
Flintshire	0·02	6·61	1·63	2·00	0·09	0·13	0·09	0·35	0·00	0·09	0·00	0·00
Glamorgan	0·02	1·55	1·73	1·66	0·06	0·19	0·13	0·12	0·00	0·01	0·00	0·25
Merionethshire	0·07	16·93	0·07	3·98	0·00	0·21	0·14	0·00	0·00	0·00	0·00	0·00
Monmouthshire	0·01	2·97	2·73	1·79	0·01	0·17	0·14	0·22	0·00	0·04	0·02	0·17
Montgomeryshire	0·06	33·81	0·34	2·12	0·00	1·09	0·00	0·00	0·00	0·00	0·00	0·00
Pembrokeshire	1·19	17·14	0·20	1·73	0·00	0·08	0·08	0·17	0·00	0·06	0·00	0·00
Radnorshire	0·14	35·36	0·55	1·66	0·00	0·00	0·00	0·00	0·00	0·00	0·00	0·14
England and Wales	0·08	4·31	1·21	2·31	0·15	0·51	0·14	0·87	0·12	0·12	0·05	0·22

Calculated from 1961 Census data on occupation (GRO 1965*b*, 1966)

* Occupation order (roman numbers) and units (arabic numbers) as in the GRO Classification (GRO 1960)

Table A4.15 Percentage of female work-force in selected occupations, England and Wales, 1961

County of residence	Occupation*				
	I	IX	X	X	XIV
	001–005	090–093	100–108	101	140
	Farmers	Leather-workers	Textile-workers	Spinners	Rubber-workers
Bedfordshire	0·44	0·16	0·34	0·01	0·14
Berkshire	0·55	0·04	0·04	0·02	0·01
Buckinghamshire	0·48	0·17	0·09	0·01	0·20
Cambridgeshire	0·66	0·05	0·03	0·00	0·00
Cheshire	0·38	0·14	1·44	0·58	0·11
Cornwall	1·18	0·00	0·17	0·03	0·00
Cumberland	1·03	1·02	1·14	0·20	0·15
Derbyshire	0·30	0·21	2·85	0·52	0·08
Devon	0·73	0·17	0·15	0·04	0·00
Dorset	0·85	0·01	0·29	0·01	0·00
Durham	0·17	0·07	0·53	0·19	0·01
Essex	0·29	0·29	0·11	0·01	0·17
Gloucestershire	0·39	0·24	0·27	0·06	0·06
Hampshire	0·44	0·02	0·03	0·00	0·02
Herefordshire	2·06	0·04	0·00	0·00	0·04
Hertfordshire	0·40	0·09	0·15	0·00	0·13
Huntingdonshire	1·15	0·17	0·07	0·03	0·24
Kent	0·87	0·03	0·04	0·00	0·06
Lancashire	0·17	0·49	4·62	1·64	0·24
Leicestershire	0·35	3·04	6·13	0·76	0·18
Lincoln. (Holland)	7·40	0·00	0·02	0·00	0·00
Lincoln. (Kesteven)	1·93	0·42	0·04	0·00	0·02
Lincoln. (Lindsey)	0·89	0·04	0·55	0·05	0·05
London and Middx.	0·05	0·21	0·10	0·01	0·05
Norfolk	1·34	1·71	0·15	0·04	0·00
Northamptonshire	0·57	8·19	0·05	0·01	0·03
Northumberland	0·38	0·04	0·16	0·01	0·01
Nottinghamshire	0·27	0·20	3·54	0·40	0·05
Oxfordshire	0·59	0·02	0·48	0·06	0·00
Rutland	1·54	0·35	0·00	0·00	0·00
Shropshire	1·65	0·00	0·23	0·03	0·09
Somerset	0·79	0·91	0·22	0·06	0·04
Staffordshire	0·24	0·55	0·51	0·15	0·21
Suffolk (East)	0·71	0·32	0·20	0·01	0·00
Suffolk (West)	1·11	0·08	0·95	0·16	0·00
Surrey	0·27	0·04	0·08	0·00	0·10
Sussex (East)	0·54	0·03	0·04	0·02	0·01
Sussex (West)	0·78	0·03	0·05	0·00	0·02
Warwickshire	0·19	0·18	0·43	0·06	0·16
Westmorland	1·52	1·62	1·01	0·18	0·00
Wight (Isle of)	0·58	0·02	0·02	0·00	0·00
Wiltshire	0·67	0·13	0·30	0·08	0·15
Worcestershire	0·80	0·15	1·43	0·26	0·03
Yorks. (East)	0·45	0·11	0·21	0·01	0·03
Yorks. (North)	0·67	0·00	0·54	0·14	0·00
Yorks. (West)	0·20	0·16	5·23	1·91	0·03
Anglesey	1·37	0·05	0·00	0·00	0·00
Breconshire	1·35	0·09	0·00	0·00	0·00
Caernarvonshire	0·53	0·00	0·04	0·00	0·02
Cardiganshire	2·29	0·00	0·00	0·00	0·00
Carmarthenshire	2·01	0·03	0·22	0·01	0·03
Denbighshire	0·78	0·03	0·54	0·03	0·00
Flintshire	0·82	0·00	0·82	0·51	0·00
Glamorgan	0·13	0·13	0·12	0·01	0·11

Table A4.15 *(cont.)*

County of residence	Occupation*				
	I	IX	X	X	XIV
	001–005	090–093	100–108	101	140
	Farmers	Leather-workers	Textile-workers	Spinners	Rubber-workers
Merionethshire	1·21	0·00	0·00	0·00	0·00
Monmouthshire	0·18	0·02	0·09	0·01	0·01
Montgomeryshire	2·29	0·34	1·03	0·00	0·00
Pembrokeshire	2·27	0·00	0·22	0·00	0·00
Radnorshire	3·87	0·00	0·00	0·00	0·00
England and Wales	0·41	0·34	1·35	0·41	0·09

Calculated from 1961 Census data on occupation (GRO 1965*b*, 1966)
* Occupation orders (roman numbers) and units (arabic numbers) as in the GRO classification (GRO 1960)

Table A4.16 Percentage of male and female work-force in selected industries, England and Wales, 1961

County of residence	Industry* Male						Female†
	II	II	II	IV	IV	VII	IV
	101	102	109	261–277	271	370	261–277
	coal-mining	stone, slate-mining	metal, etc. mining	chemicals	dyes	ship-building	chemicals
Bedfordshire	0·00	0·00	0·00	0·94	0·80	1·57	0·18
Berkshire	0·00	0·03	0·00	0·56	0·30	0·17	0·33
Buckinghamshire	0·01	0·00	0·00	2·57	0·46	0·06	1·53
Cambridgeshire	0·00	0·03	0·00	1·25	0·42	0·09	0·31
Cheshire	0·02	0·02	0·40	7·49	4·27	2·31	1·50
Cornwall	0·00	0·57	0·57	0·31	0·13	2·47	0·10
Cumberland	4·60	0·27	1·46	5·57	4·15	0·04	0·56
Derbyshire	12·77	0·86	0·14	1·64	0·59	0·01	0·33
Devon	0·00	0·40	0·01	0·35	0·18	3·22	0·08
Dorset	0·01	0·52	0·00	0·59	0·48	0·90	0·24
Durham	17·46	0·20	0·10	5·28	4·11	4·94	0·81
Essex	0·00	0·00	0·00	2·07	0·61	0·86	0·73
Gloucestershire	0·56	0·26	0·02	1·21	0·49	0·42	0·30
Hampshire	0·00	0·01	0·00	1·52	0·31	4·49	0·49
Herefordshire	0·00	0·20	0·00	0·26	0·16	0·00	0·04
Hertfordshire	0·00	0·00	0·00	2·14	0·47	0·03	1·17
Huntingdonshire	0·03	0·00	0·00	0·23	0·16	0·16	0·03
Kent	0·99	0·05	0·00	1·66	0·58	1·45	0·51
Lancashire	2·23	0·05	0·00	3·17	1·71	1·02	0·99
Leicestershire	4·44	0·41	0·13	0·57	0·07	0·02	0·31
Lincoln. (Holland)	0·00	0·00	0·03	0·48	0·48	0·05	0·02
Lincoln. (Kesteven)	0·00	0·25	0·95	0·35	0·29	0·00	0·14
Lincoln. (Lindsey)	0·01	0·06	0·62	2·52	1·90	1·18	0·24
London and Middx.	0·06	0·01	0·01	1·78	0·55	0·26	1·15
Norfolk	0·00	0·03	0·00	0·49	0·29	0·50	0·13
Northamptonshire	0·00	0·03	0·68	0·78	0·26	0·01	0·29
Northumberland	13·13	0·25	0·05	1·35	0·47	7·96	0·87
Nottinghamshire	15·95	0·05	0·24	1·39	0·08	0·04	0·81
Oxfordshire	0·01	0·06	0·10	0·14	0·08	0·10	0·01

Table A4.16 *(cont.)*

County of residence	Industry* Male						Female†
	II	II	II	IV	IV	VII	IV
	101	102	109	261–277	271	370	261–277
	coal-mining	stone, slate-mining	metal, etc. mining	chemicals	dyes	ship-building	chemicals
Rutland	0·00	0·78	1·90	0·11	0·00	0·00	0·12
Shropshire	2·95	0·37	0·00	0·23	0·11	0·00	0·02
Somerset	0·88	0·50	0·00	0·96	0·21	0·10	0·07
Staffordshire	4·96	0·05	0·05	0·93	0·58	0·01	0·30
Suffolk (East)	0·00	0·00	0·00	3·56	1·01	1·20	0·75
Suffolk (West)	0·00	0·02	0·00	0·67	0·40	0·02	0·30
Surrey	0·01	0·01	0·00	1·18	0·40	0·06	0·54
Sussex (East)	0·00	0·00	0·23	0·37	0·04	0·06	0·29
Sussex (West)	0·01	0·01	0·00	0·63	0·24	0·33	0·25
Warwickshire	1·58	0·05	0·00	1·06	0·28	0·02	0·50
Westmorland	0·00	0·73	1·41	0·24	0·04	0·28	0·04
Wight (Isle of)	0·00	0·09	0·00	0·50	0·00	6·18	0·14
Wiltshire	0·01	0·09	0·01	0·17	0·02	0·02	0·14
Worcestershire	0·11	0·06	0·04	2·17	1·16	0·03	0·57
Yorks. (East)	0·05	0·03	0·00	4·38	1·82	2·33	1·77
Yorks. (North)	0·03	0·18	0·33	5·06	0·98	1·17	0·47
Yorks. (West)	8·98	0·13	0·01	1·50	0·86	0·13	0·41
Anglesey	0·05	0·41	0·05	0·88	0·77	4·64	0·10
Breconshire	6·49	1·14	0·05	0·00	0·00	0·00	0·00
Caernarvonshire	0·00	4·52	0·00	0·05	0·00	0·44	0·02
Cardiganshire	0·00	0·25	0·00	0·05	0·05	0·05	0·00
Carmarthenshire	8·63	0·69	0·02	1·27	0·26	0·00	0·06
Denbighshire	9·38	0·60	0·02	3·02	2·65	0·00	0·28
Flintshire	1·09	0·42	0·00	1·63	0·91	0·02	0·31
Glamorgan	12·40	0·20	0·08	2·44	0·64	0·58	0·32
Merionethshire	0·00	4·59	0·00	2·19	0·00	0·07	1·21
Monmouthshire	14·78	0·30	0·00	2·99	0·97	0·30	0·65
Montgomeryshire	0·11	0·46	0·00	0·17	0·00	0·00	0·00
Pembrokeshire	0·06	0·23	0·00	0·96	0·06	1·58	0·22
Radnorshire	0·00	2·21	0·00	0·14	0·14	0·00	0·00
England and Wales	3·33	0·13	0·07	2·02	0·92	0·98	0·65

Calculated from 1961 Census data (GRO 1965*b*, 1966)

* Industry orders (roman numbers) and Minimum List Headings (arabic numbers) as in the Standard Industrial Classification (Central Statistical Office 1958)

† In the other industries shown for males, the percentages for females did not reach one per cent in any county

Table A4.17 Estimated rates of selected operations per 100 000 population by region of residence, England and Wales, 1960–61 and 1967

Hospital region	Circumcision	Salivary gland operations	Cholecystectomy	Prostatectomy	Orchidopexy	Oophorectomy	Hysterectomy
	1960–61	1967	1967	1967	1967	1967	1967
Newcastle	60	8·5	69·3	41·8	13·2	20·4	136·5
Leeds	98	12·2	69·8	47·7	19·5	17·5	130·7
Sheffield	72	9·8	52·2	37·5	11·0	19·7	107·1
East Anglia	102	8·5	55·4	49·5	22·2	15·0	87·3
NW Metropolitan	147	15·6	53·0	51·7	14·8	26·7	133·1
NE Metropolitan	136	15·9	56·1	55·8	18·3	27·7	129·5
SE Metropolitan	138	11·7	62·5	61·6	16·6	21·2	127·3
SW Metropolitan	129	10·2	60·4	47·2	23·1	25·4	159·0
Wessex	99	11·2	50·7	63·9	15·1	21·8	135·0
Oxford	87	13·3	48·5	32·9	12·7	24·9	140·3
South-western	81	9·9	61·8	67·8	15·9	20·3	145·5
Wales	68	8·0	77·5	43·0	9·2	25·7	121·7
Birmingham	77	8·9	55·3	33·8	13·9	19·4	103·0
Manchester	89	11·1	70·5	52·4	13·9	18·6	112·5
Liverpool	80	12·8	61·7	49·0	18·4	19·4	91·8
England and Wales	—	11·2	60·6	48·1	15·5	21·5	123·5

Data from Hospital In-Patient Enquiry (Ministry of Health and General Register Office 1967; Department of Health and Social Security and OPCS 1970)
– Data not available

Table A4.18 Hysterectomy ratios, women aged 25–74, by region of England and Wales, 1967–83

Region*	Hysterectomy ratio†
Newcastle/Northern	101·5
Leeds/Yorkshire	110·0
Sheffield/Trent	94·4
East Anglia	90·6
NW Metropolitan/North-west Thames	104·1
NE Metropolitan/North-east Thames	107·2
SE Metropolitan/South-east Thames	102·5
SW Metropolitan/South-west Thames	107·8
Wessex	112·5
Oxford	115·3
South-western	109·1
Birmingham/West Midlands	87·2
Manchester/North-western	96·9
Liverpool/Mersey	88·8
Wales	103·1

From Murphy *et al.* (1987)
* Regional Hospital Board Regions 1967–73, Regional Health Authority Regions 1974–83
† Age-standardized ratios: Great Britain average operation rates 1968–81 used as the standard

Table A4.19 Overcrowding of dwellings in England and Wales, 1936, 1951, and 1961

County	Per cent dwellings overcrowded, 1936	Persons per room	
		1951	1961
Bedfordshire	2·8	0·70	0·67
Berkshire	1·8	0·70	0·66
Buckinghamshire	1·5	0·69	0·66
Cambridgeshire and Isle of Ely	1·6	0·65/0·69	0·61/0·62
Cheshire	2·8	0·69	0·63
Cornwall	1·7	0·63	0·57
Cumberland	4·5	0·76	0·67
Derbyshire	2·5	0·73	0·65
Devon	3·0	0·69	0·61
Dorset	1·5	0·67	0·61
Durham	11·9	0·90	0·77
Essex	2·7	0·75	0·68
Gloucestershire	2·2	0·71	0·66
Hampshire	1·6	0·70	0·65
Herefordshire	2·8	0·71	0·64
Hertfordshire	1·4	0·70	0·67
Huntingdonshire and Peterborough	1·6	0·67/0·67	0·64/0·64
Kent	1·3	0·68	0·63
Lancashire	5·2	0·74	0·67
Leicestershire	1·7	0·69	0·63
Lincoln. (Holland)	2·5	0·70	0·63
Lincoln. (Kesteven)	1·8	0·70	0·64
Lincoln. (Lindsey)	1·6	0·69	0·64
London and Middlesex	5·7	0·83/0·74	0·77/0·67
Norfolk	2·3	0·65	0·60
Northamptonshire	1·5	0·67	0·63
Northumberland	11·1	0·86	0·76
Nottinghamshire	1·9	0·72	0·65
Oxfordshire	1·6	0·71	0·66

Table A4.19 *(cont.)*

County	Per cent dwellings overcrowded, 1936	Persons per room	
		1951	1961
Rutland	2·2	0·65	0·63
Shropshire	5·1	0·73	0·65
Somerset	1·6	0·68	0·61
Staffordshire	4·7	0·71	0·70
Suffolk (East)	1·7	0·65	0·61
Suffolk (West)	2·5	0·66	0·62
Surrey	1·2	0·69	0·64
Sussex (East)	1·8	0·66	0·60
Sussex (West)	1·0	0·64	0·60
Warwickshire	3·2	0·74	0·69
Westmorland	2·2	0·66	0·59
Wight (Isle of)	0·7	0·61	0·56
Wiltshire	1·6	0·71	0·65
Worcestershire	3·4	0·74	0·66
Yorks. (East)	2·9	0·72	0·66
Yorks. (North)	4·5	0·73	0·66
Yorks. (West)	3·6	0·76	0·67
Anglesey	9·5	0·64	0·57
Breconshire	4·5	0·69	0·60
Caernarvonshire	6·2	0·62	0·54
Cardiganshire	2·4	0·62	0·54
Carmarthenshire	4·4	0·70	0·60
Denbighshire	5·9	0·73	0·64
Flintshire	4·4	0·74	0·65
Glamorgan	3·7	0·74	0·65
Merionethshire	4·1	0·62	0·56
Monmouthshire	3·1	0·76	0·66
Montgomeryshire	3·9	0·68	0·59
Pembrokeshire	4·2	0·70	0·61
Radnorshire	2·0	0·66	0·57

1936 data recalculated from a national survey (Ministry of Health 1936); 1951 and 1961 data from the Census (GRO 1954–5, 1965*c*)

Table A4.20 Average annual total rainfall by county of England and Wales, 1955–64

County	Total rainfall (in./yr)
Bedfordshire	22·5
Berkshire	24·8
Buckinghamshire	24·0
Cambridgeshire	21·6
Cheshire	30·6
Cornwall	41·2
Cumberland	38·8
Derbyshire	32·8
Devon	38·4
Dorset	31·7
Durham	25·1
Essex	21·6
Gloucestershire	28·7
Hampshire	30·2
Herefordshire	28·5
Hertfordshire	25·5

Table A4.20 *(cont.)*

County	Total rainfall (in./yr)
Huntingdonshire	20·7
Kent	26·2
Lancashire	41·8
Leicestershire	24·6
Lincoln. (Holland) } Lincoln. (Kesteven) } Lincoln. (Lindsey)	22·6
London and Middx.	24·4
Norfolk	23·6
Northamptonshire	22·2
Northumberland	29·0
Nottinghamshire	23·9
Oxfordshire	26·3
Rutland	–
Shropshire	27·9
Somerset	33·3
Staffordshire	29·5
Suffolk (East) } Suffolk (West)	21·9
Surrey	26·0
Sussex (East) } Sussex (West)	30·6
Warwickshire	24·4
Westmorland	71·5
Wight (Isle of)	32·7
Wiltshire	28·2
Worcestershire	25·5
Yorks. (East)	24·9
Yorks. (North)	25·7
Yorks. (West)	32·0
Anglesey	34·8
Breconshire	64·6
Caernarvonshire	45·9
Cardiganshire	42·9
Carmarthenshire	41·6
Denbighshire	33·6
Flintshire	25·6
Glamorgan	41·9
Merionethshire	66·4
Monmouthshire	45·1
Montgomeryshire	63·7
Pembrokeshire	38·9
Radnorshire	39·3

– No data in published tables
Calculated from data from the Monthly Weather Reports (Meteorological Office, 1956–65)

Table A4.21 Cervical screening rates by region, England and Wales, 1967–84

Region* of screening	Mean smear rate per 1000 women aged 15–64
Newcastle/Northern	131·6
Leeds/Yorkshire	143·1
Sheffield/Trent	159·0
East Anglia	141·8
NW Metropolitan/North-west Thames	184·6
NE Metropolitan/North-east Thames	160·1
SE Metropolitan/South-east Thames	162·5
SW Metropolitan/South-west Thames	166·7
Wessex	155·0
Oxford	159·1
South-western	133·8
Birmingham/West Midlands	140·3
Manchester/North-western	195·7
Liverpool/Mersey	95·1
Wales	133·6

From Murphy *et al.* (1987)
* Regional Hospital Board Regions 1967–73, Regional Health Authority Regions 1974–84

Table A4.22 Cigarette smoking: average weekly cigarette consumption of persons aged 50 years and over, by sex and region, England and Wales, 1984 and 1986

Standard region	Cigarette smoking (weekly no. of cigarettes per capita)	
	Males aged 50+ years	Females aged 50+ years
North	42·9	28·7
Yorkshire and Humberside	41·2	27·7
North-west	36·5	27·3
East Midlands	30·3	20·6
West Midlands	32·8	24·6
East Anglia	25·6	16·1
South-east	35·3	22·0
South-west	28·0	16·7
Wales	37·9	23·1

Recalculated from General Household Survey data (OPCS 1986, 1989)

Table A4.23 Venereal disease clinic attendance rates 1963 and mortality rates 1959–63 by region, England and Wales

Hospital region	Clinic new attendance rates*				Mortality rates†	
	Gonorrhoea		Syphilis‡		Syphilis¶	
	Males	Females	Males	Females	Males	Females
Newcastle	51·6	19·5	1·7	0·2	29	13
Leeds	122·4	39·7	2·1	0·7	22	15
Sheffield	66·7	23·4	2·9	0·8	23	13
East Anglia	46·3	24·2	1·1	0·1	23	15
NW Metropolitan	404·9	85·8	15·4	1·4	26	15
NE Metropolitan	181·3	50·8	5·6	0·5	24	14
SE Metropolitan	91·7	21·5	5·4	0·7	30	15
SW Metropolitan	115·9	29·0	7·6	1·1	34	24
Wessex	60·2	23·9	2·0	0·5	24	15
Oxford	61·1	19·7	1·2	0·5	22	10
South-western	46·9	16·9	2·1	0·4	24	12
Wales	48·8	11·5	1·4	0·3	22	10
Birmingham	113·0	31·8	1·8	0·7	19	9
Manchester	122·2	36·6	1·7	0·7	28	16
Liverpool	144·1	36·6	6·3	1·4	25	12

New clinic attendances calculated from data from the Department of Health (unpublished); syphilis mortality from routine mortality statistics (GRO 1967)
* New cases seen at clinics per 100 000 population, by region of attendance
† Rates per million per annum, by region of usual residence
‡ Primary and secondary syphilis
¶ Syphilis and its sequelae (ICD7 020–029)

Table A4.24 Percentage of persons aged 3 years and over, speaking Welsh, by county, Wales, 1971

County	Per cent persons speaking Welsh	County	Per cent persons speaking Welsh
Anglesey	65·7	Glamorgan	11·7
Breconshire	22·9	Merionethshire	73·5
Caernarvonshire	61·9	Monmouthshire	2·1
Cardiganshire	67·6	Montgomeryshire	28·1
Carmarthenshire	66·5	Pembrokeshire	20·7
Denbighshire	28·1	Radnorshire	3·8
Flintshire	14·6		

From 1971 Census (OPCS 1973*a*)

Appendix 5

Numbers of cases, odds ratios, and confidence limits for each cancer site by county (Tables A5.1–A5.44), and by degree of urbanization (Table A5.45).

Table A5.1 Cancer of Lip, All Ages, 1968–85

	County	Males				Females			
		Cases	OR	95% CL		Cases	OR	95%CL	
1	Beds	71	1.624	1.285	2.051	9	1.288	0.669	2.479
2	Berks	101	1.542	1.267	1.877	17	1.488	0.923	2.397
3	Bucks	66	1.037	0.812	1.323	16	1.546	0.946	2.526
4	Cambs	13	2.598	2.148	3.142	15	2.136	1.297	3.517
5	Ches	113	0.653	0.543	0.786	18	0.563	0.355	0.892
6	Cornwall	102	1.718	1.413	2.088	14	1.308	0.773	2.213
7	Cumberland	42	1.285	0.947	1.743	4	0.691	0.260	1.836
8	Derbys	80	0.738	0.592	0.920	9	0.484	0.255	0.921
9	Devon	166	1.184	1.014	1.382	32	1.234	0.868	1.755
10	Dorset	60	1.172	0.908	1.514	19	2.076	1.331	3.239
11	Durham	154	0.943	0.803	1.108	23	0.853	0.564	1.289
12	Essex	129	0.991	0.832	1.181	24	1.077	0.718	1.616
13	Glos	132	0.999	0.840	1.188	28	1.196	0.821	1.741
14	Hants	170	0.869	0.746	1.013	32	0.952	0.669	1.355
15	Hereford	32	1.747	1.236	2.470	1	0.327	0.051	2.107
16	Herts	88	1.052	0.851	1.300	25	1.807	1.222	2.674
17	Hunt	70	3.086	2.458	3.874	5	1.294	0.538	3.109
18	Kent	169	1.108	0.950	1.293	40	1.444	1.054	1.979
19	Lancs	389	0.632	0.571	0.700	41	0.350	0.259	0.471
20	Leics	86	1.054	0.851	1.306	16	1.101	0.671	1.804
21	Lincs H	35	2.408	1.738	3.336	4	1.687	0.638	4.459
22	Lincs K	50	1.834	1.390	2.419	8	1.651	0.829	3.289
23	Lincs L	76	1.450	1.156	1.819	6	0.686	0.309	1.525
24	London	559	0.685	0.628	0.748	128	0.893	0.742	1.075
25	Norfolk	243	3.077	2.719	3.483	40	2.789	2.059	3.778
26	Northants	99	1.723	1.413	2.100	13	1.312	0.760	2.266
27	Northd	96	0.921	0.752	1.128	14	0.780	0.461	1.321
28	Notts	110	0.933	0.772	1.127	25	1.260	0.847	1.873
29	Oxon	77	1.739	1.390	2.176	15	1.987	1.204	3.280
30	Rut	6	2.107	0.953	4.659	0	0.000		
31	Salop	54	1.508	1.153	1.973	3	0.483	0.159	1.463
32	Somerset	104	1.055	0.868	1.282	22	1.227	0.805	1.871
33	Staffs	105	0.594	0.491	0.720	18	0.624	0.393	0.991
34	E Suff	137	2.660	2.255	3.137	15	1.640	0.989	2.719
35	W Suff	56	2.579	1.995	3.334	3	0.835	0.269	2.590
36	Surrey	91	0.828	0.673	1.020	21	1.058	0.687	1.630
37	E Sussex	110	1.051	0.869	1.270	15	0.662	0.399	1.099
38	W Sussex	67	0.959	0.753	1.221	23	1.634	1.085	2.462
39	Warwicks	168	0.740	0.635	0.863	27	0.705	0.482	1.031
40	Westd	6	0.615	0.277	1.365	4	2.191	0.840	5.719
41	IOW	19	1.194	0.760	1.877	4	1.318	0.495	3.513
42	Wilts	92	1.606	1.307	1.973	24	2.524	1.706	3.734
43	Worcs	65	0.840	0.658	1.074	8	0.606	0.304	1.207
44	E Yorks	85	1.323	1.067	1.640	13	1.145	0.663	1.980
45	N Yorks	59	0.754	0.583	0.975	8	0.600	0.301	1.194
46	W Yorks	290	0.639	0.568	0.718	69	0.866	0.678	1.106
47	Ang	27	3.115	2.165	4.482	3	1.883	0.616	5.750
48	Brec	11	1.699	0.942	3.065	2	1.848	0.471	7.255
49	Caer	24	1.180	0.789	1.766	6	1.456	0.654	3.238
50	Card	17	2.175	1.360	3.479	4	2.676	1.040	6.886
51	Carm	39	1.786	1.306	2.443	8	1.930	0.973	3.827
52	Den	34	1.152	0.821	1.617	4	0.690	0.260	1.832
53	Fli	21	0.817	0.531	1.255	3	0.636	0.207	1.958
54	Glam	160	1.020	0.871	1.195	32	1.190	0.837	1.692
55	Meri	13	2.379	1.396	4.056	1	0.955	0.134	6.799
56	Monm	42	0.763	0.563	1.034	9	1.002	0.519	1.931
57	Mont	15	2.445	1.488	4.017	4	3.790	1.518	9.459
58	Pemb	39	3.028	2.235	4.103	5	2.171	0.920	5.125
59	Rad	4	1.193	0.445	3.197	0	0.000		

OR = Odds ratio
CL = Confidence limits

Table A5.2 Cancer of Salivary Glands, All Ages, 1968–85

	County	Males				Females			
		Cases	OR	95% CL		Cases	OR	95% CL	
1	Beds	17	0.521	0.326	0.833	31	1.018	0.714	1.452
2	Berks	71	1.502	1.187	1.899	65	1.352	1.057	1.729
3	Bucks	52	1.122	0.853	1.477	51	1.129	0.855	1.490
4	Cambs	23	0.820	0.544	1.236	25	0.896	0.604	1.328
5	Ches	99	0.839	0.687	1.024	129	1.026	0.860	1.224
6	Cornwall	36	0.913	0.657	1.269	28	0.700	0.483	1.014
7	Cumberland	18	0.803	0.506	1.276	20	0.877	0.565	1.362
8	Derbys	76	1.029	0.819	1.292	78	1.039	0.829	1.301
9	Devon	90	0.991	0.803	1.223	69	0.743	0.586	0.942
10	Dorset	37	1.112	0.803	1.539	39	1.166	0.850	1.599
11	Durham	159	1.446	1.233	1.694	185	1.701	1.467	1.971
12	Essex	107	1.227	1.012	1.489	79	0.929	0.743	1.162
13	Glos	74	0.821	0.652	1.034	91	0.990	0.803	1.220
14	Hants	111	0.836	0.692	1.010	119	0.903	0.752	1.085
15	Hereford	10	0.810	0.435	1.510	8	0.691	0.345	1.385
16	Herts	40	0.663	0.486	0.903	47	0.784	0.588	1.044
17	Hunt	11	0.648	0.359	1.168	17	1.038	0.644	1.675
18	Kent	114	1.112	0.923	1.341	103	0.972	0.798	1.183
19	Lancs	340	0.831	0.743	0.929	334	0.775	0.693	0.867
20	Leics	63	1.110	0.864	1.426	57	0.970	0.746	1.261
21	Lincs H	9	0.909	0.471	1.754	8	0.876	0.438	1.756
22	Lincs K	16	0.857	0.524	1.403	11	0.564	0.315	1.011
23	Lincs L	36	1.005	0.723	1.397	23	0.658	0.438	0.989
24	London	506	0.925	0.842	1.016	524	0.942	0.859	1.033
25	Norfolk	83	1.538	1.238	1.911	106	1.927	1.592	2.333
26	Northants	45	1.107	0.824	1.487	46	1.130	0.844	1.514
27	Northd	110	1.578	1.306	1.907	123	1.793	1.500	2.144
28	Notts	80	0.976	0.782	1.220	67	0.841	0.660	1.071
29	Oxon	62	2.002	1.562	2.566	70	2.212	1.751	2.793
30	Rut	0	0.000			0	0.000		
31	Salop	19	0.767	0.489	1.204	25	1.000	0.674	1.483
32	Somerset	53	0.803	0.612	1.053	58	0.864	0.667	1.120
33	Staffs	137	1.112	0.937	1.320	144	1.168	0.988	1.381
34	E Suff	27	0.766	0.525	1.118	36	1.035	0.745	1.439
35	W Suff	14	0.934	0.552	1.583	22	1.559	1.027	2.369
36	Surrey	77	1.022	0.815	1.282	83	1.057	0.850	1.315
37	E Sussex	62	0.948	0.736	1.219	54	0.732	0.560	0.958
38	W Sussex	62	1.414	1.100	1.818	64	1.345	1.050	1.723
39	Warwicks	162	1.042	0.889	1.220	201	1.288	1.117	1.486
40	Westd	6	0.957	0.429	2.136	5	0.742	0.310	1.779
41	IOW	10	0.965	0.518	1.798	4	0.371	0.144	0.953
42	Wilts	36	0.885	0.636	1.230	39	0.979	0.714	1.344
43	Worcs	81	1.523	1.221	1.899	83	1.571	1.264	1.953
44	E Yorks	36	0.832	0.599	1.157	54	1.239	0.946	1.621
45	N Yorks	58	1.087	0.838	1.411	42	0.769	0.568	1.042
46	W Yorks	272	0.905	0.799	1.024	252	0.805	0.708	0.915
47	Ang	4	0.659	0.249	1.746	6	0.945	0.424	2.107
48	Brec	8	1.864	0.937	3.708	5	1.161	0.481	2.803
49	Caer	16	1.221	0.746	1.997	4	0.277	0.111	0.694
50	Card	6	1.119	0.502	2.495	5	0.875	0.365	2.102
51	Carm	15	1.004	0.604	1.671	16	0.961	0.587	1.573
52	Den	20	1.021	0.657	1.588	23	1.037	0.687	1.565
53	Fli	23	1.335	0.885	2.014	17	0.928	0.576	1.496
54	Glam	85	0.777	0.627	0.963	86	0.767	0.619	0.949
55	Meri	6	1.666	0.752	3.690	2	0.497	0.128	1.931
56	Monm	36	0.955	0.687	1.328	29	0.765	0.532	1.102
57	Mont	6	1.487	0.670	3.305	3	0.728	0.236	2.246
58	Pemb	9	0.981	0.509	1.889	5	0.510	0.215	1.210
59	Rad	6	2.885	1.332	6.250	5	2.729	1.172	6.358

OR = Odds ratio
CL = Confidence limits

Odds ratios underlined were treated as outliers in categorizing values for the maps

Table A5.3 Cancer of Tongue, All Ages, 1968–85

	County	Males				Females			
		Cases	OR	95% CL		Cases	OR	95%CL	
1	Beds	34	0.738	0.527	1.034	33	1.142	0.810	1.611
2	Berks	68	1.001	0.787	1.273	51	1.089	0.826	1.436
3	Bucks	56	0.854	0.655	1.112	53	1.238	0.944	1.624
4	Cambs	22	0.531	0.351	0.802	27	0.945	0.647	1.381
5	Ches	162	0.927	0.792	1.085	117	0.907	0.755	1.091
6	Cornwall	66	1.101	0.863	1.405	29	0.671	0.466	0.965
7	Cumberland	34	1.018	0.726	1.429	21	0.886	0.576	1.361
8	Derbys	108	0.986	0.814	1.193	60	0.793	0.614	1.023
9	Devon	128	0.912	0.765	1.088	105	1.021	0.840	1.240
10	Dorset	51	1.001	0.759	1.320	30	0.814	0.568	1.166
11	Durham	207	1.251	1.088	1.438	110	0.986	0.816	1.192
12	Essex	122	0.928	0.775	1.111	97	1.086	0.888	1.330
13	Glos	127	0.947	0.794	1.130	80	0.840	0.673	1.048
14	Hants	168	0.853	0.731	0.995	154	1.152	0.980	1.353
15	Hereford	25	1.356	0.914	2.010	7	0.568	0.273	1.182
16	Herts	69	0.793	0.625	1.006	78	1.358	1.085	1.699
17	Hunt	14	0.583	0.346	0.980	19	1.201	0.764	1.887
18	Kent	152	0.985	0.838	1.158	124	1.107	0.926	1.325
19	Lancs	664	1.116	1.029	1.211	447	1.012	0.917	1.117
20	Leics	83	0.997	0.802	1.240	60	1.010	0.782	1.305
21	Lincs H	12	0.802	0.455	1.415	7	0.727	0.347	1.523
22	Lincs K	25	0.896	0.604	1.329	15	0.757	0.456	1.256
23	Lincs L	51	0.950	0.720	1.254	39	1.099	0.801	1.508
24	London	832	1.054	0.979	1.134	632	1.130	1.038	1.230
25	Norfolk	62	0.741	0.577	0.952	68	1.154	0.907	1.467
26	Northants	49	0.823	0.621	1.092	40	0.990	0.725	1.353
27	Northd	136	1.293	1.090	1.534	64	0.875	0.683	1.120
28	Notts	118	0.982	0.817	1.179	77	0.944	0.753	1.184
29	Oxon	59	1.301	1.006	1.682	28	0.900	0.620	1.306
30	Rut	1	<u>0.341</u>	0.052	2.210	1	0.550	0.080	3.808
31	Salop	33	0.899	0.638	1.267	25	0.987	0.666	1.465
32	Somerset	101	1.024	0.840	1.248	79	1.107	0.885	1.384
33	Staffs	186	1.033	0.892	1.196	118	0.984	0.819	1.182
34	E Suff	42	0.786	0.580	1.066	36	0.982	0.707	1.365
35	W Suff	16	0.713	0.437	1.164	24	1.673	1.123	2.493
36	Surrey	88	0.785	0.635	0.969	78	0.970	0.774	1.214
37	E Sussex	124	1.217	1.018	1.456	92	1.068	0.868	1.314
38	W Sussex	62	0.903	0.702	1.161	50	0.910	0.688	1.203
39	Warwicks	203	0.873	0.759	1.005	123	0.777	0.649	0.929
40	Westd	8	0.831	0.415	1.667	3	0.407	0.136	1.218
41	IOW	17	1.072	0.665	1.730	17	1.430	0.889	2.301
42	Wilts	49	0.828	0.624	1.098	28	0.707	0.488	1.025
43	Worcs	58	0.727	0.562	0.942	36	0.661	0.477	0.917
44	E Yorks	63	0.964	0.751	1.237	55	1.197	0.917	1.562
45	N Yorks	95	1.201	0.980	1.473	48	0.881	0.662	1.172
46	W Yorks	474	1.065	0.969	1.170	324	1.012	0.903	1.134
47	Ang	8	0.888	0.443	1.780	2	0.308	0.083	1.141
48	Brec	9	1.369	0.711	2.638	3	0.677	0.219	2.092
49	Caer	17	0.834	0.518	1.344	14	0.861	0.509	1.457
50	Card	11	1.390	0.768	2.514	5	0.823	0.342	1.981
51	Carm	39	1.746	1.276	2.389	19	1.109	0.706	1.743
52	Den	24	0.809	0.541	1.209	14	0.601	0.357	1.010
53	Fli	26	1.009	0.685	1.486	14	0.732	0.434	1.237
54	Glam	175	1.092	0.938	1.270	119	1.068	0.890	1.283
55	Meri	3	0.538	0.176	1.643	7	1.659	0.794	3.469
56	Monm	57	1.018	0.783	1.323	32	0.862	0.608	1.221
57	Mont	7	1.132	0.537	2.384	1	0.231	0.038	1.388
58	Pemb	19	1.408	0.896	2.211	10	1.048	0.562	1.952
59	Rad	4	1.212	0.452	3.247	2	0.987	0.246	3.961

OR = Odds ratio
CL = Confidence limits

Odds ratios underlined were treated as outliers in categorizing values for the maps

Table A5.4 Cancer of Mouth, All Ages, 1968–85

	County	Males				Females			
		Cases	OR	95% CL		Cases	OR	95%CL	
1	Beds	39	0.627	0.459	0.858	28	0.857	0.591	1.244
2	Berks	57	0.615	0.475	0.797	49	0.930	0.701	1.233
3	Bucks	74	0.836	0.664	1.052	46	0.951	0.711	1.273
4	Cambs	28	0.496	0.344	0.714	38	1.187	0.862	1.635
5	Ches	279	1.189	1.055	1.341	158	1.096	0.935	1.285
6	Cornwall	58	0.700	0.540	0.906	37	0.762	0.552	1.053
7	Cumberland	42	0.924	0.681	1.253	26	0.977	0.664	1.438
8	Derbys	151	1.016	0.864	1.195	97	1.146	0.937	1.402
9	Devon	176	0.914	0.786	1.062	110	0.948	0.784	1.146
10	Dorset	53	0.755	0.576	0.990	42	1.015	0.748	1.376
11	Durham	372	1.689	1.522	1.874	143	1.145	0.968	1.353
12	Essex	124	0.686	0.574	0.819	83	0.821	0.660	1.020
13	Glos	140	0.763	0.645	0.902	78	0.726	0.580	0.907
14	Hants	188	0.696	0.603	0.805	99	0.645	0.529	0.786
15	Hereford	32	1.269	0.895	1.800	12	0.868	0.492	1.530
16	Herts	77	0.652	0.522	0.816	55	0.844	0.646	1.101
17	Hunt	20	0.617	0.399	0.954	9	0.503	0.265	0.957
18	Kent	194	0.921	0.798	1.062	139	1.103	0.931	1.307
19	Lancs	1 137	1.465	1.375	1.560	583	1.195	1.095	1.304
20	Leics	117	1.040	0.865	1.250	68	1.018	0.801	1.295
21	Lincs H	19	0.933	0.593	1.468	15	1.376	0.829	2.284
22	Lincs K	24	0.629	0.422	0.937	23	1.031	0.684	1.556
23	Lincs L	59	0.806	0.624	1.043	31	0.769	0.541	1.095
24	London	937	0.850	0.794	0.910	658	1.031	0.949	1.120
25	Norfolk	90	0.788	0.640	0.970	69	1.037	0.817	1.316
26	Northants	50	0.617	0.468	0.814	34	0.745	0.532	1.043
27	Northd	233	1.647	1.446	1.876	113	1.386	1.150	1.671
28	Notts	167	1.026	0.879	1.197	65	0.702	0.550	0.897
29	Oxon	54	0.872	0.666	1.141	39	1.120	0.817	1.537
30	Rut	4	1.015	0.378	2.727	1	0.491	0.072	3.358
31	Salop	32	0.638	0.451	0.901	31	1.088	0.763	1.551
32	Somerset	99	0.728	0.597	0.888	55	0.678	0.520	0.884
33	Staffs	284	1.178	1.045	1.327	143	1.059	0.896	1.252
34	E Suff	47	0.641	0.482	0.854	51	1.240	0.941	1.636
35	W Suff	26	0.852	0.579	1.254	13	0.796	0.461	1.371
36	Surrey	122	0.802	0.670	0.959	77	0.848	0.676	1.062
37	E Sussex	120	0.845	0.705	1.013	102	1.054	0.865	1.283
38	W Sussex	61	0.641	0.499	0.824	70	1.138	0.898	1.443
39	Warwicks	329	1.055	0.944	1.179	156	0.879	0.749	1.032
40	Westd	17	1.298	0.804	2.095	3	0.362	0.122	1.072
41	IOW	19	0.874	0.556	1.375	14	1.036	0.612	1.754
42	Wilts	53	0.658	0.503	0.861	39	0.877	0.639	1.202
43	Worcs	121	1.132	0.945	1.356	52	0.851	0.647	1.119
44	E Yorks	85	0.954	0.769	1.183	51	0.983	0.745	1.297
45	N Yorks	122	1.136	0.949	1.360	65	1.063	0.832	1.359
46	W Yorks	737	1.237	1.146	1.335	374	1.040	0.935	1.156
47	Ang	13	1.064	0.615	1.840	6	0.819	0.368	1.825
48	Brec	5	0.550	0.231	1.311	1	0.201	0.034	1.174
49	Caer	31	1.114	0.781	1.590	13	0.709	0.412	1.221
50	Card	9	0.826	0.428	1.592	6	0.877	0.393	1.957
51	Carm	36	1.175	0.845	1.634	20	1.031	0.664	1.602
52	Den	54	1.342	1.025	1.756	33	1.264	0.897	1.781
53	Fli	35	0.999	0.715	1.395	26	1.215	0.825	1.788
54	Glam	206	0.942	0.819	1.082	151	1.208	1.027	1.421
55	Meri	8	1.054	0.524	2.119	3	0.629	0.204	1.937
56	Monm	62	0.811	0.631	1.042	33	0.788	0.559	1.109
57	Mont	14	1.670	0.988	2.823	7	1.447	0.690	3.033
58	Pemb	22	1.203	0.790	1.833	16	1.497	0.917	2.443
59	Rad	10	2.234	1.210	4.124	2	0.875	0.218	3.510

OR = Odds ratio
CL = Confidence limits

Table A5.5 Cancer of Pharynx, All Ages, 1968–85

	County	Males				Females			
		Cases	OR	95% CL		Cases	OR	95%CL	
1	Beds	52	0.850	0.646	1.118	44	1.145	0.850	1.543
2	Berks	79	0.874	0.699	1.092	45	0.732	0.546	0.981
3	Bucks	94	1.090	0.888	1.338	48	0.846	0.636	1.124
4	Cambs	39	0.708	0.517	0.970	37	0.995	0.719	1.376
5	Ches	274	1.179	1.044	1.331	221	1.313	1.147	1.502
6	Cornwall	63	0.773	0.603	0.992	59	1.053	0.814	1.362
7	Cumberland	40	0.888	0.650	1.213	19	0.602	0.385	0.941
8	Derbys	123	0.832	0.696	0.995	84	0.836	0.673	1.037
9	Devon	178	0.940	0.809	1.092	112	0.839	0.696	1.012
10	Dorset	54	0.781	0.597	1.022	42	0.875	0.646	1.187
11	Durham	236	1.052	0.924	1.199	145	0.964	0.817	1.137
12	Essex	133	0.748	0.630	0.888	84	0.716	0.577	0.888
13	Glos	174	0.968	0.832	1.126	107	0.862	0.711	1.044
14	Hants	196	0.739	0.642	0.852	146	0.831	0.705	0.980
15	Hereford	41	1.659	1.220	2.255	19	1.183	0.753	1.859
16	Herts	84	0.723	0.583	0.896	68	0.887	0.698	1.127
17	Hunt	31	0.976	0.684	1.392	29	1.389	0.964	2.001
18	Kent	193	0.929	0.805	1.073	129	0.877	0.736	1.045
19	Lancs	970	1.225	1.144	1.310	751	1.324	1.225	1.430
20	Leics	109	0.980	0.810	1.185	68	0.867	0.682	1.101
21	Lincs H	12	0.591	0.337	1.037	17	1.316	0.816	2.120
22	Lincs K	31	0.829	0.582	1.181	25	0.956	0.644	1.418
23	Lincs L	56	0.773	0.594	1.007	37	0.779	0.564	1.076
24	London	1 162	1.108	1.041	1.180	659	0.866	0.798	0.940
25	Norfolk	121	1.080	0.902	1.295	117	1.526	1.271	1.833
26	Northants	42	0.526	0.390	0.709	40	0.755	0.553	1.031
27	Northd	144	1.007	0.853	1.189	97	0.993	0.812	1.215
28	Notts	124	0.764	0.640	0.913	95	0.876	0.715	1.073
29	Oxon	49	0.803	0.606	1.065	34	0.839	0.598	1.176
30	Rut	4	1.034	0.385	2.775	5	2.122	0.894	5.033
31	Salop	56	1.142	0.877	1.489	29	0.861	0.597	1.241
32	Somerset	132	0.995	0.837	1.183	54	0.577	0.443	0.753
33	Staffs	285	1.189	1.056	1.340	187	1.150	0.993	1.332
34	E Suff	50	0.695	0.527	0.918	37	0.775	0.561	1.071
35	W Suff	25	0.828	0.558	1.229	13	0.683	0.397	1.174
36	Surrey	134	0.897	0.755	1.065	104	0.990	0.815	1.203
37	E Sussex	140	1.010	0.853	1.195	119	1.097	0.914	1.317
38	W Sussex	102	1.106	0.909	1.347	70	1.010	0.797	1.280
39	Warwicks	415	1.362	1.233	1.505	236	1.133	0.994	1.292
40	Westd	6	0.459	0.210	1.005	9	0.943	0.489	1.819
41	IOW	14	0.648	0.384	1.093	5	0.318	0.138	0.730
42	Wilts	49	0.618	0.467	0.817	26	0.496	0.340	0.724
43	Worcs	135	1.27	1.077	1.517	90	1.250	1.014	1.540
44	E Yorks	70	0.791	0.625	1.001	66	1.086	0.851	1.386
45	N Yorks	109	1.024	0.846	1.238	78	1.083	0.865	1.356
46	W Yorks	555	0.912	0.836	0.995	398	0.933	0.842	1.034
47	Ang	15	1.242	0.746	2.067	13	1.519	0.882	2.615
48	Brec	15	1.682	1.015	2.790	10	1.719	0.929	3.182
49	Caer	28	1.017	0.700	1.478	29	1.392	0.966	2.006
50	Card	7	0.653	0.312	1.366	7	0.879	0.418	1.848
51	Carm	30	0.983	0.685	1.410	32	1.386	0.979	1.963
52	Den	34	0.848	0.605	1.190	31	1.019	0.715	1.453
53	Fli	24	0.689	0.462	1.029	15	0.596	0.361	0.986
54	Glam	223	1.031	0.902	1.179	190	1.278	1.105	1.478
55	Meri	2	0.263	0.072	0.951	8	1.446	0.723	2.891
56	Monm	80	1.062	0.851	1.326	67	1.361	1.069	1.732
57	Mont	13	1.581	0.916	2.727	14	2.517	1.509	4.198
58	Pemb	21	1.155	0.750	1.778	14	1.093	0.646	1.852
59	Rad	9	2.043	1.070	3.904	5	1.893	0.794	4.511

OR = Odds ratio
CL = Confidence limits

Table A5.6 Cancers of Tongue, Mouth, and Pharynx, All Ages, 1968–85

	County	Males				Females			
		Cases	OR	95% CL		Cases	OR	95% CL	
1	Beds	136	0.748	0.631	0.887	111	1.040	0.861	1.256
2	Berks	222	0.826	0.722	0.945	155	0.900	0.767	1.056
3	Bucks	238	0.926	0.813	1.055	148	0.935	0.794	1.101
4	Cambs	90	0.544	0.442	0.668	102	0.975	0.801	1.187
5	Ches	754	1.103	1.024	1.188	537	1.141	1.046	1.245
6	Cornwall	191	0.792	0.685	0.915	136	0.859	0.725	1.019
7	Cumberland	127	0.960	0.803	1.146	74	0.844	0.671	1.063
8	Derbys	411	0.947	0.858	1.046	262	0.940	0.831	1.063
9	Devon	520	0.930	0.851	1.016	356	0.945	0.850	1.051
10	Dorset	170	0.832	0.714	0.970	127	0.941	0.789	1.122
11	Durham	868	1.346	1.255	1.442	422	1.021	0.925	1.125
12	Essex	408	0.775	0.702	0.856	284	0.862	0.766	0.971
13	Glos	475	0.892	0.813	0.979	295	0.843	0.751	0.947
14	Hants	609	0.775	0.715	0.841	429	0.866	0.786	0.954
15	Hereford	103	1.426	1.170	1.738	39	0.862	0.628	1.183
16	Herts	244	0.707	0.622	0.803	217	1.020	0.891	1.168
17	Hunt	66	0.695	0.545	0.887	60	1.029	0.796	1.330
18	Kent	577	0.942	0.866	1.025	416	1.011	0.916	1.116
19	Lancs	2 944	1.283	1.233	1.335	1 900	1.190	1.134	1.250
20	Leics	341	1.043	0.935	1.163	213	0.974	0.850	1.117
21	Lincs H	47	0.787	0.589	1.051	42	1.177	0.867	1.599
22	Lincs K	84	0.755	0.608	0.938	68	0.932	0.732	1.185
23	Lincs L	185	0.867	0.749	1.005	115	0.871	0.724	1.048
24	London	3 119	0.993	0.956	1.032	2 083	0.995	0.950	1.043
25	Norfolk	286	0.860	0.764	0.968	259	1.201	1.060	1.360
26	Northants	149	0.627	0.534	0.737	121	0.813	0.679	0.973
27	Northd	540	1.308	1.199	1.428	289	1.072	0.953	1.206
28	Notts	457	0.962	0.876	1.057	261	0.863	0.763	0.977
29	Oxon	168	0.934	0.800	1.090	104	0.913	0.752	1.109
30	Rut	9	0.778	0.401	1.510	8	1.209	0.600	2.437
31	Salop	129	0.886	0.743	1.057	89	0.951	0.770	1.174
32	Somerset	354	0.900	0.809	1.001	212	0.805	0.702	0.923
33	Staffs	799	1.137	1.058	1.222	468	1.048	0.955	1.151
34	E Suff	154	0.721	0.614	0.846	132	0.984	0.828	1.170
35	W Suff	74	0.830	0.658	1.046	52	0.978	0.743	1.288
36	Surrey	375	0.846	0.763	0.939	276	0.934	0.828	1.053
37	E Sussex	401	0.979	0.885	1.083	330	1.060	0.949	1.184
38	W Sussex	233	0.847	0.743	0.966	192	0.966	0.836	1.115
39	Warwicks	989	1.093	1.024	1.167	536	0.920	0.843	1.003
40	Westd	35	0.914	0.652	1.281	16	0.590	0.362	0.962
41	IOW	55	0.867	0.662	1.134	41	0.932	0.684	1.270
42	Wilts	168	0.714	0.612	0.832	96	0.655	0.536	0.800
43	Worcs	323	1.036	0.926	1.158	185	0.921	0.796	1.066
44	E Yorks	241	0.928	0.815	1.056	185	1.093	0.944	1.266
45	N Yorks	354	1.137	1.022	1.266	207	1.033	0.899	1.187
46	W Yorks	1 883	1.071	1.021	1.124	1 175	0.994	0.936	1.056
47	Ang	36	1.011	0.724	1.411	23	0.961	0.636	1.452
48	Brec	32	1.228	0.862	1.750	14	0.859	0.507	1.456
49	Caer	83	1.027	0.824	1.279	62	1.048	0.814	1.348
50	Card	31	0.984	0.687	1.409	20	0.895	0.575	1.394
51	Carm	110	1.243	1.026	1.505	73	1.147	0.909	1.448
52	Den	122	1.039	0.867	1.246	90	1.057	0.857	1.303
53	Fli	101	0.990	0.811	1.209	65	0.926	0.724	1.184
54	Glam	642	1.011	0.933	1.095	497	1.212	1.107	1.326
55	Meri	14	0.624	0.369	1.055	18	1.162	0.728	1.854
56	Monm	208	0.936	0.815	1.076	143	1.044	0.884	1.233
57	Mont	37	1.542	1.108	2.145	24	1.534	1.025	2.298
58	Pemb	68	1.286	1.008	1.641	45	1.280	0.953	1.721
59	Rad	24	1.885	1.253	2.834	9	1.213	0.627	2.347

OR = Odds ratio
CL = Confidence limits

Table A5.7 Cancer of Nasopharynx, All Ages, 1968–85

	County	Males				Females			
		Cases	OR	95% CL		Cases	OR	95%CL	
1	Beds	13	0.707	0.410	1.220	4	0.444	0.171	1.154
2	Berks	20	0.752	0.484	1.169	12	0.846	0.478	1.495
3	Bucks	26	1.016	0.689	1.497	16	1.203	0.733	1.973
4	Cambs	26	1.774	1.209	2.603	9	1.095	0.568	2.113
5	Ches	61	0.937	0.726	1.210	26	0.689	0.468	1.014
6	Cornwall	10	0.476	0.259	0.875	8	0.670	0.336	1.337
7	Cumberland	12	0.971	0.550	1.716	5	0.733	0.305	1.760
8	Derbys	46	1.138	0.849	1.525	15	0.666	0.401	1.106
9	Devon	36	0.754	0.543	1.048	28	1.008	0.693	1.468
10	Dorset	12	0.680	0.386	1.198	5	0.489	0.207	1.156
11	Durham	65	1.049	0.819	1.343	38	1.150	0.832	1.590
12	Essex	40	0.842	0.616	1.151	23	0.909	0.601	1.373
13	Glos	51	1.054	0.797	1.392	23	0.845	0.559	1.277
14	Hants	66	0.934	0.730	1.194	37	0.952	0.686	1.321
15	Hereford	1	0.151	0.028	0.821	1	0.286	0.046	1.797
16	Herts	31	0.926	0.649	1.321	21	1.209	0.785	1.863
17	Hunt	13	1.409	0.817	2.430	6	1.259	0.566	2.805
18	Kent	63	1.143	0.889	1.470	33	1.045	0.739	1.478
19	Lancs	237	1.077	0.940	1.233	161	1.320	1.118	1.558
20	Leics	22	0.709	0.466	1.077	14	0.806	0.476	1.366
21	Lincs H	7	1.304	0.621	2.735	5	1.778	0.747	4.231
22	Lincs K	7	0.698	0.333	1.461	5	0.864	0.358	2.087
23	Lincs L	16	0.815	0.499	1.333	5	0.475	0.201	1.119
24	London	461	1.720	1.553	1.906	204	1.307	1.124	1.520
25	Norfolk	27	0.923	0.631	1.351	19	1.144	0.727	1.802
26	Northants	11	0.496	0.277	0.887	7	0.579	0.278	1.205
27	Northd	44	1.126	0.835	1.518	20	0.950	0.611	1.479
28	Notts	33	0.725	0.514	1.022	22	0.929	0.609	1.417
29	Oxon	24	1.419	0.949	2.121	3	0.319	0.109	0.934
30	Rut	2	1.843	0.470	7.221	1	1.883	0.274	2.969
31	Salop	12	0.882	0.498	1.561	3	0.401	0.134	1.200
32	Somerset	22	0.625	0.412	0.949	12	0.599	0.341	1.052
33	Staffs	65	0.929	0.726	1.190	30	0.809	0.563	1.162
34	E Suff	20	1.079	0.695	1.678	11	1.064	0.587	1.928
35	W Suff	8	0.976	0.486	1.960	6	1.402	0.630	3.121
36	Surrey	32	0.771	0.544	1.093	21	0.903	0.587	1.390
37	E Sussex	33	0.992	0.702	1.400	12	0.540	0.308	0.946
38	W Sussex	7	0.304	0.151	0.613	11	0.762	0.422	1.377
39	Warwicks	88	1.007	0.813	1.248	53	1.135	0.861	1.495
40	Westd	1	0.301	0.048	1.907	1	0.496	0.073	3.390
41	IOW	6	1.108	0.496	2.472	6	1.818	0.824	4.010
42	Wilts	10	0.450	0.246	0.824	11	0.923	0.509	1.672
43	Worcs	29	0.970	0.671	1.400	17	1.069	0.662	1.726
44	E Yorks	20	0.857	0.551	1.331	17	1.303	0.807	2.103
45	N Yorks	21	0.707	0.461	1.085	17	1.057	0.655	1.707
46	W Yorks	130	0.777	0.650	0.928	87	0.941	0.756	1.171
47	Ang	1	0.300	0.047	1.901	1	0.514	0.075	3.526
48	Brec	1	0.412	0.060	2.829	0	0.000		
49	Caer	8	1.140	0.569	2.283	5	1.161	0.482	2.794
50	Card	5	1.739	0.731	4.139	0	0.000		
51	Carm	6	0.720	0.324	1.599	6	1.184	0.531	2.640
52	Den	12	1.138	0.644	2.009	7	1.060	0.504	2.229
53	Fli	4	0.429	0.165	1.112	8	1.444	0.720	2.895
54	Glam	56	0.926	0.710	1.208	34	1.024	0.728	1.441
55	Meri	1	0.511	0.075	3.498	2	1.677	0.420	6.687
56	Monm	16	0.763	0.467	1.247	12	1.061	0.601	1.875
57	Mont	1	0.467	0.069	3.178	0	0.000		
58	Pemb	2	0.389	0.102	1.480	2	0.688	0.173	2.734
59	Rad	2	1.886	0.481	7.393	0	0.000		

OR = Odds ratio
CL = Confidence limits

Odds ratios underlined were treated as outliers in categorizing values for the maps

Table A5.8 Cancer of Oesophagus, All Ages, 1968–85

	County	Males				Females			
		Cases	OR	95% CL		Cases	OR	95% CL	
1	Beds	276	0.991	0.877	1.120	206	1.037	0.901	1.193
2	Berks	301	0.707	0.629	0.793	297	0.902	0.802	1.013
3	Bucks	321	0.792	0.708	0.887	258	0.864	0.762	0.979
4	Cambs	229	0.876	0.766	1.001	187	0.916	0.791	1.062
5	Ches	1 301	1.214	1.146	1.286	1 059	1.186	1.114	1.263
6	Cornwall	392	1.006	0.907	1.115	363	1.181	1.062	1.314
7	Cumberland	234	1.120	0.980	1.280	213	1.297	1.129	1.490
8	Derbys	640	0.926	0.855	1.004	476	0.898	0.818	0.984
9	Devon	914	0.999	0.934	1.070	780	1.035	0.962	1.113
10	Dorset	353	1.068	0.958	1.191	233	0.865	0.759	0.987
11	Durham	1 018	0.975	0.914	1.040	748	0.969	0.899	1.043
12	Essex	847	1.016	0.947	1.090	631	0.982	0.906	1.064
13	Glos	772	0.906	0.842	0.975	669	0.988	0.914	1.069
14	Hants	1 270	1.024	0.966	1.085	968	1.007	0.943	1.075
15	Hereford	132	1.117	0.935	1.334	93	1.058	0.859	1.304
16	Herts	528	0.997	0.912	1.089	381	0.950	0.856	1.053
17	Hunt	153	1.035	0.878	1.220	95	0.859	0.699	1.055
18	Kent	1 022	1.044	0.979	1.113	780	0.963	0.895	1.035
19	Lancs	4 298	1.162	1.124	1.201	3 538	1.154	1.113	1.196
20	Leics	559	1.080	0.990	1.178	428	1.025	0.929	1.130
21	Lincs H	92	0.959	0.776	1.184	84	1.245	1.000	1.552
22	Lincs K	199	1.140	0.986	1.317	143	1.026	0.867	1.215
23	Lincs L	397	1.187	1.071	1.316	264	1.059	0.935	1.199
24	London	4 683	0.930	0.901	0.960	3 798	0.923	0.891	0.956
25	Norfolk	577	1.082	0.994	1.179	383	0.900	0.812	0.997
26	Northants	251	0.662	0.583	0.751	213	0.738	0.644	0.846
27	Northd	645	0.963	0.889	1.044	502	0.974	0.890	1.066
28	Notts	670	0.884	0.817	0.956	506	0.875	0.800	0.958
29	Oxon	199	0.683	0.593	0.788	158	0.717	0.612	0.840
30	Rut	27	1.515	1.021	2.247	17	1.363	0.835	2.224
31	Salop	250	1.091	0.959	1.241	185	1.045	0.901	1.211
32	Somerset	564	0.880	0.808	0.959	448	0.857	0.779	0.942
33	Staffs	1 090	0.984	0.925	1.048	888	1.099	1.026	1.176
34	E Suff	322	0.940	0.840	1.053	253	0.955	0.842	1.084
35	W Suff	148	1.040	0.879	1.229	99	0.967	0.790	1.184
36	Surrey	642	0.919	0.848	0.996	495	0.860	0.785	0.941
37	E Sussex	689	1.013	0.937	1.095	660	1.014	0.937	1.097
38	W Sussex	472	1.049	0.954	1.152	412	1.002	0.907	1.107
39	Warwicks	1 365	0.949	0.898	1.004	1 063	0.976	0.917	1.039
40	Westd	76	1.235	0.977	1.560	72	1.384	1.091	1.755
41	IOW	104	1.005	0.824	1.227	97	1.114	0.908	1.367
42	Wilts	368	0.999	0.898	1.111	253	0.912	0.804	1.035
43	Worcs	522	1.063	0.972	1.163	387	1.028	0.928	1.139
44	E Yorks	420	1.008	0.913	1.114	330	1.006	0.900	1.125
45	N Yorks	574	1.171	1.075	1.276	396	1.044	0.944	1.156
46	W Yorks	2 641	0.926	0.889	0.964	1 895	0.816	0.779	0.856
47	Ang	63	1.110	0.858	1.435	60	1.332	1.026	1.727
48	Brec	50	1.186	0.889	1.581	41	1.339	0.976	1.835
49	Caer	152	1.161	0.983	1.370	185	1.592	1.371	1.849
50	Card	54	1.065	0.808	1.405	57	1.332	1.019	1.741
51	Carm	156	1.103	0.937	1.298	158	1.339	1.141	1.572
52	Den	213	1.121	0.974	1.289	228	1.399	1.223	1.600
53	Fli	187	1.146	0.987	1.331	159	1.182	1.008	1.388
54	Glam	1 058	1.056	0.991	1.125	946	1.239	1.159	1.324
55	Meri	50	1.417	1.061	1.891	47	1.594	1.187	2.139
56	Monm	359	1.023	0.918	1.139	300	1.181	1.051	1.327
57	Mont	32	0.795	0.557	1.135	45	1.492	1.105	2.015
58	Pemb	100	1.200	0.978	1.471	69	1.049	0.824	1.336
59	Rad	24	1.109	0.731	1.681	17	1.172	0.719	1.912

OR = Odds ratio
CL = Confidence limits

Table A5.9 Cancer of Stomach, All Ages, 1968–85

County		Males				Females			
		Cases	OR	95% CL		Cases	OR	95% CL	
1	Beds	967	1.000	0.932	1.073	529	0.884	0.807	0.968
2	Berks	1 317	0.899	0.847	0.955	801	0.802	0.745	0.863
3	Bucks	1 368	0.983	0.926	1.043	810	0.906	0.842	0.976
4	Cambs	707	0.761	0.702	0.825	470	0.753	0.684	0.829
5	Ches	4 039	1.063	1.026	1.101	2 870	1.060	1.018	1.103
6	Cornwall	1 208	0.869	0.816	0.925	811	0.855	0.794	0.920
7	Cumberland	849	1.162	1.077	1.255	557	1.128	1.031	1.234
8	Derbys	2 574	1.076	1.030	1.125	1 700	1.083	1.029	1.141
9	Devon	2 806	0.858	0.823	0.894	1 875	0.804	0.766	0.844
10	Dorset	858	0.716	0.666	0.771	580	0.701	0.643	0.764
11	Durham	4 269	1.196	1.155	1.238	3 187	1.436	1.382	1.493
12	Essex	2 721	0.922	0.884	0.962	1 691	0.863	0.819	0.908
13	Glos	2 697	0.904	0.867	0.943	1 766	0.855	0.813	0.899
14	Hants	3 398	0.762	0.734	0.791	2 095	0.701	0.670	0.734
15	Hereford	322	0.761	0.676	0.857	216	0.804	0.698	0.927
16	Herts	1 639	0.883	0.836	0.931	1 032	0.856	0.802	0.914
17	Hunt	472	0.904	0.818	0.999	270	0.810	0.714	0.919
18	Kent	3 218	0.926	0.891	0.963	2 097	0.847	0.809	0.887
19	Lancs	15 363	1.192	1.170	1.215	11 620	1.292	1.265	1.320
20	Leics	1 817	0.996	0.946	1.049	1 159	0.919	0.864	0.977
21	Lincs H	295	0.871	0.768	0.987	179	0.872	0.746	1.019
22	Lincs K	570	0.920	0.840	1.008	335	0.793	0.708	0.888
23	Lincs L	1 065	0.891	0.834	0.953	754	1.007	0.933	1.088
24	London	16 943	0.970	0.953	0.988	11 804	0.960	0.941	0.981
25	Norfolk	1 746	0.916	0.869	0.965	1 053	0.813	0.762	0.867
26	Northants	1 432	1.110	1.047	1.177	856	1.000	0.930	1.075
27	Northd	2 373	1.020	0.975	1.067	1 790	1.179	1.121	1.241
28	Notts	2 595	0.985	0.944	1.029	1 593	0.922	0.875	0.972
29	Oxon	925	0.921	0.857	0.990	556	0.842	0.770	0.920
30	Rut	59	0.907	0.683	1.203	33	0.861	0.599	1.237
31	Salop	891	1.115	1.035	1.201	475	0.886	0.805	0.975
32	Somerset	1 882	0.829	0.789	0.872	1 224	0.765	0.721	0.812
33	Staffs	5 097	1.368	1.325	1.413	3 190	1.362	1.311	1.416
34	E Suff	917	0.751	0.699	0.806	642	0.792	0.730	0.860
35	W Suff	415	0.812	0.730	0.903	224	0.714	0.622	0.819
36	Surrey	1 906	0.770	0.733	0.809	1 350	0.772	0.729	0.817
37	E Sussex	1 938	0.789	0.751	0.829	1 494	0.731	0.693	0.772
38	W Sussex	1 221	0.749	0.704	0.797	941	0.734	0.686	0.785
39	Warwicks	5 186	1.046	1.014	1.079	3 337	1.033	0.995	1.072
40	Westd	206	0.931	0.799	1.083	131	0.806	0.672	0.967
41	IOW	243	0.645	0.563	0.739	153	0.561	0.477	0.661
42	Wilts	1 071	0.821	0.768	0.876	665	0.789	0.728	0.855
43	Worcs	1 706	0.993	0.941	1.047	1 175	1.049	0.986	1.115
44	E Yorks	1 511	1.035	0.978	1.096	1 036	1.055	0.987	1.127
45	N Yorks	1 900	1.107	1.052	1.165	1 313	1.165	1.098	1.235
46	W Yorks	10 251	1.041	1.018	1.065	7 441	1.107	1.079	1.136
47	Ang	245	1.236	1.071	1.427	150	1.099	0.925	1.306
48	Brec	137	0.904	0.751	1.089	101	1.076	0.870	1.330
49	Caer	622	1.368	1.249	1.498	520	1.473	1.340	1.619
50	Card	203	1.140	0.974	1.334	171	1.333	1.133	1.570
51	Carm	587	1.193	1.088	1.308	417	1.175	1.058	1.304
52	Den	788	1.183	1.093	1.281	597	1.206	1.106	1.317
53	Fli	661	1.146	1.051	1.250	484	1.198	1.087	1.320
54	Glam	3 871	1.108	1.069	1.149	2 631	1.150	1.103	1.199
55	Meri	158	1.250	1.045	1.496	133	1.489	1.234	1.796
56	Monm	1 468	1.210	1.141	1.283	886	1.169	1.089	1.256
57	Mont	156	1.127	0.943	1.346	91	0.972	0.779	1.213
58	Pemb	309	1.049	0.925	1.189	190	0.953	0.818	1.111
59	Rad	68	0.880	0.677	1.144	40	0.909	0.655	1.261

OR = Odds ratio
CL = Confidence limits

Table A5.10 Cancers of Colon and Rectum, All Ages, 1968–85

	County	Males				Females			
		Cases	OR	95% CL		Cases	OR	95% CL	
1	Beds	1 499	1.029	0.969	1.092	1 597	1.110	1.047	1.176
2	Berks	2 251	1.023	0.974	1.075	2 495	1.050	1.003	1.100
3	Bucks	2 020	0.951	0.903	1.001	2 194	1.010	0.962	1.061
4	Cambs	1 385	1.013	0.952	1.079	1 432	0.970	0.914	1.031
5	Ches	5 871	1.030	0.999	1.062	6 812	1.040	1.011	1.070
6	Cornwall	1 925	0.923	0.876	0.973	2 199	0.980	0.934	1.029
7	Cumberland	1 226	1.125	1.052	1.203	1 324	1.105	1.037	1.178
8	Derbys	3 752	1.045	1.006	1.086	3 723	0.966	0.931	1.003
9	Devon	4 679	0.959	0.927	0.992	5 394	0.993	0.962	1.024
10	Dorset	1 707	0.962	0.910	1.018	1 884	0.969	0.919	1.021
11	Durham	5 693	1.053	1.020	1.086	5 473	0.964	0.935	0.994
12	Essex	3 936	0.878	0.846	0.910	4 446	0.950	0.918	0.983
13	Glos	4 478	1.007	0.973	1.043	4 745	0.966	0.935	0.999
14	Hants	6 119	0.920	0.893	0.947	6 806	0.971	0.945	0.999
15	Hereford	702	1.137	1.040	1.243	694	1.109	1.016	1.211
16	Herts	2 503	0.892	0.852	0.933	2 840	0.970	0.929	1.012
17	Hunt	765	0.972	0.894	1.057	773	0.962	0.887	1.043
18	Kent	4 857	0.925	0.895	0.956	5 814	0.995	0.965	1.025
19	Lancs	20 459	1.040	1.022	1.058	23 339	1.031	1.015	1.047
20	Leics	2 683	0.973	0.930	1.018	2 924	0.957	0.918	0.999
21	Lincs H	534	1.072	0.969	1.187	503	1.012	0.913	1.121
22	Lincs K	1 056	1.157	1.076	1.244	1 035	1.022	0.952	1.098
23	Lincs L	1 834	1.034	0.979	1.091	1 863	1.028	0.975	1.084
24	London	23 221	0.861	0.847	0.875	28 233	0.948	0.935	0.962
25	Norfolk	2 959	1.047	1.002	1.093	3 074	1.003	0.963	1.046
26	Northants	2 099	1.080	1.026	1.136	2 186	1.068	1.017	1.122
27	Northd	3 438	0.979	0.941	1.018	3 708	0.984	0.948	1.022
28	Notts	3 947	0.999	0.962	1.036	4 162	0.999	0.964	1.035
29	Oxon	1 592	1.067	1.006	1.131	1 635	1.036	0.979	1.096
30	Rut	91	0.931	0.734	1.181	83	0.888	0.694	1.135
31	Salop	1 456	1.238	1.164	1.318	1 409	1.106	1.040	1.176
32	Somerset	3 086	0.907	0.870	0.946	3 642	0.973	0.936	1.010
33	Staffs	6 641	1.182	1.148	1.217	6 683	1.139	1.107	1.172
34	E Suff	1 811	1.008	0.954	1.064	1 927	1.014	0.963	1.069
35	W Suff	800	1.071	0.986	1.163	815	1.109	1.023	1.203
36	Surrey	3 468	0.943	0.906	0.980	4 145	1.001	0.966	1.038
37	E Sussex	3 718	1.028	0.989	1.069	5 108	1.114	1.078	1.151
38	W Sussex	2 385	0.988	0.942	1.037	3 209	1.109	1.065	1.156
39	Warwicks	8 371	1.145	1.116	1.176	8 191	1.040	1.013	1.067
40	Westd	315	0.945	0.830	1.076	410	1.083	0.966	1.214
41	IOW	569	1.038	0.941	1.145	592	0.931	0.848	1.021
42	Wilts	1 991	1.030	0.977	1.085	2 033	1.010	0.960	1.063
43	Worcs	3 019	1.200	1.149	1.253	2 903	1.069	1.024	1.115
44	E Yorks	2 102	0.952	0.905	1.001	2 319	0.970	0.925	1.017
45	N Yorks	2 931	1.149	1.100	1.201	2 870	1.042	0.998	1.087
46	W Yorks	15 270	1.036	1.016	1.057	16 164	0.979	0.961	0.997
47	Ang	313	1.042	0.913	1.189	341	1.037	0.917	1.173
48	Brec	236	1.062	0.912	1.237	203	0.890	0.760	1.041
49	Caer	746	1.074	0.985	1.170	965	1.138	1.056	1.227
50	Card	277	1.035	0.899	1.190	305	0.965	0.848	1.099
51	Carm	816	1.113	1.026	1.208	799	0.905	0.836	0.980
52	Den	1 085	1.086	1.012	1.166	1 139	0.942	0.881	1.008
53	Fli	875	1.006	0.930	1.088	958	0.974	0.905	1.048
54	Glam	5 199	0.985	0.954	1.018	5 133	0.893	0.865	0.922
55	Meri	204	1.091	0.927	1.283	204	0.923	0.789	1.081
56	Monm	1 760	0.947	0.897	1.001	1 748	0.926	0.877	0.977
57	Mont	255	1.259	1.085	1.460	217	0.982	0.843	1.145
58	Pemb	414	0.928	0.829	1.039	460	0.958	0.862	1.064
59	Rad	120	1.052	0.851	1.301	111	1.057	0.850	1.315

OR = Odds ratio
CL = Confidence limits

Table A5.11 Cancer of Liver, All Ages, 1968–85

	County	Males				Females			
		Cases	OR	95% CL		Cases	OR	95% CL	
1	Beds	75	1.042	0.829	1.311	39	0.898	0.654	1.233
2	Berks	69	0.637	0.503	0.807	48	0.679	0.512	0.902
3	Bucks	107	1.044	0.862	1.265	46	0.716	0.536	0.957
4	Cambs	55	0.837	0.641	1.092	34	0.793	0.566	1.112
5	Ches	289	1.044	0.928	1.175	201	1.054	0.915	1.214
6	Cornwall	61	0.621	0.484	0.798	52	0.807	0.614	1.061
7	Cumberland	48	0.896	0.674	1.192	25	0.709	0.479	1.050
8	Derbys	158	0.904	0.771	1.059	167	1.511	1.296	1.762
9	Devon	177	0.774	0.667	0.899	143	0.922	0.781	1.090
10	Dorset	50	0.600	0.455	0.791	47	0.847	0.635	1.129
11	Durham	251	0.944	0.832	1.072	181	1.101	0.949	1.278
12	Essex	234	1.117	0.980	1.274	139	1.034	0.874	1.225
13	Glos	218	1.020	0.891	1.168	145	1.023	0.867	1.207
14	Hants	264	0.836	0.740	0.946	170	0.836	0.717	0.974
15	Hereford	26	0.870	0.591	1.282	8	0.432	0.220	0.848
16	Herts	106	0.773	0.638	0.936	90	1.052	0.854	1.297
17	Hunt	29	0.761	0.528	1.097	13	0.547	0.320	0.936
18	Kent	190	0.759	0.657	0.877	164	0.975	0.834	1.139
19	Lancs	1 145	1.218	1.145	1.297	719	1.107	1.023	1.197
20	Leics	118	0.888	0.740	1.066	91	1.030	0.837	1.269
21	Lincs H	24	0.994	0.664	1.490	15	1.048	0.629	1.745
22	Lincs K	34	0.763	0.544	1.069	37	1.268	0.917	1.754
23	Lincs L	81	0.944	0.757	1.177	61	1.151	0.893	1.483
24	London	1 600	1.326	1.256	1.400	927	1.107	1.032	1.188
25	Norfolk	63	0.462	0.362	0.588	54	0.606	0.464	0.790
26	Northants	60	0.630	0.489	0.811	58	0.957	0.738	1.241
27	Northd	197	1.170	1.014	1.348	99	0.912	0.747	1.113
28	Notts	158	0.821	0.701	0.962	134	1.110	0.935	1.319
29	Oxon	64	0.880	0.687	1.127	27	0.577	0.397	0.839
30	Rut	2	0.426	0.111	1.641	2	0.739	0.185	2.954
31	Salop	39	0.663	0.484	0.907	33	0.872	0.619	1.230
32	Somerset	131	0.819	0.689	0.974	93	0.865	0.704	1.062
33	Staffs	262	0.914	0.808	1.035	128	0.718	0.603	0.855
34	E Suff	60	0.699	0.542	0.900	26	0.469	0.322	0.683
35	W Suff	35	0.969	0.694	1.355	31	1.433	1.006	2.041
36	Surrey	149	0.840	0.714	0.989	98	0.813	0.666	0.993
37	E Sussex	144	0.861	0.729	1.016	105	0.796	0.656	0.966
38	W Sussex	89	0.799	0.648	0.985	56	0.664	0.511	0.863
39	Warwicks	366	0.997	0.897	1.108	185	0.788	0.681	0.912
40	Westd	11	0.706	0.391	1.276	4	0.362	0.141	0.928
41	IOW	23	0.890	0.589	1.344	20	1.112	0.715	1.730
42	Wilts	55	0.580	0.446	0.755	42	0.706	0.521	0.956
43	Worcs	89	0.698	0.566	0.860	61	0.757	0.588	0.974
44	E Yorks	78	0.740	0.592	0.925	60	0.873	0.677	1.126
45	N Yorks	111	0.878	0.727	1.060	65	0.799	0.625	1.020
46	W Yorks	775	1.091	1.013	1.175	545	1.157	1.059	1.263
47	Ang	15	1.037	0.622	1.728	15	1.540	0.928	2.555
48	Brec	14	1.309	0.771	2.220	12	1.860	1.061	3.259
49	Caer	47	1.440	1.079	1.922	29	1.184	0.821	1.706
50	Card	8	0.624	0.313	1.244	12	1.313	0.744	2.316
51	Carm	39	1.080	0.787	1.484	40	1.574	1.154	2.146
52	Den	77	1.631	1.303	2.042	53	1.534	1.171	2.010
53	Fli	68	1.659	1.306	2.108	51	1.795	1.365	2.360
54	Glam	315	1.237	1.105	1.386	191	1.162	1.005	1.342
55	Meri	11	1.219	0.671	2.214	19	3.076	1.994	4.744
56	Monm	117	1.315	1.095	1.580	84	1.530	1.234	1.897
57	Mont	13	1.322	0.764	2.287	7	1.087	0.516	2.291
58	Pemb	40	1.885	1.382	2.570	38	2.732	2.005	3.723
59	Rad	5	0.929	0.384	2.248	4	1.327	0.496	3.547

OR = Odds ratio
CL = Confidence limits

Table A5.12 Cancer of Gallbladder, All Ages, 1968–85

	County	Males				Females			
		Cases	OR	95% CL		Cases	OR	95%CL	
1	Beds	88	1.426	1.155	1.761	106	1.189	0.980	1.442
2	Berks	99	1.058	0.866	1.291	154	1.055	0.898	1.238
3	Bucks	90	1.003	0.814	1.236	130	0.981	0.824	1.168
4	Cambs	57	0.976	0.751	1.269	84	0.921	0.742	1.144
5	Ches	255	1.044	0.921	1.184	379	0.927	0.837	1.028
6	Cornwall	81	0.920	0.738	1.147	123	0.880	0.736	1.053
7	Cumberland	50	1.060	0.801	1.403	79	1.056	0.844	1.321
8	Derbys	174	1.132	0.973	1.317	262	1.109	0.980	1.255
9	Devon	183	0.882	0.761	1.022	271	0.795	0.704	0.897
10	Dorset	51	0.674	0.512	0.887	102	0.845	0.695	1.029
11	Durham	287	1.243	1.104	1.400	393	1.133	1.024	1.254
12	Essex	172	0.913	0.784	1.062	219	0.754	0.659	0.862
13	Glos	176	0.923	0.794	1.073	308	1.019	0.909	1.143
14	Hants	223	0.788	0.689	0.900	341	0.782	0.702	0.872
15	Hereford	21	0.780	0.508	1.198	45	1.148	0.853	1.543
16	Herts	108	0.909	0.751	1.101	167	0.933	0.799	1.088
17	Hunt	27	0.806	0.551	1.178	31	0.622	0.438	0.884
18	Kent	206	0.928	0.807	1.067	337	0.928	0.832	1.035
19	Lancs	862	1.016	0.946	1.091	1 369	0.963	0.910	1.019
20	Leics	126	1.079	0.903	1.288	211	1.127	0.983	1.293
21	Lincs H	10	0.460	0.251	0.844	27	0.875	0.598	1.280
22	Lincs K	33	0.830	0.589	1.171	62	0.990	0.769	1.273
23	Lincs L	57	0.744	0.573	0.967	85	0.750	0.605	0.929
24	London	1 120	1.006	0.944	1.072	1 794	0.987	0.938	1.038
25	Norfolk	105	0.865	0.713	1.050	194	1.021	0.885	1.178
26	Northants	95	1.142	0.931	1.400	164	1.299	1.112	1.518
27	Northd	167	1.120	0.960	1.307	236	1.018	0.894	1.160
28	Notts	205	1.224	1.065	1.408	303	1.183	1.054	1.328
29	Oxon	87	1.367	1.105	1.691	117	1.214	1.010	1.459
30	Rut	2	0.476	0.122	1.860	2	0.349	0.093	1.312
31	Salop	40	0.769	0.563	1.050	95	1.194	0.974	1.465
32	Somerset	148	1.035	0.878	1.219	218	0.939	0.821	1.075
33	Staffs	297	1.212	1.079	1.362	483	1.331	1.214	1.459
34	E Suff	74	0.961	0.763	1.211	113	0.957	0.794	1.154
35	W Suff	17	0.524	0.328	0.838	40	0.864	0.632	1.182
36	Surrey	145	0.929	0.787	1.096	238	0.933	0.820	1.062
37	E Sussex	127	0.819	0.687	0.976	261	0.893	0.789	1.011
38	W Sussex	89	0.867	0.703	1.070	179	0.975	0.840	1.132
39	Warwicks	379	1.197	1.079	1.328	657	1.370	1.266	1.483
40	Westd	9	0.635	0.331	1.217	28	1.183	0.813	1.722
41	IOW	16	0.680	0.417	1.111	31	0.782	0.549	1.115
42	Wilts	71	0.854	0.675	1.080	131	1.057	0.888	1.258
43	Worcs	127	1.154	0.967	1.378	195	1.152	0.999	1.329
44	E Yorks	89	0.949	0.769	1.171	121	0.817	0.682	0.979
45	N Yorks	112	1.007	0.834	1.215	190	1.114	0.963	1.287
46	W Yorks	694	1.104	1.021	1.195	1 094	1.079	1.013	1.148
47	Ang	13	1.014	0.586	1.754	28	1.362	0.937	1.981
48	Brec	4	0.412	0.159	1.070	13	0.922	0.533	1.596
49	Caer	29	0.973	0.674	1.404	54	1.007	0.769	1.319
50	Card	7	0.607	0.291	1.269	14	0.708	0.418	1.197
51	Carm	21	0.655	0.427	1.004	38	0.694	0.504	0.955
52	Den	36	0.831	0.598	1.155	46	0.609	0.456	0.812
53	Fli	33	0.885	0.628	1.249	48	0.780	0.586	1.037
54	Glam	211	0.932	0.813	1.070	321	0.909	0.813	1.017
55	Meri	6	0.735	0.331	1.632	9	0.652	0.339	1.252
56	Monm	69	0.873	0.688	1.108	118	1.019	0.849	1.224
57	Mont	7	0.778	0.370	1.635	10	0.721	0.388	1.341
58	Pemb	8	0.419	0.214	0.823	23	0.762	0.505	1.150
59	Rad	1	0.201	0.034	1.173	7	1.061	0.502	2.242

OR = Odds ratio
CL = Confidence limits

Odds ratios underlined were treated as outliers in categorizing values for the maps

Table A5.13 Cancer of Pancreas, All Ages, 1968–85

	County	Males Cases	OR	95% CL		Females Cases	OR	95% CL	
1	Beds	365	0.950	0.853	1.058	311	0.986	0.879	1.107
2	Berks	630	1.104	1.017	1.199	615	1.207	1.111	1.312
3	Bucks	577	1.052	0.965	1.146	489	1.051	0.959	1.153
4	Cambs	311	0.860	0.766	0.966	311	0.968	0.863	1.087
5	Ches	1 445	0.959	0.908	1.013	1 422	0.992	0.940	1.048
6	Cornwall	495	0.915	0.834	1.003	418	0.844	0.764	0.932
7	Cumberland	304	1.055	0.937	1.187	293	1.120	0.994	1.262
8	Derbys	950	1.002	0.937	1.072	827	0.991	0.923	1.064
9	Devon	1 194	0.939	0.884	0.997	1 151	0.963	0.906	1.023
10	Dorset	419	0.907	0.820	1.003	372	0.871	0.784	0.968
11	Durham	1 435	1.001	0.948	1.058	1 240	1.015	0.957	1.076
12	Essex	1 113	0.964	0.906	1.026	1 039	1.028	0.965	1.096
13	Glos	1 068	0.908	0.853	0.968	1 002	0.935	0.876	0.998
14	Hants	1 454	0.834	0.790	0.881	1 410	0.922	0.873	0.974
15	Hereford	133	0.801	0.672	0.956	142	1.022	0.861	1.214
16	Herts	727	0.998	0.924	1.077	593	0.938	0.863	1.020
17	Hunt	200	0.977	0.845	1.130	191	1.105	0.953	1.281
18	Kent	1 536	1.145	1.086	1.208	1 421	1.125	1.065	1.189
19	Lancs	5 373	1.036	1.005	1.067	5 053	1.019	0.989	1.051
20	Leics	662	0.917	0.846	0.993	639	0.963	0.889	1.045
21	Lincs H	137	1.038	0.870	1.238	112	1.037	0.856	1.257
22	Lincs K	223	0.914	0.797	1.048	228	1.038	0.907	1.188
23	Lincs L	484	1.040	0.947	1.143	376	0.948	0.853	1.052
24	London	7 151	1.056	1.029	1.084	6 558	1.031	1.003	1.059
25	Norfolk	694	0.933	0.863	1.009	729	1.095	1.015	1.182
26	Northants	522	1.022	0.933	1.118	430	0.955	0.865	1.053
27	Northd	910	0.989	0.924	1.059	823	1.010	0.941	1.085
28	Notts	1 034	0.999	0.936	1.065	912	1.005	0.939	1.076
29	Oxon	367	0.930	0.835	1.035	372	1.093	0.983	1.215
30	Rut	20	0.778	0.495	1.223	25	1.270	0.844	1.910
31	Salop	317	0.996	0.887	1.119	291	1.037	0.920	1.169
32	Somerset	806	0.912	0.848	0.980	762	0.927	0.861	0.998
33	Staffs	1 662	1.104	1.048	1.162	1 339	1.039	0.982	1.099
34	E Suff	428	0.903	0.817	0.997	400	0.957	0.864	1.060
35	W Suff	195	0.989	0.853	1.146	151	0.928	0.787	1.095
36	Surrey	978	1.025	0.959	1.095	919	1.026	0.958	1.098
37	E Sussex	1 082	1.161	1.089	1.237	1 124	1.103	1.038	1.174
38	W Sussex	650	1.043	0.961	1.131	713	1.108	1.026	1.197
39	Warwicks	1 955	0.993	0.947	1.041	1 625	0.939	0.892	0.988
40	Westd	78	0.898	0.712	1.132	95	1.145	0.929	1.412
41	IOW	122	0.842	0.700	1.014	152	1.101	0.933	1.300
42	Wilts	478	0.937	0.853	1.029	409	0.932	0.843	1.031
43	Worcs	684	1.009	0.933	1.092	591	0.987	0.907	1.074
44	E Yorks	595	1.039	0.955	1.131	581	1.131	1.038	1.231
45	N Yorks	707	1.037	0.959	1.121	617	1.028	0.947	1.116
46	W Yorks	3 890	0.998	0.965	1.033	3 474	0.962	0.928	0.997
47	Ang	86	1.097	0.878	1.371	66	0.906	0.707	1.162
48	Brec	51	0.862	0.648	1.146	47	0.954	0.710	1.280
49	Caer	189	1.038	0.893	1.206	160	0.838	0.714	0.984
50	Card	77	1.108	0.877	1.401	53	0.757	0.574	0.999
51	Carm	172	0.871	0.746	1.018	161	0.837	0.714	0.981
52	Den	233	0.875	0.765	1.000	200	0.748	0.649	0.863
53	Fli	202	0.879	0.761	1.015	185	0.852	0.734	0.989
54	Glam	1 367	0.986	0.932	1.043	1 146	0.924	0.870	0.982
55	Meri	48	0.959	0.713	1.290	36	0.733	0.524	1.027
56	Monm	496	1.029	0.938	1.129	444	1.099	0.998	1.212
57	Mont	56	1.020	0.775	1.342	39	0.791	0.572	1.092
58	Pemb	114	0.980	0.808	1.187	102	0.969	0.792	1.185
59	Rad	24	0.791	0.523	1.196	16	0.673	0.408	1.112

OR = Odds ratio
CL = Confidence limits

Table A5.14 Cancers of Nose, Ear, and Nasal Sinuses, All Ages, 1968–85

County	Males				Females			
	Cases	OR	95% CL		Cases	OR	95%CL	
1 Beds	39	1.146	0.835	1.572	21	0.895	0.582	1.375
2 Berks	53	1.055	0.804	1.385	32	0.847	0.598	1.200
3 Bucks	89	1.871	1.520	2.303	48	1.393	1.048	1.852
4 Cambs	25	0.830	0.560	1.231	25	1.096	0.739	1.625
5 Ches	108	0.834	0.689	1.010	88	0.849	0.687	1.050
6 Cornwall	37	0.840	0.608	1.162	34	0.993	0.708	1.393
7 Cumberland	24	0.972	0.650	1.454	15	0.791	0.477	1.313
8 Derbys	99	1.232	1.009	1.505	56	0.923	0.708	1.203
9 Devon	101	0.990	0.812	1.207	82	1.003	0.805	1.250
10 Dorset	34	0.911	0.650	1.278	24	0.817	0.547	1.221
11 Durham	88	0.705	0.571	0.871	75	0.831	0.661	1.045
12 Essex	110	1.147	0.948	1.387	94	1.327	1.081	1.628
13 Glos	113	1.155	0.958	1.393	78	1.029	0.822	1.289
14 Hants	125	0.867	0.725	1.036	107	0.994	0.819	1.205
15 Hereford	21	1.551	1.011	2.379	3	0.304	0.105	0.887
16 Herts	77	1.209	0.964	1.516	41	0.881	0.647	1.199
17 Hunt	21	1.190	0.774	1.830	13	1.016	0.589	1.754
18 Kent	121	1.071	0.894	1.285	95	1.060	0.864	1.301
19 Lancs	429	0.959	0.868	1.061	370	1.050	0.942	1.171
20 Leics	55	0.896	0.686	1.170	59	1.247	0.964	1.614
21 Lincs H	4	0.362	0.141	0.928	12	1.547	0.880	2.719
22 Lincs K	27	1.328	0.909	1.940	8	0.502	0.254	0.992
23 Lincs L	27	0.681	0.467	0.993	36	1.263	0.909	1.754
24 London	590	1.008	0.924	1.100	478	1.058	0.960	1.166
25 Norfolk	70	1.151	0.908	1.459	46	0.972	0.726	1.301
26 Northants	65	1.504	1.178	1.921	30	0.924	0.644	1.324
27 Northd	64	0.814	0.636	1.042	50	0.851	0.643	1.126
28 Notts	100	1.131	0.927	1.381	68	1.041	0.819	1.325
29 Oxon	38	1.133	0.822	1.561	29	1.165	0.808	1.680
30 Rut	3	1.407	0.454	4.365	3	2.101	0.691	6.387
31 Salop	18	0.663	0.418	1.051	18	0.884	0.556	1.406
32 Somerset	68	0.939	0.738	1.194	49	0.857	0.646	1.136
33 Staffs	149	1.117	0.948	1.316	91	0.937	0.760	1.154
34 E Suff	38	0.977	0.709	1.346	29	0.989	0.686	1.427
35 W Suff	17	1.031	0.639	1.663	11	0.945	0.522	1.709
36 Surrey	93	1.138	0.926	1.399	74	1.155	0.917	1.455
37 E Sussex	87	1.177	0.951	1.456	69	1.012	0.796	1.285
38 W Sussex	39	0.780	0.569	1.070	38	0.870	0.632	1.199
39 Warwicks	163	0.951	0.813	1.113	117	0.925	0.769	1.113
40 Westd	2	0.284	0.077	1.041	4	0.685	0.258	1.818
41 IOW	12	1.035	0.586	1.828	12	1.252	0.710	2.209
42 Wilts	46	1.062	0.793	1.421	37	1.168	0.844	1.616
43 Worcs	58	0.988	0.762	1.281	50	1.155	0.873	1.528
44 E Yorks	43	0.894	0.662	1.209	36	0.978	0.703	1.359
45 N Yorks	58	0.990	0.763	1.284	38	0.867	0.630	1.195
46 W Yorks	333	1.009	0.902	1.129	269	1.053	0.929	1.193
47 Ang	4	0.599	0.227	1.583	5	0.954	0.396	2.297
48 Brec	7	1.436	0.684	3.014	3	0.852	0.274	2.644
49 Caer	8	0.535	0.270	1.060	8	0.619	0.311	1.232
50 Card	7	1.201	0.571	2.527	5	1.028	0.427	2.477
51 Carm	17	1.021	0.633	1.646	16	1.158	0.708	1.895
52 Den	21	0.967	0.629	1.487	9	0.482	0.254	0.914
53 Fli	13	0.683	0.397	1.175	12	0.786	0.446	1.384
54 Glam	106	0.887	0.731	1.076	87	0.968	0.782	1.198
55 Meri	6	1.470	0.660	3.270	4	1.184	0.443	3.160
56 Monm	30	0.720	0.503	1.031	27	0.900	0.616	1.315
57 Mont	2	0.442	0.114	1.704	2	0.580	0.147	2.284
58 Pemb	12	1.194	0.677	2.108	3	0.387	0.130	1.151
59 Rad	1	0.415	0.062	2.775	2	1.245	0.311	4.981

OR = Odds ratio
CL = Confidence limits

Odds ratios underlined were treated as outliers in categorizing values for the maps

Table A5.15 Cancer of Larynx, All Ages, 1968–85

	County	Males				Females			
		Cases	OR	95% CL		Cases	OR	95% CL	
1	Beds	197	0.998	0.864	1.151	31	0.842	0.591	1.200
2	Berks	274	0.949	0.841	1.072	50	0.861	0.651	1.138
3	Bucks	291	1.057	0.939	1.190	47	0.871	0.653	1.161
4	Cambs	138	0.783	0.661	0.928	23	0.654	0.435	0.983
5	Ches	755	0.998	0.926	1.074	181	1.127	0.971	1.308
6	Cornwall	172	0.656	0.564	0.763	27	0.508	0.351	0.737
7	Cumberland	134	0.920	0.774	1.094	36	1.214	0.874	1.687
8	Derbys	497	1.053	0.961	1.153	89	0.935	0.758	1.154
9	Devon	470	0.773	0.705	0.849	95	0.762	0.622	0.933
10	Dorset	194	0.884	0.765	1.021	33	0.733	0.520	1.031
11	Durham	767	1.056	0.981	1.137	180	1.269	1.093	1.474
12	Essex	607	1.087	1.001	1.180	99	0.903	0.740	1.103
13	Glos	509	0.876	0.801	0.958	91	0.776	0.631	0.955
14	Hants	829	0.995	0.927	1.068	153	0.931	0.792	1.094
15	Hereford	68	0.848	0.665	1.080	10	0.656	0.354	1.217
16	Herts	359	0.960	0.863	1.068	65	0.890	0.697	1.138
17	Hunt	93	0.913	0.742	1.124	17	0.853	0.529	1.374
18	Kent	680	1.030	0.953	1.114	126	0.914	0.765	1.091
19	Lancs	3 047	1.187	1.141	1.234	706	1.315	1.214	1.424
20	Leics	327	0.911	0.815	1.019	64	0.862	0.673	1.104
21	Lincs H	61	0.937	0.725	1.211	11	0.893	0.493	1.617
22	Lincs K	108	0.903	0.744	1.095	20	0.806	0.520	1.251
23	Lincs L	239	1.034	0.908	1.178	33	0.732	0.520	1.030
24	London	3 735	1.107	1.068	1.147	728	1.040	0.961	1.126
25	Norfolk	316	0.875	0.782	0.980	61	0.833	0.647	1.072
26	Northants	253	1.003	0.883	1.138	35	0.699	0.502	0.974
27	Northd	475	1.030	0.939	1.131	112	1.217	1.008	1.468
28	Notts	492	0.946	0.863	1.036	99	0.965	0.791	1.179
29	Oxon	175	0.898	0.772	1.046	29	0.754	0.524	1.087
30	Rut	11	0.897	0.492	1.638	2	0.884	0.221	3.542
31	Salop	96	0.597	0.488	0.729	16	0.498	0.307	0.807
32	Somerset	367	0.864	0.778	0.960	57	0.652	0.503	0.846
33	Staffs	813	1.032	0.961	1.109	138	0.874	0.738	1.036
34	E Suff	158	0.686	0.586	0.803	37	0.827	0.598	1.143
35	W Suff	83	0.858	0.689	1.069	20	1.120	0.721	1.741
36	Surrey	430	0.893	0.810	0.984	97	0.977	0.799	1.195
37	E Sussex	393	0.898	0.811	0.994	97	0.971	0.794	1.188
38	W Sussex	228	0.777	0.681	0.887	53	0.828	0.631	1.086
39	Warwicks	962	0.947	0.886	1.011	170	0.846	0.725	0.986
40	Westd	42	1.025	0.752	1.398	7	0.782	0.372	1.642
41	IOW	59	0.854	0.658	1.108	13	0.889	0.515	1.535
42	Wilts	221	0.874	0.764	1.000	48	0.974	0.732	1.295
43	Worcs	320	0.923	0.825	1.033	59	0.853	0.659	1.103
44	E Yorks	353	1.266	1.136	1.410	65	1.132	0.886	1.447
45	N Yorks	359	1.048	0.942	1.166	77	1.128	0.900	1.414
46	W Yorks	988	1.021	0.974	1.070	452	1.142	1.037	1.259
47	Ang	35	0.893	0.637	1.251	4	0.492	0.188	1.288
48	Brec	36	1.251	0.894	1.751	7	1.273	0.606	2.677
49	Caer	92	1.053	0.854	1.299	18	0.925	0.581	1.471
50	Card	29	0.851	0.587	1.233	6	0.804	0.361	1.791
51	Carm	88	0.885	0.715	1.096	30	1.363	0.952	1.951
52	Den	121	0.949	0.790	1.138	33	1.156	0.820	1.629
53	Fli	102	0.919	0.754	1.121	25	1.063	0.716	1.576
54	Glam	750	1.075	0.997	1.158	181	1.279	1.102	1.483
55	Meri	19	0.778	0.493	1.230	4	0.765	0.287	2.040
56	Monm	220	0.897	0.783	1.027	54	1.151	0.879	1.507
57	Mont	15	0.562	0.339	0.932	7	1.322	0.630	2.775
58	Pemb	70	1.189	0.935	1.513	12	0.984	0.558	1.738
59	Rad	9	0.628	0.326	1.209	3	1.201	0.386	3.734

OR = Odds ratio
CL = Confidence limits

Table A5.16 Cancer of Lung, Ages 0–44, 1968–85

	County	Males				Females			
		Cases	OR	95% CL		Cases	OR	95% CL	
1	Beds	50	0.595	0.443	0.799	38	1.235	0.884	1.725
2	Berks	73	0.621	0.486	0.793	32	0.603	0.423	0.860
3	Bucks	84	0.742	0.591	0.932	44	0.920	0.676	1.252
4	Cambs	37	0.642	0.457	0.903	19	0.730	0.461	1.156
5	Ches	305	1.262	1.110	1.435	139	1.278	1.069	1.529
6	Cornwall	44	0.635	0.463	0.870	22	0.681	0.441	1.049
7	Cumberland	44	0.893	0.647	1.231	28	1.568	1.056	2.329
8	Derbys	149	0.955	0.800	1.139	47	0.673	0.502	0.904
9	Devon	89	0.574	0.460	0.715	41	0.600	0.438	0.821
10	Dorset	34	0.534	0.375	0.760	20	0.790	0.501	1.244
11	Durham	340	1.524	1.347	1.725	154	1.583	1.334	1.880
12	Essex	140	0.824	0.689	0.985	78	1.070	0.845	1.354
13	Glos	138	0.802	0.670	0.962	42	0.513	0.378	0.697
14	Hants	200	0.726	0.625	0.844	94	0.794	0.643	0.980
15	Hereford	19	0.788	0.485	1.279	3	0.311	0.104	0.929
16	Herts	114	0.853	0.698	1.041	54	0.883	0.668	1.167
17	Hunt	36	0.878	0.616	1.254	15	0.803	0.476	1.353
18	Kent	173	0.858	0.728	1.011	91	1.047	0.842	1.301
19	Lancs	1 160	1.627	1.516	1.745	485	1.507	1.362	1.667
20	Leics	129	1.049	0.866	1.270	45	0.871	0.643	1.179
21	Lincs H	14	0.842	0.482	1.471	4	0.531	0.198	1.425
22	Lincs K	30	0.804	0.548	1.179	16	0.924	0.560	1.527
23	Lincs L	69	1.013	0.782	1.312	21	0.687	0.442	1.069
24	London	1 001	0.876	0.815	0.942	537	1.168	1.061	1.287
25	Norfolk	78	0.762	0.600	0.969	29	0.585	0.404	0.847
26	Northants	76	0.859	0.672	1.099	26	0.654	0.440	0.972
27	Northd	163	1.275	1.071	1.517	100	1.740	1.408	2.152
28	Notts	167	0.978	0.828	1.156	74	1.110	0.872	1.414
29	Oxon	40	0.534	0.385	0.740	29	0.930	0.637	1.358
30	Rut	2	0.483	0.122	1.908	2	0.967	0.221	4.238
31	Salop	56	1.102	0.823	1.477	17	0.725	0.443	1.186
32	Somerset	81	0.635	0.505	0.800	20	0.334	0.219	0.512
33	Staffs	345	1.261	1.118	1.423	123	1.011	0.838	1.221
34	E Suff	30	0.439	0.305	0.633	20	0.632	0.403	0.992
35	W Suff	23	0.771	0.497	1.197	7	0.488	0.232	1.027
36	Surrey	133	0.783	0.651	0.940	56	0.783	0.596	1.028
37	E Sussex	77	0.756	0.594	0.961	32	0.679	0.474	0.971
38	W Sussex	58	0.817	0.619	1.077	21	0.618	0.399	0.957
39	Warwicks	334	1.035	0.917	1.167	122	0.828	0.686	0.999
40	Westd	9	0.810	0.397	1.656	3	0.575	0.181	1.829
41	IOW	10	0.538	0.280	1.036	9	1.185	0.588	2.390
42	Wilts	60	0.689	0.528	0.899	22	0.548	0.359	0.837
43	Worcs	122	1.032	0.847	1.257	37	0.817	0.583	1.145
44	E Yorks	99	1.207	0.969	1.504	46	1.255	0.923	1.707
45	N Yorks	143	1.305	1.085	1.570	67	1.384	1.071	1.788
46	W Yorks	716	1.288	1.183	1.403	291	1.157	1.020	1.312
47	Ang	16	1.438	0.818	2.528	5	0.873	0.349	2.183
48	Brec	7	1.004	0.449	2.247	1	0.253	0.041	1.556
49	Caer	33	1.471	0.992	2.179	9	0.814	0.414	1.603
50	Card	8	0.879	0.422	1.832	2	0.524	0.129	2.130
51	Carm	24	0.881	0.567	1.370	10	0.665	0.352	1.255
52	Den	29	0.919	0.620	1.360	16	0.886	0.532	1.476
53	Fli	29	0.822	0.558	1.213	14	0.960	0.552	1.668
54	Glam	189	0.864	0.739	1.010	86	0.863	0.691	1.078
55	Meri	8	1.111	0.525	2.352	0	0.000		
56	Monm	69	0.908	0.702	1.175	29	0.715	0.492	1.039
57	Mont	1	0.145	0.025	0.840	2	0.607	0.153	2.410
58	Pemb	11	0.474	0.257	0.876	8	0.849	0.419	1.724
59	Rad	6	1.756	0.689	4.474	0	0.000		

OR = Odds ratio
CL = Confidence limits

Odds ratios underlined were treated as outliers in categorizing values for the maps

Table A5.17 Cancer of Lung, Ages 45+, 1968–85

	County	Males				Females			
		Cases	OR	95% CL		Cases	OR	95% CL	
1	Beds	3 420	0.950	0.907	0.994	879	0.945	0.878	1.016
2	Berks	4 971	0.930	0.895	0.966	1 553	1.071	1.013	1.132
3	Bucks	5 055	0.994	0.957	1.033	1 505	1.128	1.066	1.194
4	Cambs	2 844	0.853	0.812	0.896	796	0.880	0.816	0.949
5	Ches	14 575	1.042	1.018	1.066	4 206	1.016	0.982	1.051
6	Cornwall	3 458	0.680	0.652	0.710	1 046	0.744	0.697	0.795
7	Cumberland	2 397	0.883	0.837	0.932	653	0.844	0.776	0.917
8	Derbys	8 181	0.922	0.895	0.950	1 956	0.793	0.755	0.832
9	Devon	8 849	0.744	0.723	0.764	2 807	0.844	0.811	0.879
10	Dorset	3 180	0.741	0.709	0.776	983	0.820	0.766	0.877
11	Durham	14 850	1.115	1.090	1.141	3 816	1.047	1.011	1.086
12	Essex	10 463	0.976	0.950	1.002	2 964	1.048	1.007	1.092
13	Glos	9 708	0.885	0.861	0.909	2 473	0.809	0.775	0.845
14	Hants	13 668	0.855	0.836	0.875	4 194	0.986	0.954	1.020
15	Hereford	1 115	0.725	0.672	0.782	313	0.783	0.694	0.882
16	Herts	6 921	1.014	0.981	1.048	2 028	1.119	1.066	1.175
17	Hunt	1 810	0.955	0.897	1.018	484	0.963	0.873	1.063
18	Kent	12 989	1.032	1.007	1.058	4 010	1.130	1.091	1.170
19	Lancs	55 890	1.169	1.154	1.183	15 939	1.124	1.104	1.145
20	Leics	5 934	0.881	0.851	0.912	1 433	0.740	0.699	0.782
21	Lincs H	991	0.799	0.736	0.867	237	0.733	0.639	0.840
22	Lincs K	2 120	0.941	0.887	0.997	633	0.994	0.912	1.084
23	Lincs L	4 198	0.961	0.922	1.002	1 065	0.916	0.857	0.978
24	London	73 451	1.184	1.171	1.197	22 784	1.335	1.314	1.357
25	Norfolk	6 373	0.920	0.889	0.951	1 665	0.871	0.826	0.918
26	Northants	4 371	0.919	0.883	0.957	1 191	0.933	0.876	0.993
27	Northd	9 893	1.162	1.130	1.196	2 850	1.208	1.159	1.260
28	Notts	9 326	0.962	0.935	0.989	2 473	0.934	0.894	0.975
29	Oxon	3 194	0.872	0.832	0.914	1 013	1.046	0.976	1.120
30	Rut	209	0.896	0.746	1.077	66	1.170	0.894	1.531
31	Salop	2 855	0.965	0.918	1.015	652	0.785	0.722	0.853
32	Somerset	6 256	0.760	0.736	0.785	1 679	0.726	0.690	0.764
33	Staffs	16 203	1.138	1.113	1.164	3 189	0.794	0.764	0.825
34	E Suff	3 696	0.839	0.804	0.877	940	0.801	0.747	0.858
35	W Suff	1 549	0.837	0.783	0.895	443	0.956	0.863	1.059
36	Surrey	8 340	0.931	0.904	0.959	2 835	1.127	1.082	1.175
37	E Sussex	8 092	0.936	0.909	0.965	2 829	1.048	1.005	1.092
38	W Sussex	5 442	0.953	0.918	0.988	1 853	1.085	1.032	1.142
39	Warwicks	19 287	1.039	1.019	1.060	4 773	0.935	0.906	0.965
40	Westd	658	0.825	0.746	0.913	182	0.763	0.652	0.892
41	IOW	1 132	0.838	0.775	0.907	329	0.837	0.744	0.941
42	Wilts	3 964	0.834	0.800	0.869	1 164	0.920	0.863	0.980
43	Worcs	6 402	1.004	0.970	1.039	1 549	0.866	0.820	0.915
44	E Yorks	5 917	1.113	1.074	1.155	1 609	1.085	1.027	1.146
45	N Yorks	6 944	1.098	1.062	1.135	2 023	1.169	1.113	1.228
46	W Yorks	36 987	1.014	0.999	1.029	9 801	0.937	0.916	0.958
47	Ang	655	0.882	0.795	0.978	173	0.813	0.691	0.955
48	Brec	400	0.705	0.622	0.800	84	0.574	0.459	0.719
49	Caer	1 609	0.949	0.887	1.015	346	0.654	0.585	0.731
50	Card	479	0.726	0.647	0.815	104	0.512	0.420	0.625
51	Carm	1 295	0.687	0.641	0.737	272	0.462	0.409	0.522
52	Den	2 095	0.844	0.797	0.894	568	0.749	0.686	0.819
53	Fli	1 962	0.922	0.868	0.980	535	0.864	0.788	0.948
54	Glam	11 179	0.845	0.824	0.866	2 850	0.761	0.731	0.792
55	Meri	368	0.782	0.684	0.894	94	0.670	0.541	0.831
56	Monm	4 164	0.911	0.874	0.949	941	0.776	0.724	0.832
57	Mont	371	0.722	0.633	0.824	93	0.663	0.535	0.823
58	Pemb	855	0.772	0.707	0.842	201	0.632	0.546	0.731
59	Rad	149	0.532	0.439	0.644	51	0.756	0.562	1.016

OR = Odds ratio
CL = Confidence limits

Odds ratios underlined were treated as outliers in categorizing values for the maps

Table A5.18 Cancer of Pleura, All Ages, 1968–85

	County	Males				Females			
		Cases	OR	95% CL		Cases	OR	95%CL	
1	Beds	19	0.544	0.349	0.849	8	0.810	0.405	1.622
2	Berks	44	0.872	0.648	1.175	6	0.382	0.176	0.827
3	Bucks	68	1.417	1.115	1.801	17	1.182	0.733	1.908
4	Cambs	13	0.430	0.254	0.731	10	1.067	0.572	1.988
5	Ches	201	1.567	1.361	1.805	40	0.928	0.677	1.271
6	Cornwall	34	0.775	0.553	1.086	9	0.637	0.333	1.222
7	Cumberland	9	0.357	0.190	0.668	1	0.126	0.024	0.656
8	Derbys	55	0.666	0.511	0.867	20	0.785	0.505	1.220
9	Devon	174	1.762	1.515	2.048	13	0.387	0.229	0.656
10	Dorset	15	0.402	0.246	0.656	1	0.082	0.018	0.381
11	Durham	183	1.474	1.271	1.709	67	1.800	1.412	2.294
12	Essex	111	1.157	0.958	1.398	30	1.027	0.715	1.476
13	Glos	67	0.669	0.526	0.851	18	0.573	0.362	0.907
14	Hants	261	1.895	1.674	2.145	32	0.719	0.507	1.020
15	Hereford	5	0.365	0.157	0.847	3	0.742	0.240	2.297
16	Herts	63	0.965	0.752	1.239	22	1.139	0.747	1.736
17	Hunt	15	0.847	0.510	1.408	4	0.744	0.280	1.979
18	Kent	169	1.517	1.301	1.769	41	1.121	0.821	1.530
19	Lancs	599	1.370	1.257	1.494	210	1.497	1.293	1.733
20	Leics	30	0.480	0.338	0.683	26	1.324	0.899	1.951
21	Lincs H	3	0.269	0.093	0.772	1	0.306	0.048	1.952
22	Lincs K	5	0.243	0.108	0.544	3	0.454	0.151	1.370
23	Lincs L	24	0.598	0.402	0.891	5	0.416	0.177	0.974
24	London	603	1.014	0.930	1.106	250	1.413	1.232	1.620
25	Norfolk	58	0.947	0.730	1.229	18	0.923	0.580	1.470
26	Northants	23	0.522	0.349	0.782	9	0.672	0.350	1.289
27	Northd	186	2.419	2.096	2.793	34	1.395	0.993	1.958
28	Notts	55	0.606	0.465	0.788	46	1.717	1.283	2.297
29	Oxon	16	0.473	0.293	0.765	11	1.072	0.592	1.942
30	Rut	1	0.471	0.069	3.210	0	0.000		
31	Salop	8	0.291	0.152	0.559	3	0.351	0.119	1.036
32	Somerset	51	0.705	0.535	0.928	18	0.773	0.486	1.229
33	Staffs	71	0.504	0.400	0.634	29	0.688	0.477	0.993
34	E Suff	50	1.300	0.983	1.719	7	0.585	0.280	1.218
35	W Suff	16	0.970	0.593	1.589	4	0.826	0.310	2.202
36	Surrey	56	0.670	0.515	0.871	15	0.564	0.341	0.931
37	E Sussex	54	0.737	0.564	0.964	12	0.441	0.254	0.767
38	W Sussex	36	0.736	0.530	1.021	14	0.813	0.480	1.376
39	Warwicks	124	0.694	0.581	0.829	29	0.535	0.373	0.769
40	Westd	3	0.430	0.143	1.291	3	1.261	0.407	3.910
41	IOW	21	1.819	1.189	2.784	1	0.255	0.041	1.568
42	Wilts	41	0.942	0.692	1.283	11	0.829	0.458	1.501
43	Worcs	33	0.545	0.388	0.764	7	0.378	0.185	0.773
44	E Yorks	31	0.635	0.447	0.902	11	0.715	0.396	1.292
45	N Yorks	72	1.217	0.963	1.538	14	0.763	0.451	1.290
46	W Yorks	313	0.924	0.823	1.037	124	1.179	0.980	1.419
47	Ang	7	1.042	0.495	2.193	2	0.917	0.229	3.675
48	Brec	2	0.400	0.105	1.528	1	0.678	0.096	4.761
49	Caer	10	0.670	0.361	1.244	3	0.574	0.187	1.758
50	Card	1	0.172	0.030	0.967	3	1.509	0.489	4.657
51	Carm	12	0.701	0.399	1.235	6	1.020	0.457	2.275
52	Den	8	0.367	0.188	0.714	5	0.649	0.272	1.553
53	Fli	8	0.419	0.214	0.821	7	1.105	0.526	2.323
54	Glam	84	0.683	0.550	0.847	41	1.077	0.789	1.471
55	Meri	5	1.215	0.504	2.927	3	2.144	0.707	6.497
56	Monm	29	0.683	0.475	0.983	12	0.949	0.537	1.676
57	Mont	2	0.447	0.116	1.731	1	0.707	0.101	4.972
58	Pemb	8	0.774	0.387	1.549	4	1.219	0.457	3.250
59	Rad	1	0.420	0.063	2.809	0	0.000		

OR = Odds ratio
CL = Confidence limits

Odds ratios underlined were treated as outliers in categorizing values for the maps

Table A5.19 Cancer of Bone, Ages 0–24, 1968–85

	County	Males				Females			
		Cases	OR	95% CL		Cases	OR	95% CL	
1	Beds	14	0.817	0.459	1.453	18	1.819	1.080	3.064
2	Berks	19	0.754	0.460	1.237	15	0.921	0.540	1.570
3	Bucks	26	1.108	0.717	1.712	10	0.504	0.269	0.943
4	Cambs	13	1.208	0.636	2.295	7	0.810	0.359	1.826
5	Ches	47	1.058	0.767	1.461	42	1.271	0.907	1.780
6	Cornwall	15	1.031	0.600	1.775	6	0.635	0.263	1.533
7	Cumberland	13	1.491	0.798	2.786	3	0.480	0.149	1.549
8	Derbys	27	0.998	0.659	1.511	18	0.754	0.460	1.237
9	Devon	30	1.035	0.692	1.546	22	0.978	0.618	1.547
10	Dorset	10	0.919	0.479	1.765	7	0.829	0.374	1.834
11	Durham	37	1.037	0.720	1.494	37	1.269	0.883	1.825
12	Essex	32	0.963	0.648	1.431	32	1.542	1.040	2.285
13	Glos	21	0.678	0.428	1.074	27	1.069	0.709	1.610
14	Hants	46	0.991	0.719	1.365	48	1.205	0.885	1.641
15	Hereford	3	0.672	0.211	2.137	9	3.006	1.367	6.609
16	Herts	21	0.839	0.532	1.324	17	0.914	0.551	1.515
17	Hunt	4	0.450	0.164	1.233	11	2.795	1.412	5.531
18	Kent	30	0.811	0.552	1.191	31	1.038	0.696	1.546
19	Lancs	136	1.034	0.851	1.256	119	1.177	0.954	1.452
20	Leics	31	1.486	0.988	2.235	18	1.074	0.656	1.758
21	Lincs H	3	0.759	0.236	2.443	3	0.929	0.284	3.043
22	Lincs K	6	0.932	0.381	2.275	9	1.525	0.743	3.131
23	Lincs L	19	1.433	0.841	2.442	6	0.521	0.230	1.180
24	London	196	1.005	0.852	1.185	150	1.014	0.842	1.222
25	Norfolk	23	1.296	0.820	2.048	17	1.285	0.753	2.191
26	Northants	18	1.153	0.681	1.952	10	0.659	0.344	1.264
27	Northd	27	0.941	0.623	1.421	12	0.709	0.389	1.293
28	Notts	24	0.669	0.434	1.031	30	1.447	0.979	2.138
29	Oxon	16	1.247	0.723	2.148	6	0.517	0.225	1.187
30	Rut	2	2.211	0.475	10.286	1	2.408	0.347	16.719
31	Salop	12	1.185	0.619	2.269	3	0.397	0.125	1.255
32	Somerset	18	0.723	0.438	1.193	16	0.960	0.564	1.634
33	Staffs	53	1.156	0.849	1.575	29	0.778	0.527	1.148
34	E Suff	4	0.348	0.131	0.927	16	1.654	0.959	2.854
35	W Suff	3	0.455	0.141	1.464	1	0.198	0.037	1.049
36	Surrey	27	0.942	0.617	1.439	24	1.065	0.687	1.652
37	E Sussex	16	0.880	0.503	1.538	12	0.892	0.489	1.628
38	W Sussex	13	0.914	0.503	1.664	12	1.222	0.684	2.182
39	Warwicks	49	0.859	0.632	1.169	50	1.002	0.739	1.359
40	Westd	3	1.431	0.436	4.694	2	1.324	0.262	6.682
41	IOW	3	1.153	0.306	4.350	0	0.000		
42	Wilts	17	0.979	0.578	1.657	14	0.942	0.531	1.672
43	Worcs	20	1.013	0.626	1.641	14	0.996	0.572	1.735
44	E Yorks	13	0.917	0.499	1.686	7	0.675	0.311	1.464
45	N Yorks	16	0.782	0.454	1.348	16	1.006	0.588	1.719
46	W Yorks	125	1.187	0.968	1.457	66	0.759	0.580	0.993
47	Ang	2	0.873	0.197	3.858	1	0.377	0.056	2.549
48	Brec	0	0.000			1	1.765	0.254	12.269
49	Caer	4	0.942	0.317	2.803	0	0.000		
50	Card	0	0.000			0	0.000		
51	Carm	3	0.541	0.167	1.755	5	1.231	0.495	3.062
52	Den	2	<u>0.214</u>	0.065	0.710	4	0.650	0.229	1.844
53	Fli	13	2.245	1.195	4.217	11	1.669	0.866	3.215
54	Glam	53	1.277	0.942	1.732	30	0.903	0.611	1.335
55	Meri	2	1.705	0.312	9.313	0	0.000		
56	Monm	22	1.548	0.940	2.548	12	0.900	0.484	1.673
57	Mont	1	0.981	0.159	6.033	0	0.000		
58	Pemb	7	2.337	0.962	5.677	3	0.897	0.262	3.069
59	Rad	0	0.000			0	0.000		

OR = Odds ratio
CL = Confidence limits

Odds ratios underlined were treated as outliers in categorizing values for the maps

Table A5.20 Cancer of Bone, Ages 25+, 1968–85

	County	Males				Females			
		Cases	OR	95% CL		Cases	OR	95% CL	
1	Beds	20	0.782	0.503	1.216	18	0.942	0.593	1.498
2	Berks	30	0.784	0.547	1.125	25	0.812	0.547	1.205
3	Bucks	30	0.805	0.562	1.154	15	0.533	0.323	0.879
4	Cambs	18	0.801	0.502	1.277	15	0.822	0.495	1.366
5	Ches	114	1.228	1.018	1.482	90	1.103	0.893	1.362
6	Cornwall	22	0.700	0.461	1.064	23	0.859	0.569	1.295
7	Cumberland	10	0.559	0.303	1.031	7	0.468	0.227	0.966
8	Derbys	60	1.023	0.792	1.322	51	1.053	0.798	1.391
9	Devon	62	0.850	0.661	1.094	64	1.025	0.799	1.314
10	Dorset	17	0.631	0.393	1.014	21	0.928	0.604	1.427
11	Durham	77	0.853	0.680	1.070	60	0.830	0.642	1.072
12	Essex	77	1.096	0.873	1.375	60	1.066	0.824	1.378
13	Glos	57	0.786	0.605	1.021	55	0.916	0.701	1.196
14	Hants	100	0.937	0.767	1.144	105	1.237	1.017	1.503
15	Hereford	9	0.917	0.476	1.767	5	0.654	0.273	1.565
16	Herts	52	1.085	0.824	1.429	48	1.291	0.970	1.719
17	Hunt	10	0.735	0.396	1.367	7	0.667	0.319	1.398
18	Kent	70	0.842	0.664	1.068	64	0.911	0.711	1.168
19	Lancs	403	1.288	1.160	1.431	279	1.008	0.890	1.142
20	Leics	48	1.051	0.790	1.400	43	1.134	0.838	1.534
21	Lincs H	4	0.508	0.194	1.328	3	0.502	0.164	1.533
22	Lincs K	19	1.278	0.814	2.005	10	0.797	0.428	1.484
23	Lincs L	22	0.764	0.502	1.163	15	0.664	0.401	1.100
24	London	435	0.998	0.901	1.105	358	0.992	0.886	1.109
25	Norfolk	35	0.799	0.572	1.116	27	0.720	0.493	1.052
26	Northants	38	1.156	0.837	1.596	23	0.882	0.584	1.331
27	Northd	49	0.869	0.655	1.154	37	0.806	0.582	1.115
28	Notts	51	0.774	0.587	1.021	52	1.006	0.764	1.325
29	Oxon	17	0.675	0.420	1.083	14	0.678	0.402	1.142
30	Rut	1	0.598	0.082	4.386	0	0.000		
31	Salop	26	1.323	0.899	1.948	15	0.928	0.558	1.542
32	Somerset	41	0.779	0.572	1.060	41	0.921	0.676	1.255
33	Staffs	80	0.797	0.638	0.996	71	0.904	0.713	1.144
34	E Suff	20	0.709	0.457	1.098	15	0.653	0.394	1.082
35	W Suff	13	1.080	0.625	1.867	8	0.863	0.431	1.727
36	Surrey	77	1.289	1.028	1.617	52	1.021	0.775	1.345
37	E Sussex	44	0.838	0.623	1.129	44	0.851	0.632	1.147
38	W Sussex	26	0.736	0.500	1.083	31	0.932	0.653	1.329
39	Warwicks	92	0.727	0.591	0.895	91	0.900	0.730	1.110
40	Westd	2	0.394	0.102	1.527	4	0.879	0.330	2.344
41	IOW	9	1.074	0.558	2.068	8	1.103	0.551	2.210
42	Wilts	34	1.046	0.744	1.469	26	1.023	0.694	1.507
43	Worcs	36	0.828	0.596	1.152	25	0.716	0.483	1.061
44	E Yorks	31	0.898	0.630	1.281	34	1.184	0.844	1.662
45	N Yorks	32	0.744	0.525	1.053	24	0.682	0.457	1.017
46	W Yorks	239	1.004	0.879	1.146	187	0.920	0.793	1.068
47	Ang	9	1.874	0.980	3.585	7	1.719	0.825	3.584
48	Brec	3	0.880	0.283	2.734	3	1.054	0.340	3.273
49	Caer	25	2.364	1.609	3.471	13	1.312	0.762	2.260
50	Card	8	1.931	0.967	3.857	5	1.313	0.547	3.153
51	Carm	19	1.589	1.014	2.491	18	1.659	1.048	2.628
52	Den	31	2.042	1.442	2.891	35	2.396	1.733	3.314
53	Fli	19	1.373	0.875	2.156	19	1.615	1.032	2.530
54	Glam	153	1.810	1.541	2.127	133	1.908	1.606	2.267
55	Meri	5	1.737	0.729	4.139	4	1.502	0.566	3.986
56	Monm	38	1.260	0.915	1.735	38	1.603	1.166	2.203
57	Mont	10	3.154	1.739	5.723	1	0.377	0.057	2.481
58	Pemb	4	0.544	0.207	1.431	17	2.765	1.746	4.379
59	Rad	0	0.000			0	0.000		

OR = Odds ratio
CL = Confidence limits

Table A5.21 Cancer of Soft Tissues, All Ages, 1968–85

	County	Males				Females			
		Cases	OR	95% CL		Cases	OR	95% CL	
1	Beds	47	0.713	0.535	0.950	60	1.034	0.800	1.335
2	Berks	92	0.938	0.762	1.156	95	1.036	0.842	1.275
3	Bucks	108	1.152	0.948	1.400	79	0.927	0.741	1.160
4	Cambs	58	1.077	0.829	1.400	63	1.211	0.942	1.558
5	Ches	209	0.907	0.789	1.042	212	0.900	0.785	1.033
6	Cornwall	78	1.031	0.822	1.292	77	1.051	0.839	1.318
7	Cumberland	32	0.719	0.507	1.020	44	1.034	0.765	1.397
8	Derbys	162	1.136	0.970	1.330	135	0.960	0.809	1.140
9	Devon	202	1.190	1.033	1.371	187	1.091	0.942	1.263
10	Dorset	61	0.961	0.744	1.241	66	1.042	0.816	1.330
11	Durham	236	1.097	0.962	1.250	202	0.968	0.841	1.114
12	Essex	171	0.989	0.848	1.154	193	1.204	1.042	1.392
13	Glos	201	1.161	1.007	1.339	182	1.060	0.914	1.230
14	Hants	254	0.984	0.867	1.117	260	1.058	0.933	1.199
15	Hereford	26	1.093	0.738	1.619	30	1.367	0.948	1.970
16	Herts	120	1.006	0.837	1.208	114	1.028	0.852	1.240
17	Hunt	30	0.871	0.604	1.256	30	0.978	0.681	1.404
18	Kent	199	0.987	0.855	1.138	166	0.833	0.713	0.972
19	Lancs	760	0.972	0.901	1.049	754	0.958	0.888	1.034
20	Leics	93	0.834	0.678	1.025	109	0.992	0.818	1.203
21	Lincs H	15	0.777	0.466	1.296	15	0.870	0.525	1.442
22	Lincs K	30	0.831	0.578	1.193	35	0.984	0.704	1.376
23	Lincs L	66	0.942	0.736	1.205	61	0.911	0.704	1.178
24	London	1 018	0.956	0.894	1.022	1 049	1.019	0.954	1.089
25	Norfolk	97	0.919	0.750	1.126	113	1.084	0.898	1.309
26	Northants	100	1.251	1.023	1.529	110	1.443	1.192	1.748
27	Northd	128	0.921	0.772	1.100	118	0.906	0.754	1.088
28	Notts	144	0.893	0.756	1.055	151	1.016	0.863	1.196
29	Oxon	62	0.986	0.764	1.272	75	1.242	0.987	1.564
30	Rut	2	0.490	0.125	1.925	1	0.277	0.041	1.862
31	Salop	38	0.770	0.558	1.063	40	0.845	0.618	1.156
32	Somerset	141	1.110	0.938	1.313	156	1.274	1.086	1.495
33	Staffs	210	0.850	0.740	0.977	190	0.810	0.700	0.936
34	E Suff	92	1.387	1.126	1.709	64	0.980	0.764	1.258
35	W Suff	30	0.986	0.684	1.422	26	0.946	0.643	1.392
36	Surrey	138	0.937	0.791	1.111	136	0.924	0.778	1.097
37	E Sussex	107	0.886	0.731	1.074	110	0.801	0.663	0.969
38	W Sussex	86	1.045	0.842	1.296	76	0.830	0.661	1.042
39	Warwicks	302	0.984	0.876	1.105	272	0.912	0.807	1.031
40	Westd	11	0.922	0.508	1.673	16	1.276	0.777	2.095
41	IOW	31	1.611	1.127	2.304	29	1.437	0.997	2.070
42	Wilts	89	1.105	0.894	1.366	97	1.286	1.051	1.574
43	Worcs	106	0.987	0.811	1.200	90	0.893	0.724	1.102
44	E Yorks	101	1.241	1.017	1.515	80	0.984	0.787	1.229
45	N Yorks	115	1.106	0.918	1.333	120	1.184	0.987	1.421
46	W Yorks	595	1.032	0.948	1.123	583	1.008	0.926	1.099
47	Ang	11	0.920	0.508	1.665	13	1.049	0.603	1.824
48	Brec	10	1.187	0.634	2.222	5	0.647	0.270	1.548
49	Caer	27	1.081	0.741	1.578	27	0.990	0.675	1.452
50	Card	7	0.671	0.321	1.403	12	1.082	0.610	1.919
51	Carm	33	1.128	0.799	1.592	38	1.194	0.863	1.652
52	Den	42	1.108	0.814	1.509	47	1.131	0.845	1.512
53	Fli	46	1.368	1.019	1.836	41	1.160	0.851	1.581
54	Glam	221	1.028	0.897	1.177	191	0.916	0.792	1.058
55	Meri	9	1.269	0.662	2.432	11	1.499	0.820	2.739
56	Monm	71	0.947	0.747	1.200	73	1.008	0.797	1.273
57	Mont	7	0.895	0.420	1.908	4	0.501	0.187	1.338
58	Pemb	21	1.186	0.771	1.826	20	1.084	0.690	1.704
59	Rad	9	2.359	1.214	4.581	3	0.880	0.284	2.723

OR = Odds ratio
CL = Confidence limits

Odds ratios underlined were treated as outliers in categorizing values for the maps

Table A5.22 Malignant Melanoma of Skin, All Ages, 1968–85

	County	Males				Females			
		Cases	OR	95% CL		Cases	OR	95% CL	
1	Beds	92	1.014	0.823	1.249	155	0.964	0.820	1.134
2	Berks	180	1.382	1.189	1.606	301	1.198	1.064	1.348
3	Bucks	170	1.332	1.142	1.553	296	1.267	1.125	1.427
4	Cambs	94	1.269	1.032	1.560	235	1.687	1.477	1.928
5	Ches	289	0.900	0.800	1.014	586	0.897	0.824	0.976
6	Cornwall	198	2.007	1.742	2.313	355	1.822	1.635	2.031
7	Cumberland	57	0.944	0.726	1.228	157	1.359	1.155	1.598
8	Derbys	215	1.074	0.936	1.232	343	0.874	0.783	0.976
9	Devon	347	1.528	1.371	1.703	757	1.718	1.594	1.852
10	Dorset	133	1.576	1.325	1.874	293	1.801	1.599	2.029
11	Durham	199	0.637	0.553	0.733	414	0.694	0.629	0.766
12	Essex	253	1.086	0.957	1.233	364	0.830	0.747	0.923
13	Glos	273	1.145	1.014	1.294	649	1.412	1.302	1.531
14	Hants	529	1.548	1.417	1.692	955	1.468	1.372	1.570
15	Hereford	43	1.340	0.989	1.814	53	0.900	0.681	1.189
16	Herts	150	0.899	0.764	1.058	336	1.077	0.964	1.205
17	Hunt	61	1.320	1.023	1.704	95	1.098	0.891	1.352
18	Kent	324	1.198	1.071	1.341	597	1.118	1.028	1.216
19	Lancs	748	0.657	0.610	0.708	1 499	0.666	0.631	0.702
20	Leics	145	0.936	0.793	1.104	262	0.861	0.761	0.975
21	Lincs H	22	0.846	0.554	1.289	35	0.759	0.543	1.061
22	Lincs K	50	1.005	0.758	1.332	83	0.830	0.666	1.034
23	Lincs L	88	0.916	0.741	1.133	137	0.767	0.647	0.908
24	London	1 380	0.925	0.873	0.980	2 552	0.886	0.849	0.925
25	Norfolk	169	1.187	1.017	1.385	374	1.327	1.194	1.475
26	Northants	113	1.020	0.845	1.230	228	1.085	0.948	1.242
27	Northd	151	0.785	0.667	0.923	326	0.899	0.803	1.005
28	Notts	197	0.882	0.765	1.017	307	0.743	0.662	0.833
29	Oxon	110	1 293	1.069	1.565	173	1.033	0.886	1.204
30	Rut	8	1.499	0.743	3.025	8	0.866	0.432	1.738
31	Salop	74	1.113	0.882	1.404	149	1.154	0.976	1.364
32	Somerset	230	1.353	1.184	1.545	528	1.603	1.466	1.753
33	Staffs	249	0.709	0.625	0.804	514	0.773	0.707	0.845
34	E Suff	105	1.143	0.940	1.390	213	1.218	1.059	1.401
35	W Suff	50	1.269	0.956	1.684	67	0.917	0.718	1.171
36	Surrey	310	1.547	1.379	1.735	527	1.325	1.211	1.450
37	E Sussex	213	1.319	1.149	1.513	550	1.592	1.459	1.737
38	W Sussex	145	1.313	1.112	1.550	323	1.401	1.251	1.568
39	Warwicks	383	0.887	0.800	0.983	789	0.958	0.890	1.031
40	Westd	9	0.558	0.293	1.066	52	1.555	1.171	2.064
41	IOW	40	1.509	1.101	2.068	90	1.762	1.425	2.178
42	Wilts	139	1.272	1.073	1.506	264	1.300	1.147	1.473
43	Worcs	131	0.881	0.740	1.048	258	0.930	0.821	1.055
44	E Yorks	652	0.924	0.761	1.122	164	0.722	0.617	0.843
45	N Yorks	124	0.849	0.710	1.015	248	0.875	0.770	0.994
46	W Yorks	652	0.796	0.735	0.862	1 293	0.803	0.758	0.850
47	Ang	7	0.417	0.200	0.871	32	0.993	0.696	1.417
48	Brec	14	1.245	0.731	2.121	11	0.483	0.269	0.867
49	Caer	33	0.977	0.692	1.379	65	0.915	0.715	1.171
50	Card	16	1.141	0.693	1.877	26	0.902	0.610	1.335
51	Carm	47	1.168	0.875	1.560	90	1.042	0.842	1.289
52	Den	40	0.783	0.574	1.070	80	0.704	0.565	0.878
53	Fli	43	0.932	0.688	1.262	77	0.824	0.657	1.035
54	Glam	289	0.976	0.867	1.098	543	0.938	0.860	1.024
55	Meri	7	0.732	0.349	1.537	29	1.452	0.997	2.115
56	Monm	88	0.856	0.692	1.059	152	0.767	0.653	0.901
57	Mont	11	1.054	0.579	1.918	16	0.773	0.471	1.271
58	Pemb	29	1.149	0.792	1.667	53	1.040	0.788	1.374
59	Rad	4	0.742	0.280	1.962	7	0.747	0.355	1.571

OR = Odds ratio
CL = Confidence limits

Table A5.23 Cancer of Breast, Females, by Age, 1968–85

	County	Ages 0–44				Ages 45+			
		Cases	OR	95% CL		Cases	OR	95% CL	
1	Beds	459	1.091	0.951	1.251	2 374	1.177	1.121	1.236
2	Berks	714	1.013	0.908	1.130	4 100	1.107	1.064	1.152
3	Bucks	660	1.039	0.928	1.163	3 609	1.042	1.000	1.086
4	Cambs	338	0.957	0.818	1.120	2 316	1.039	0.987	1.094
5	Ches	1 569	1.067	0.990	1.149	9 928	0.949	0.926	0.973
6	Cornwall	348	0.799	0.690	0.924	3 189	0.947	0.907	0.988
7	Cumberland	238	0.954	0.794	1.146	1 537	0.785	0.739	0.834
8	Derbys	940	1.026	0.933	1.128	6 119	1.009	0.978	1.041
9	Devon	841	0.945	0.856	1.043	8 071	1.017	0.989	1.045
10	Dorset	350	1.022	0.874	1.195	3 082	1.081	1.033	1.130
11	Durham	1 321	0.967	0.894	1.047	7 980	0.855	0.832	0.878
12	Essex	1 029	1.045	0.954	1.144	7 702	1.102	1.071	1.134
13	Glos	1 031	0.968	0.885	1.058	7 563	1.012	0.983	1.041
14	Hants	1 627	1.037	0.964	1.115	11 144	1.069	1.043	1.094
15	Hereford	125	1.042	0.810	1.341	1 076	1.114	1.032	1.201
16	Herts	797	0.966	0.872	1.071	5 078	1.087	1.049	1.126
17	Hunt	208	0.827	0.684	1.000	1 211	0.958	0.893	1.028
18	Kent	1 225	1.055	0.970	1.147	9 167	1.038	1.012	1.066
19	Lancs	4 639	1.014	0.970	1.060	32 769	0.905	0.892	0.917
20	Leics	790	1.135	1.020	1.263	5 419	1.154	1.115	1.195
21	Lincs H	126	1.395	1.060	1.835	720	0.896	0.818	0.980
22	Lincs K	234	1.033	0.858	1.245	1 596	1.009	0.949	1.073
23	Lincs L	430	1.105	0.959	1.274	2 794	0.968	0.924	1.014
24	London	6 184	0.974	0.936	1.012	46 538	1.034	1.021	1.047
25	Norfolk	660	1.015	0.906	1.138	4 989	1.077	1.040	1.116
26	Northants	511	0.984	0.867	1.117	3 548	1.130	1.084	1.179
27	Northd	739	0.932	0.840	1.035	5 071	0.841	0.813	0.870
28	Notts	985	1.101	1.002	1.210	6 679	1.014	0.983	1.045
29	Oxon	372	0.870	0.754	1.004	2 673	1.099	1.047	1.153
30	Rut	22	0.832	0.469	1.475	152	1.090	0.892	1.332
31	Salop	324	1.055	0.896	1.242	2 152	1.061	1.005	1.119
32	Somerset	714	0.933	0.839	1.037	5 951	1.078	1.044	1.113
33	Staffs	1 744	1.078	1.003	1.158	10 370	1.038	1.013	1.064
34	E Suff	365	0.887	0.766	1.027	3 122	1.103	1.055	1.153
35	W Suff	180	0.963	0.778	1.192	1 193	1.069	0.996	1.148
36	Surrey	1 038	1.096	0.999	1.202	7 238	1.129	1.095	1.163
37	E Sussex	606	0.976	0.869	1.097	6 665	1.036	1.006	1.068
38	W Sussex	400	0.873	0.758	1.006	4 204	1.016	0.978	1.055
39	Warwicks	1 889	0.973	0.910	1.040	13 113	1.030	1.007	1.053
40	Westd	66	0.913	0.638	1.305	573	0.998	0.901	1.104
41	IOW	99	0.991	0.743	1.322	1 012	1.098	1.016	1.186
42	Wilts	485	0.920	0.810	1.045	3 370	1.085	1.040	1.133
43	Worcs	649	1.081	0.963	1.212	4 654	1.061	1.023	1.100
44	E Yorks	470	0.939	0.824	1.069	3 287	0.884	0.848	0.922
45	N Yorks	640	0.953	0.851	1.066	3 821	0.860	0.827	0.894
46	W Yorks	3 594	1.051	1.000	1.106	24 098	0.923	0.908	0.938
47	Ang	67	0.882	0.625	1.244	476	0.922	0.825	1.029
48	Brec	51	0.965	0.646	1.441	336	0.944	0.827	1.078
49	Caer	156	1.060	0.835	1.344	1 291	1.039	0.970	1.112
50	Card	52	0.991	0.659	1.490	505	1.059	0.950	1.180
51	Carm	154	0.762	0.613	0.948	1 291	0.921	0.861	0.984
52	Den	238	1.003	0.836	1.204	1 998	1.106	1.047	1.169
53	Fli	202	1.048	0.856	1.283	1 495	0.996	0.936	1.061
54	Glam	1 270	0.959	0.885	1.039	8 362	0.914	0.889	0.938
55	Meri	43	1.117	0.720	1.733	395	1.203	1.061	1.364
56	Monm	418	0.798	0.700	0.910	2 856	0.951	0.908	0.996
57	Mont	41	0.925	0.594	1.441	354	1.059	0.931	1.206
58	Pemb	107	0.829	0.639	1.076	763	0.980	0.896	1.071
59	Rad	16	0.823	0.402	1.684	165	1.033	0.852	1.252

OR = Odds ratio
CL = Confidence limits

Table A5.24 Cancer of Breast, All Ages, 1968–85

	County	Males				Females			
		Cases	OR	95% CL		Cases	OR	95% CL	
1	Beds	35	1.439	1.032	2.007	3 193	1.167	1.114	1.222
2	Berks	35	0.957	0.685	1.337	4 814	1.096	1.056	1.137
3	Bucks	41	1.171	0.860	1.595	4 269	1.042	1.002	1.083
4	Cambs	20	0.893	0.575	1.388	2 654	1.031	0.982	1.082
5	Ches	80	0.843	0.675	1.052	11 497	0.960	0.938	0.983
6	Cornwall	35	1.057	0.756	1.476	3 537	0.934	0.897	0.973
7	Cumberland	9	0.492	0.259	0.936	1 775	0.800	0.755	0.847
8	Derbys	58	0.974	0.751	1.264	7 059	1.011	0.981	1.041
9	Devon	75	0.966	0.768	1.215	8 912	1.011	0.985	1.038
10	Dorset	26	0.919	0.624	1.353	3 432	1.076	1.031	1.123
11	Durham	81	0.894	0.716	1.115	9 301	0.866	0.844	0.888
12	Essex	70	0.976	0.770	1.238	8 731	1.097	1.067	1.127
13	Glos	80	1.101	0.881	1.376	8 594	1.008	0.981	1.035
14	Hants	142	1.345	1.137	1.592	12 771	1.065	1.042	1.090
15	Hereford	12	1.179	0.668	2.081	1 201	1.107	1.030	1.191
16	Herts	44	0.950	0.705	1.280	5 875	1.073	1.038	1.110
17	Hunt	6	0.462	0.211	1.010	1 419	0.942	0.882	1.006
18	Kent	88	1.044	0.845	1.292	10 392	1.040	1.014	1.066
19	Lancs	291	0.878	0.778	0.991	37 408	0.914	0.902	0.926
20	Leics	51	1.134	0.860	1.497	6 209	1.152	1.115	1.191
21	Lincs H	3	0.365	0.123	1.083	846	0.934	0.858	1.018
22	Lincs K	14	0.922	0.545	1.560	1 830	1.012	0.954	1.072
23	Lincs L	24	0.821	0.549	1.227	3 224	0.980	0.938	1.025
24	London	444	1.038	0.939	1.148	52 722	1.028	1.016	1.041
25	Norfolk	41	0.894	0.657	1.218	5 649	1.072	1.036	1.108
26	Northants	20	0.618	0.399	0.956	4 059	1.115	1.071	1.160
27	Northd	47	0.813	0.610	1.085	5 810	0.849	0.822	0.877
28	Notts	48	0.732	0.551	0.973	7 664	1.021	0.992	1.051
29	Oxon	25	1.010	0.681	1.499	3 045	1.072	1.024	1.122
30	Rut	1	0.630	0.090	4.410	174	1.059	0.876	1.279
31	Salop	14	0.700	0.415	1.181	2 476	1.060	1.008	1.116
32	Somerset	43	0.787	0.583	1.064	6 665	1.065	1.033	1.098
33	Staffs	81	0.833	0.668	1.039	12 114	1.042	1.018	1.067
34	E Suff	26	0.889	0.604	1.309	3 487	1.082	1.037	1.129
35	W Suff	20	1.642	1.060	2.542	1 373	1.058	0.989	1.132
36	Surrey	90	1.514	1.228	1.865	8 276	1.125	1.094	1.158
37	E Sussex	91	1.610	1.308	1.982	7 271	1.032	1.003	1.063
38	W Sussex	49	1.289	0.972	1.710	4 604	1.006	0.970	1.043
39	Warwicks	119	0.956	0.795	1.148	15 002	1.024	1.003	1.046
40	Westd	1	0.187	0.033	1.077	639	0.991	0.899	1.093
41	IOW	8	0.909	0.454	1.822	1 111	1.090	1.012	1.175
42	Wilts	45	1.417	1.056	1.901	3 855	1.067	1.024	1.111
43	Worcs	34	0.792	0.565	1.110	5 303	1.063	1.026	1.100
44	E Yorks	39	1.094	0.797	1.502	3 757	0.889	0.854	0.925
45	N Yorks	45	1.049	0.781	1.409	4 461	0.869	0.837	0.902
46	W Yorks	241	0.988	0.866	1.128	27 692	0.934	0.920	0.949
47	Ang	6	1.222	0.548	2.725	543	0.918	0.826	1.019
48	Brec	4	1.101	0.411	2.945	387	0.946	0.834	1.073
49	Caer	7	0.622	0.298	1.297	1 447	1.040	0.974	1.111
50	Card	4	0.918	0.344	2.451	557	1.054	0.949	1.171
51	Carm	12	0.978	0.554	1.726	1 445	0.906	0.849	0.966
52	Den	15	0.919	0.553	1.527	2 236	1.097	1.041	1.157
53	Fli	17	1.203	0.746	1.940	1 697	1.001	0.942	1.063
54	Glam	105	1.215	1.000	1.476	9 632	0.918	0.895	0.942
55	Meri	4	1.308	0.490	3.490	438	1.196	1.060	1.349
56	Monm	33	1.087	0.771	1.534	3 274	0.933	0.894	0.975
57	Mont	2	0.587	0.149	2.317	395	1.048	0.925	1.187
58	Pemb	7	0.954	0.454	2.006	870	0.963	0.885	1.048
59	Rad	2	1.082	0.270	4.342	181	1.016	0.844	1.224

OR = Odds ratio
CL = Confidence limits

Odds ratios underlined were treated as outliers in categorizing values for the maps

Table A5.25 Cancer of Cervix Uteri, All Ages, 1968–85

	County	Cases	OR	95% CL	
1	Beds	522	0.921	0.839	1.011
2	Berks	741	0.828	0.767	0.895
3	Bucks	695	0.829	0.766	0.898
4	Cambs	398	0.781	0.703	0.867
5	Ches	2 540	1.090	1.044	1.139
6	Cornwall	730	1.010	0.933	1.094
7	Cumberland	397	0.951	0.856	1.056
8	Derbys	1 247	0.899	0.846	0.954
9	Devon	1 478	0.900	0.852	0.952
10	Dorset	553	0.917	0.837	1.003
11	Durham	2 198	1.062	1.014	1.112
12	Essex	1 300	0.844	0.796	0.895
13	Glos	1 487	0.884	0.837	0.935
14	Hants	2 304	0.976	0.933	1.021
15	Hereford	230	1.100	0.955	1.268
16	Herts	939	0.837	0.781	0.897
17	Hunt	304	0.990	0.876	1.120
18	Kent	1 779	0.923	0.877	0.971
19	Lancs	9 699	1.305	1.275	1.337
20	Leics	1 146	1.062	0.996	1.132
21	Lincs H	167	0.986	0.835	1.164
22	Lincs K	329	0.929	0.827	1.043
23	Lincs L	777	1.226	1.134	1.326
24	London	8 673	0.845	0.825	0.866
25	Norfolk	1 029	1.007	0.941	1.076
26	Northants	703	0.940	0.867	1.020
27	Northd	1 229	0.951	0.896	1.011
28	Notts	1 544	1.062	1.005	1.122
29	Oxon	420	0.704	0.636	0.779
30	Rut	30	0.896	0.607	1.323
31	Salop	467	1.010	0.914	1.115
32	Somerset	923	0.758	0.708	0.813
33	Staffs	2 531	1.068	1.023	1.116
34	E Suff	512	0.811	0.739	0.890
35	W Suff	255	0.964	0.841	1.105
36	Surrey	1 085	0.755	0.709	0.804
37	E Sussex	1 048	0.826	0.774	0.882
38	W Sussex	592	0.716	0.658	0.779
39	Warwicks	3 053	1.026	0.986	1.068
40	Westd	100	0.813	0.659	1.002
41	IOW	158	0.826	0.698	0.976
42	Wilts	666	0.909	0.837	0.987
43	Worcs	945	0.939	0.876	1.007
44	E Yorks	869	1.079	1.003	1.161
45	N Yorks	1 183	1.177	1.104	1.254
46	W Yorks	6 518	1.180	1.147	1.213
47	Ang	165	1.481	1.250	1.755
48	Brec	77	0.957	0.750	1.220
49	Caer	259	1.009	0.883	1.153
50	Card	101	0.980	0.793	1.212
51	Carm	405	1.316	1.181	1.467
52	Den	493	1.219	1.103	1.346
53	Fli	421	1.250	1.120	1.396
54	Glam	2 335	1.141	1.091	1.194
55	Meri	81	1.109	0.872	1.410
56	Monm	690	0.967	0.891	1.050
57	Mont	82	1.124	0.887	1.425
58	Pemb	254	1.380	1.197	1.591
59	Rad	34	1.011	0.702	1.455

OR = Odds ratio
CL = Confidence limits

Table A5.26 Cancer of Placenta, All Ages, 1968–85

	County	Cases	OR	95% CL	
1	Beds	5	1.475	0.610	3.571
2	Berks	5	0.987	0.405	2.408
3	Bucks	5	1.067	0.438	2.597
4	Cambs	0	0.000		
5	Ches	14	1.222	0.712	2.097
6	Cornwall	2	0.658	0.165	2.628
7	Cumberland	0	0.000		
8	Derbys	6	0.843	0.377	1.885
9	Devon	4	0.609	0.229	1.620
10	Dorset	0	0.000		
11	Durham	15	1.441	0.856	2.426
12	Essex	6	0.847	0.377	1.904
13	Glos	6	0.698	0.311	1.565
14	Hants	9	0.687	0.354	1.331
15	Hereford	1	1.174	0.167	8.262
16	Herts	3	0.489	0.161	1.491
17	Hunt	2	1.165	0.287	4.722
18	Kent	8	0.937	0.462	1.899
19	Lancs	35	1.043	0.734	1.482
20	Leics	10	1.732	0.921	3.258
21	Lincs H	0	0.000		
22	Lincs K	1	0.600	0.086	4.176
23	Lincs L	5	1.594	0.655	3.879
24	London	46	0.863	0.633	1.177
25	Norfolk	6	1.294	0.573	2.925
26	Northants	8	1.945	0.966	3.918
27	Northd	4	0.691	0.258	1.853
28	Notts	8	1.180	0.582	2.394
29	Oxon	2	0.491	0.124	1.938
30	Rut	0	0.000		
31	Salop	7	3.024	1.453	6.296
32	Somerset	0	0.000		
33	Staffs	22	1.889	1.229	2.904
34	E Suff	3	1.013	0.322	3.185
35	W Suff	1	0.739	0.106	5.149
36	Surrey	8	1.175	0.581	2.376
37	E Sussex	3	0.629	0.204	1.943
38	W Sussex	4	1.135	0.424	3.041
39	Warwicks	14	0.891	0.521	1.525
40	Westd	1	1.988	0.293	13.489
41	IOW	0	0.000		
42	Wilts	2	0.497	0.127	1.936
43	Worcs	3	0.574	0.186	1.774
44	E Yorks	10	2.982	1.620	5.491
45	N Yorks	7	1.323	0.624	2.804
46	W Yorks	28	1.064	0.721	1.570
47	Ang	0	0.000		
48	Brec	0	0.000		
49	Caer	2	2.012	0.499	8.122
50	Card	1	1.950	0.282	13.461
51	Carm	0	0.000		
52	Den	3	1.480	0.473	4.634
53	Fli	0	0.000		
54	Glam	3	1.225	0.703	2.134
55	Meri	0	0.000		
56	Monm	2	0.556	0.142	2.179
57	Mont	2	6.431	1.872	22.095
58	Pemb	0	0.000		
59	Rad	0	0.000		

OR = Odds ratio
CL = Confidence limits

Odds ratios underlined were treated as outliers in categorizing values for the maps

Table A5.27 Cancer of Corpus Uteri, All Ages, 1968–85

	County	Cases	OR	95% CL	
1	Beds	589	1.214	1.113	1.323
2	Berks	848	1.102	1.026	1.184
3	Bucks	802	1.116	1.037	1.202
4	Cambs	543	1.175	1.074	1.286
5	Ches	2 029	0.937	0.894	0.981
6	Cornwall	861	1.247	1.160	1.339
7	Cumberland	361	0.910	0.816	1.014
8	Derbys	1 381	1.092	1.032	1.156
9	Devon	1 931	1.188	1.132	1.247
10	Dorset	717	1.220	1.128	1.319
11	Durham	1 491	0.760	0.721	0.802
12	Essex	1 495	1.026	0.972	1.083
13	Glos	1 687	1.087	1.033	1.145
14	Hants	2 229	1.022	0.977	1.068
15	Hereford	263	1.326	1.165	1.509
16	Herts	953	0.970	0.907	1.038
17	Hunt	300	1.137	1.008	1.283
18	Kent	2 001	1.096	1.046	1.149
19	Lancs	6 077	0.791	0.770	0.813
20	Leics	1 182	1.213	1.141	1.289
21	Lincs H	216	1.336	1.158	1.542
22	Lincs K	374	1.139	1.022	1.268
23	Lincs L	614	1.028	0.945	1.118
24	London	9 148	0.963	0.941	0.986
25	Norfolk	1 171	1.219	1.147	1.297
26	Northants	801	1.217	1.130	1.311
27	Northd	971	0.767	0.719	0.820
28	Notts	1 378	1.000	0.945	1.058
29	Oxon	542	1.065	0.974	1.165
30	Rut	31	1.020	0.702	1.483
31	Salop	500	1.185	1.079	1.301
32	Somerset	1 394	1.220	1.153	1.291
33	Staffs	2 253	1.074	1.027	1.122
34	E Suff	681	1.153	1.064	1.249
35	W Suff	269	1.140	1.004	1.295
36	Surrey	1 343	1.006	0.950	1.065
37	E Sussex	1 363	1.028	0.971	1.087
38	W Sussex	817	0.959	0.892	1.032
39	Warwicks	2 894	1.092	1.050	1.136
40	Westd	110	0.919	0.756	1.118
41	IOW	218	1.139	0.989	1.311
42	Wilts	727	1.114	1.031	1.204
43	Worcs	1 109	1.222	1.147	1.301
44	E Yorks	670	0.863	0.797	0.935
45	N Yorks	746	0.804	0.746	0.867
46	W Yorks	4 937	0.910	0.883	0.938
47	Ang	108	1.000	0.820	1.221
48	Brec	90	1.255	1.008	1.562
49	Caer	274	1.066	0.941	1.209
50	Card	117	1.196	0.987	1.450
51	Carm	369	1.282	1.149	1.430
52	Den	363	0.951	0.853	1.060
53	Fli	254	0.802	0.705	0.912
54	Glam	1 870	0.983	0.936	1.031
55	Meri	74	1.072	0.842	1.365
56	Monm	626	0.997	0.918	1.084
57	Mont	63	0.886	0.684	1.148
58	Pemb	163	1.017	0.865	1.196
59	Rad	44	1.362	0.995	1.865

OR = Odds ratio
CL = Confidence limits

Table A5.28 Cancer of Ovary, All Ages, 1968–85

	County	Cases	OR	95% CL	
1	Beds	548	0.967	0.884	1.057
2	Berks	857	0.959	0.893	1.031
3	Bucks	970	1.177	1.099	1.260
4	Cambs	541	1.026	0.937	1.122
5	Ches	2 502	1.032	0.989	1.077
6	Cornwall	777	0.995	0.923	1.072
7	Cumberland	438	0.978	0.885	1.081
8	Derbys	1 478	1.025	0.970	1.083
9	Devon	1 973	1.095	1.044	1.149
10	Dorset	823	1.270	1.180	1.368
11	Durham	1 934	0.879	0.838	0.922
12	Essex	1 767	1.087	1.033	1.143
13	Glos	1 747	0.998	0.949	1.049
14	Hants	2 450	0.993	0.951	1.036
15	Hereford	250	1.118	0.979	1.276
16	Herts	1 143	1.019	0.958	1.085
17	Hunt	327	1.072	0.955	1.204
18	Kent	2 272	1.118	1.070	1.169
19	Lancs	7 389	0.870	0.849	0.893
20	Leics	1 238	1.110	1.045	1.179
21	Lincs H	206	1.132	0.978	1.310
22	Lincs K	374	0.997	0.895	1.111
23	Lincs L	671	0.992	0.915	1.075
24	London	10 809	1.028	1.006	1.051
25	Norfolk	1 290	1.201	1.132	1.274
26	Northants	750	0.989	0.916	1.067
27	Northd	1 191	0.846	0.796	0.898
28	Notts	1 479	0.954	0.904	1.008
29	Oxon	619	1.058	0.972	1.151
30	Rut	43	1.281	0.928	1.767
31	Salop	528	1.101	1.005	1.206
32	Somerset	1 309	1.016	0.958	1.076
33	Staffs	2 605	1.086	1.041	1.132
34	E Suff	715	1.080	0.998	1.168
35	W Suff	281	1.049	0.926	1.188
36	Surrey	1 699	1.144	1.087	1.205
37	E Sussex	1 637	1.150	1.092	1.212
38	W Sussex	1 097	1.199	1.126	1.278
39	Warwicks	3 044	1.004	0.966	1.043
40	Westd	137	1.040	0.871	1.242
41	IOW	239	1.137	0.994	1.302
42	Wilts	724	0.966	0.894	1.044
43	Worcs	1 073	1.033	0.968	1.101
44	E Yorks	748	0.859	0.796	0.927
45	N Yorks	987	0.943	0.882	1.008
46	W Yorks	5 728	0.944	0.918	0.972
47	Ang	106	0.861	0.705	1.052
48	Brec	89	1.071	0.858	1.338
49	Caer	270	0.943	0.830	1.070
50	Card	89	0.783	0.629	0.975
51	Carm	291	0.871	0.771	0.983
52	Den	388	0.903	0.813	1.004
53	Fli	325	0.920	0.820	1.032
54	Glam	1 845	0.842	0.802	0.884
55	Meri	67	0.844	0.654	1.089
56	Monm	653	0.897	0.826	0.973
57	Mont	71	0.886	0.693	1.133
58	Pemb	187	1.009	0.866	1.176
59	Rad	45	1.237	0.902	1.697

OR = Odds ratio
CL = Confidence limits

Table A5.29 Cancers of Vagina and Vulva, All Ages, 1968–85

	County	Cases	OR	95% CL	
1	Beds	100	0.790	0.648	0.963
2	Berks	196	0.951	0.824	1.096
3	Bucks	189	1.013	0.876	1.171
4	Cambs	103	0.809	0.666	0.984
5	Ches	571	1.013	0.931	1.103
6	Cornwall	202	1.056	0.918	1.216
7	Cumberland	101	0.973	0.798	1.187
8	Derbys	384	1.175	1.060	1.302
9	Devon	453	0.976	0.888	1.072
10	Dorset	174	1.058	0.910	1.232
11	Durham	539	1.123	1.029	1.225
12	Essex	355	0.886	0.797	0.986
13	Glos	406	0.965	0.873	1.066
14	Hants	566	0.943	0.867	1.027
15	Hereford	56	1.029	0.789	1.343
16	Herts	222	0.879	0.769	1.005
17	Hunt	64	0.923	0.720	1.183
18	Kent	437	0.868	0.788	0.955
19	Lancs	2 021	1.044	0.997	1.095
20	Leics	298	1.149	1.023	1.291
21	Lincs H	35	0.824	0.590	1.152
22	Lincs K	99	1.145	0.937	1.400
23	Lincs L	172	1.108	0.952	1.291
24	London	2 171	0.838	0.801	0.877
25	Norfolk	357	1.380	1.241	1.535
26	Northants	173	0.972	0.835	1.131
27	Northd	326	1.020	0.913	1.140
28	Notts	382	1.073	0.968	1.189
29	Oxon	132	0.967	0.813	1.150
30	Rut	15	1.933	1.162	3.218
31	Salop	144	1.312	1.111	1.550
32	Somerset	328	1.026	0.918	1.146
33	Staffs	552	1.080	0.991	1.177
34	E Suff	209	1.292	1.125	1.484
35	W Suff	76	1.198	0.953	1.507
36	Surrey	337	0.947	0.849	1.057
37	E Sussex	331	0.827	0.741	0.923
38	W Sussex	195	0.768	0.666	0.886
39	Warwicks	708	1.042	0.966	1.125
40	Westd	29	0.883	0.610	1.278
41	IOW	62	1.159	0.900	1.493
42	Wilts	195	1.132	0.981	1.307
43	Worcs	238	1.011	0.888	1.151
44	E Yorks	210	1.033	0.900	1.186
45	N Yorks	246	1.036	0.912	1.176
46	W Yorks	1 468	1.045	0.990	1.104
47	Ang	20	0.695	0.447	1.080
48	Brec	30	1.570	1.093	2.255
49	Caer	72	0.980	0.775	1.239
50	Card	33	1.233	0.872	1.743
51	Carm	105	1.421	1.170	1.726
52	Den	100	0.969	0.794	1.183
53	Fli	90	1.070	0.868	1.321
54	Glam	513	1.060	0.970	1.159
55	Meri	23	1.234	0.816	1.867
56	Monm	180	1.121	0.966	1.301
57	Mont	18	0.943	0.590	1.505
58	Pemb	38	0.913	0.662	1.260
59	Rad	10	1.114	0.593	2.092

OR = Odds ratio
CL = Confidence limits

Odds ratios underlined were treated as outliers in categorizing values for the maps

Table A5.30 Cancer of Prostate, All Ages, 1968–85

	County	Cases	OR	95% CL	
1	Beds	1 162	1.225	1.143	1.312
2	Berks	1 559	1.025	0.967	1.086
3	Bucks	1 439	0.994	0.936	1.055
4	Cambs	1 277	1.308	1.223	1.398
5	Ches	3 930	0.992	0.956	1.029
6	Cornwall	1 812	1.193	1.129	1.261
7	Cumberland	709	0.909	0.834	0.989
8	Derbys	2 516	0.995	0.950	1.041
9	Devon	4 443	1.222	1.179	1.267
10	Dorset	1 539	1.171	1.103	1.244
11	Durham	2 956	0.781	0.750	0.814
12	Essex	3 062	0.948	0.909	0.989
13	Glos	3 268	1.028	0.987	1.070
14	Hants	4 972	1.033	0.999	1.068
15	Hereford	537	1.172	1.059	1.298
16	Herts	1 937	1.044	0.991	1.100
17	Hunt	560	1.031	0.936	1.135
18	Kent	3 584	0.937	0.901	0.974
19	Lancs	12 506	0.894	0.876	0.914
20	Leics	1 984	1.019	0.967	1.073
21	Lincs H	353	0.959	0.848	1.084
22	Lincs K	701	1.046	0.958	1.141
23	Lincs L	1 296	1.031	0.967	1.099
24	London	17 635	0.967	0.949	0.985
25	Norfolk	2 602	1.275	1.217	1.336
26	Northants	1 525	1.100	1.037	1.168
27	Northd	2 094	0.848	0.807	0.890
28	Notts	2 868	1.048	1.003	1.094
29	Oxon	1 173	1.102	1.030	1.180
30	Rut	65	0.886	0.667	1.175
31	Salop	932	1.095	1.015	1.182
32	Somerset	3 171	1.292	1.238	1.349
33	Staffs	3 444	0.905	0.870	0.940
34	E Suff	1 573	1.190	1.121	1.263
35	W Suff	621	1.139	1.037	1.252
36	Surrey	2 847	1.130	1.081	1.180
37	E Sussex	3 271	1.154	1.107	1.204
38	W Sussex	2 002	1.068	1.013	1.125
39	Warwicks	5 115	1.023	0.990	1.057
40	Westd	280	1.115	0.968	1.284
41	IOW	453	1.106	0.990	1.235
42	Wilts	1 674	1.219	1.150	1.292
43	Worcs	1 810	1.029	0.974	1.086
44	E Yorks	1 546	0.982	0.927	1.041
45	N Yorks	1 605	0.877	0.829	0.929
46	W Yorks	9 867	0.949	0.926	0.971
47	Ang	228	1.071	0.917	1.249
48	Brec	134	0.827	0.681	1.004
49	Caer	451	0.857	0.771	0.953
50	Card	213	1.076	0.917	1.261
51	Carm	490	0.940	0.847	1.042
52	Den	588	0.773	0.705	0.847
53	Fli	559	0.870	0.790	0.957
54	Glam	3 047	0.827	0.793	0.861
55	Meri	146	1.030	0.849	1.249
56	Monm	1 218	0.959	0.898	1.023
57	Mont	155	0.976	0.812	1.174
58	Pemb	259	0.862	0.749	0.991
59	Rad	77	0.876	0.679	1.129

OR = Odds ratio
CL = Confidence limits

Table A5.31 Cancer of Testis, by Age, 1968–85

	County	Ages 0–49				Ages 50+			
		Cases	OR	95% CL		Cases	OR	95% CL	
1	Beds	110	0.927	0.749	1.147	16	0.842	0.515	1.377
2	Berks	216	1.300	1.113	1.519	29	1.078	0.747	1.556
3	Bucks	193	1.149	0.977	1.351	30	1.166	0.812	1.674
4	Cambs	103	1.125	0.899	1.409	17	1.074	0.665	1.735
5	Ches	410	1.203	1.073	1.348	80	1.138	0.910	1.424
6	Cornwall	86	0.851	0.675	1.074	20	0.870	0.560	1.351
7	Cumberland	53	0.838	0.622	1.128	13	0.960	0.555	1.659
8	Derbys	238	1.064	0.917	1.234	44	1.016	0.753	1.370
9	Devon	262	1.193	1.037	1.373	55	1.057	0.808	1.382
10	Dorset	98	1.179	0.939	1.481	28	1.492	1.028	2.163
11	Durham	266	0.811	0.709	0.928	54	0.774	0.591	1.013
12	Essex	242	0.941	0.817	1.084	50	0.976	0.737	1.293
13	Glos	277	1.052	0.918	1.205	52	0.991	0.752	1.305
14	Hants	448	1.104	0.991	1.231	83	1.098	0.881	1.368
15	Hereford	36	1.142	0.801	1.628	11	1.537	0.852	2.774
16	Herts	217	1.101	0.946	1.280	30	0.839	0.585	1.204
17	Hunt	64	1.010	0.763	1.337	11	1.189	0.657	2.150
18	Kent	347	1.188	1.050	1.344	73	1.234	0.977	1.559
19	Lancs	1 136	0.995	0.929	1.066	228	0.918	0.800	1.053
20	Leics	216	1.183	1.015	1.379	39	1.196	0.870	1.643
21	Lincs H	30	1.114	0.741	1.676	3	0.507	0.167	1.537
22	Lincs K	50	0.939	0.692	1.274	11	0.997	0.550	1.806
23	Lincs L	112	1.107	0.896	1.369	20	0.939	0.604	1.461
24	London	1 425	0.780	0.734	0.830	303	0.937	0.830	1.058
25	Norfolk	193	1.374	1.163	1.622	41	1.305	0.958	1.778
26	Northants	147	1.099	0.915	1.320	16	0.688	0.421	1.123
27	Northd	158	0.767	0.644	0.915	31	0.706	0.496	1.005
28	Notts	232	0.906	0.784	1.048	39	0.809	0.589	1.111
29	Oxon	120	1.126	0.917	1.383	13	0.734	0.426	1.266
30	Rut	13	1.723	0.845	3.514	0	0.000		
31	Salop	81	1.142	0.890	1.466	19	1.323	0.842	2.081
32	Somerset	191	1.017	0.864	1.195	48	1.294	0.972	1.723
33	Staffs	425	1.071	0.960	1.195	68	0.906	0.711	1.154
34	E Suff	100	1.077	0.864	1.342	30	1.493	1.041	2.140
35	W Suff	57	1.344	0.990	1.823	19	2.231	1.432	3.475
36	Surrey	303	1.381	1.211	1.575	63	1.431	1.114	1.838
37	E Sussex	167	1.187	0.997	1.413	42	1.132	0.833	1.538
38	W Sussex	117	1.163	0.945	1.432	35	1.417	1.015	1.979
39	Warwicks	423	0.882	0.791	0.985	96	0.997	0.812	1.224
40	Westd	19	1.385	0.854	2.248	3	0.827	0.265	2.578
41	IOW	20	0.741	0.464	1.182	9	1.531	0.798	2.937
42	Wilts	133	0.983	0.813	1.189	31	1.344	0.942	1.916
43	Worcs	149	0.868	0.724	1.039	33	1.023	0.725	1.445
44	E Yorks	112	0.969	0.786	1.195	20	0.781	0.502	1.213
45	N Yorks	159	1.012	0.847	1.208	25	0.774	0.522	1.148
46	W Yorks	870	1.048	0.969	1.134	165	0.906	0.773	1.063
47	Ang	18	1.042	0.623	1.742	3	0.858	0.276	2.673
48	Brec	8	0.704	0.325	1.525	5	1.954	0.815	4.683
49	Caer	22	0.743	0.475	1.164	14	1.789	1.063	3.010
50	Card	14	0.895	0.503	1.596	5	1.611	0.670	3.876
51	Carm	39	0.955	0.674	1.353	14	1.476	0.873	2.496
52	Den	35	0.674	0.473	0.960	13	1.141	0.660	1.971
53	Fli	44	0.856	0.615	1.192	5	0.520	0.218	1.236
54	Glam	293	0.873	0.766	0.995	49	0.737	0.556	0.977
55	Meri	3	0.285	0.090	0.905	0	0.000		
56	Monm	96	0.845	0.674	1.059	17	0.736	0.458	1.184
57	Mont	10	1.048	0.526	2.087	5	2.213	0.933	5.249
58	Pemb	25	0.872	0.555	1.369	4	0.724	0.271	1.939
59	Rad	5	1.053	0.397	2.797	1	0.851	0.120	6.032

OR = Odds ratio
CL = Confidence limits

Odds ratios underlined were treated as outliers in categorizing values for the maps

Table A5.32 Cancer of Penis, All Ages, 1968–85

	County	Cases	OR	95% CL	
1	Beds	39	1.074	0.782	1.474
2	Berks	58	1.061	0.818	1.377
3	Bucks	52	1.006	0.767	1.320
4	Cambs	20	0.593	0.384	0.916
5	Ches	143	1.025	0.867	1.211
6	Cornwall	61	1.240	0.962	1.598
7	Cumberland	27	1.006	0.688	1.471
8	Derbys	87	0.985	0.796	1.219
9	Devon	117	1.012	0.841	1.217
10	Dorset	41	0.974	0.715	1.326
11	Durham	154	1.164	0.991	1.367
12	Essex	82	0.762	0.613	0.948
13	Glos	101	0.930	0.763	1.133
14	Hants	142	0.884	0.748	1.046
15	Hereford	20	1.325	0.853	2.056
16	Herts	65	0.944	0.738	1.206
17	Hunt	19	0.983	0.625	1.545
18	Kent	100	0.790	0.648	0.963
19	Lancs	518	1.086	0.991	1.190
20	Leics	77	1.151	0.918	1.443
21	Lincs H	18	1.496	0.942	2.375
22	Lincs K	23	1.061	0.709	1.588
23	Lincs L	49	1.135	0.855	1.505
24	London	561	0.861	0.788	0.941
25	Norfolk	85	1.257	1.013	1.559
26	Northants	52	1.084	0.824	1.426
27	Northd	107	1.267	1.046	1.536
28	Notts	114	1.187	0.985	1.430
29	Oxon	30	0.808	0.564	1.158
30	Rut	2	0.834	0.208	3.349
31	Salop	34	1.149	0.819	1.613
32	Somerset	66	0.810	0.635	1.033
33	Staffs	153	1.079	0.917	1.268
34	E Suff	45	1.032	0.768	1.386
35	W Suff	23	1.268	0.841	1.912
36	Surrey	17	0.798	0.632	1.008
37	E Sussex	66	0.775	0.608	0.987
38	W Sussex	42	0.729	0.538	0.987
39	Warwicks	173	0.942	0.809	1.098
40	Westd	7	0.881	0.419	1.854
41	IOW	6	0.456	0.209	0.998
42	Wilts	51	1.069	0.810	1.410
43	Worcs	61	0.965	0.749	1.244
44	E Yorks	51	0.963	0.730	1.270
45	N Yorks	54	0.861	0.659	1.124
46	W Yorks	417	1.177	1.064	1.302
47	Ang	13	1.801	1.048	3.093
48	Brec	7	1.318	0.627	2.771
49	Caer	19	1.145	0.728	1.799
50	Card	1	<u>0.153</u>	0.028	0.834
51	Carm	13	0.775	0.459	1.310
52	Den	26	1.072	0.728	1.578
53	Fli	30	1.429	0.998	2.046
54	Glam	149	1.166	0.990	1.374
55	Meri	3	0.659	0.213	2.035
56	Monm	52	1.187	0.905	1.558
57	Mont	7	1.372	0.653	2.884
58	Pemb	7	0.739	0.370	1.478
59	Rad	1	<u>0.360</u>	0.055	2.365

OR = Odds ratio
CL = Confidence limits

Odds ratios underlined were treated as outliers in categorizing values for the maps

Table A5.33 Cancer of Scrotum, All Ages, 1968–85

	County	Cases	OR	95% CL	
1	Beds	11	1.414	0.782	2.557
2	Berks	5	0.425	0.181	0.998
3	Bucks	5	0.444	0.189	1.044
4	Cambs	3	0.414	0.138	1.244
5	Ches	47	1.584	1.184	2.118
6	Cornwall	3	0.278	0.096	0.802
7	Cumberland	3	0.513	0.168	1.561
8	Derbys	29	1.540	1.067	2.223
9	Devon	12	0.472	0.271	0.825
10	Dorset	7	0.766	0.365	1.610
11	Durham	24	0.828	0.553	1.241
12	Essex	18	0.778	0.488	1.238
13	Glos	11	0.465	0.260	0.830
14	Hants	17	0.486	0.304	0.777
15	Hereford	6	1.837	0.832	4.055
16	Herts	6	0.402	0.185	0.873
17	Hunt	0	0.000		
18	Kent	17	0.621	0.386	0.998
19	Lancs	212	2.304	1.988	2.670
20	Leics	15	1.038	0.623	1.730
21	Lincs H	2	0.758	0.190	3.026
22	Lincs K	4	0.820	0.308	2.187
23	Lincs L	13	1.393	0.808	2.403
24	London	107	0.749	0.613	0.915
25	Norfolk	2	0.134	0.041	0.435
26	Northants	9	0.874	0.453	1.685
27	Northd	15	0.810	0.486	1.347
28	Notts	19	0.911	0.578	1.434
29	Oxon	2	0.250	0.069	0.903
30	Rut	1	1.956	0.284	13.456
31	Salop	1	0.156	0.028	0.856
32	Somerset	9	0.510	0.268	0.971
33	Staffs	51	1.696	1.282	2.242
34	E Suff	4	0.423	0.163	1.097
35	W Suff	2	0.507	0.130	1.978
36	Surrey	8	0.410	0.209	0.803
37	E Sussex	6	0.319	0.149	0.682
38	W Sussex	7	0.564	0.271	1.174
39	Warwicks	91	2.430	1.971	2.997
40	Westd	0	0.000		
41	IOW	5	1.773	0.744	4.225
42	Wilts	6	0.583	0.264	1.289
43	Worcs	23	1.700	1.129	2.560
44	E Yorks	6	0.519	0.236	1.143
45	N Yorks	5	0.360	0.155	0.835
46	W Yorks	105	1.386	1.133	1.696
47	Ang	0	0.000		
48	Brec	0	0.000		
49	Caer	0	0.000		
50	Card	0	0.000		
51	Carm	4	1.020	0.382	2.725
52	Den	4	0.759	0.285	2.020
53	Fli	5	1.100	0.457	2.652
54	Glam	22	0.784	0.514	1.196
55	Meri	1	1.007	0.142	7.156
56	Monm	5	0.511	0.216	1.212
57	Mont	1	0.912	0.128	6.490
58	Pemb	1	0.427	0.064	2.864
59	Rad	0	0.000		

OR = Odds ratio
CL = Confidence limits

Table A5.34 Cancer of Bladder, All Ages, 1968–85

	County	Males				Females			
		Cases	OR	95% CL		Cases	OR	95% CL	
1	Beds	891	1.102	1.024	1.185	257	0.941	0.829	1.067
2	Berks	1 326	1.089	1.026	1.156	469	1.063	0.967	1.167
3	Bucks	1 167	0.994	0.933	1.059	403	1.001	0.905	1.107
4	Cambs	790	1.039	0.962	1.122	262	0.953	0.841	1.080
5	Ches	2 983	0.926	0.890	0.963	1 189	0.963	0.907	1.022
6	Cornwall	1 066	0.921	0.862	0.984	358	0.847	0.761	0.942
7	Cumberland	531	0.851	0.776	0.933	210	0.923	0.803	1.061
8	Derbys	2 102	1.045	0.997	1.096	797	1.118	1.040	1.203
9	Devon	2 519	0.924	0.885	0.965	936	0.918	0.859	0.981
10	Dorset	908	0.918	0.855	0.986	308	0.845	0.753	0.948
11	Durham	2 992	0.980	0.942	1.020	1 052	0.994	0.933	1.059
12	Essex	2 386	0.965	0.923	1.009	828	0.953	0.887	1.023
13	Glos	2 676	1.086	1.041	1.133	931	1.022	0.956	1.093
14	Hants	3 779	1.034	0.998	1.072	1 276	0.982	0.927	1.040
15	Hereford	265	0.743	0.653	0.846	99	0.824	0.674	1.009
16	Herts	1 563	1.011	0.957	1.068	578	1.068	0.981	1.163
17	Hunt	427	0.980	0.883	1.087	141	0.939	0.792	1.113
18	Kent	2 912	1.003	0.963	1.045	1 032	0.942	0.884	1.004
19	Lancs	10 926	0.979	0.958	1.000	4 473	1.056	1.023	1.091
20	Leics	1 426	0.925	0.874	0.979	532	0.932	0.853	1.017
21	Lincs H	247	0.874	0.764	1.001	78	0.832	0.662	1.044
22	Lincs K	490	0.943	0.856	1.039	166	0.870	0.744	1.017
23	Lincs L	927	0.928	0.865	0.996	354	1.041	0.935	1.160
24	London	16 174	1.135	1.114	1.156	6 048	1.129	1.098	1.162
25	Norfolk	1 371	0.856	0.808	0.907	472	0.814	0.741	0.893
26	Northants	1 171	1.079	1.013	1.150	363	0.939	0.844	1.045
27	Northd	2 026	1.040	0.991	1.091	793	1.142	1.062	1.228
28	Notts	2 463	1.128	1.079	1.179	826	1.063	0.990	1.142
29	Oxon	902	1.080	1.004	1.161	317	1.085	0.968	1.216
30	Rut	37	0.663	0.470	0.934	18	1.043	0.646	1.685
31	Salop	480	0.694	0.631	0.764	165	0.669	0.573	0.781
32	Somerset	1 875	1.001	0.952	1.052	680	0.974	0.901	1.053
33	Staffs	2 938	0.902	0.867	0.939	1 016	0.897	0.841	0.956
34	E Suff	938	0.926	0.863	0.994	334	0.936	0.838	1.046
35	W Suff	386	0.911	0.817	1.016	138	0.993	0.836	1.179
36	Surrey	1 960	0.959	0.913	1.007	751	0.974	0.904	1.049
37	E Sussex	2 221	1.105	1.054	1.158	956	1.113	1.041	1.190
38	W Sussex	1 516	1.144	1.081	1.210	595	1.094	1.006	1.190
39	Warwicks	3 650	0.861	0.831	0.892	1 290	0.857	0.810	0.907
40	Westd	160	0.853	0.720	1.010	61	0.846	0.654	1.095
41	IOW	318	1.041	0.922	1.176	117	0.988	0.820	1.192
42	Wilts	1 236	1.150	1.080	1.224	394	1.051	0.949	1.165
43	Worcs	1 120	0.761	0.714	0.811	369	0.702	0.632	0.779
44	E Yorks	1 368	1.126	1.061	1.195	470	1.060	0.965	1.164
45	N Yorks	1 409	0.967	0.913	1.024	493	0.948	0.866	1.039
46	W Yorks	8 897	1.084	1.059	1.111	3 532	1.169	1.128	1.212
47	Ang	120	0.699	0.577	0.846	44	0.695	0.515	0.938
48	Brec	103	0.810	0.658	0.998	33	0.772	0.546	1.092
49	Caer	260	0.649	0.571	0.739	113	0.690	0.572	0.833
50	Card	93	0.601	0.485	0.745	33	0.547	0.389	0.770
51	Carm	375	0.894	0.801	0.999	119	0.710	0.592	0.853
52	Den	429	0.742	0.670	0.821	159	0.694	0.592	0.813
53	Fli	359	0.726	0.650	0.811	127	0.675	0.566	0.806
54	Glam	2 850	0.962	0.923	1.002	950	0.884	0.828	0.945
55	Meri	58	0.528	0.404	0.690	19	0.449	0.288	0.699
56	Monm	1 095	1.071	1.003	1.144	333	0.945	0.846	1.056
57	Mont	69	0.576	0.451	0.737	33	0.783	0.553	1.109
58	Pemb	198	0.792	0.682	0.920	61	0.661	0.513	0.852
59	Rad	39	0.592	0.426	0.823	10	0.490	0.264	0.907

OR = Odds ratio
CL = Confidence limits

Odds ratios underlined were treated as outliers in categorizing values for the maps

Table A5.35 Cancer of Kidney, All Ages, 1968–85

	County	Males				Females			
		Cases	OR	95% CL		Cases	OR	95% CL	
1	Beds	244	1.048	0.920	1.193	113	0.882	0.731	1.063
2	Berks	352	1.021	0.917	1.138	216	1.070	0.933	1.227
3	Bucks	365	1.114	1.002	1.239	200	1.083	0.940	1.248
4	Cambs	202	0.991	0.859	1.142	107	0.874	0.721	1.059
5	Ches	866	0.981	0.916	1.052	536	0.971	0.890	1.059
6	Cornwall	304	1.020	0.908	1.145	154	0.838	0.713	0.985
7	Cumberland	166	0.977	0.836	1.143	111	1.097	0.908	1.326
8	Derbys	522	0.939	0.859	1.026	317	0.973	0.869	1.090
9	Devon	682	0.983	0.909	1.063	432	1.000	0.908	1.102
10	Dorset	288	1.150	1.021	1.296	154	0.984	0.838	1.155
11	Durham	859	1.017	0.948	1.090	601	1.255	1.155	1.363
12	Essex	649	0.984	0.908	1.066	384	0.992	0.895	1.099
13	Glos	661	0.980	0.906	1.061	368	0.905	0.816	1.005
14	Hants	993	1.016	0.952	1.084	553	0.964	0.884	1.050
15	Hereford	102	1.106	0.905	1.351	53	0.999	0.760	1.314
16	Herts	450	1.026	0.932	1.130	237	0.951	0.835	1.083
17	Hunt	136	1.138	0.957	1.353	69	1.003	0.790	1.273
18	Kent	762	0.981	0.911	1.056	488	1.023	0.934	1.121
19	Lancs	2 877	0.931	0.895	0.969	1 888	0.991	0.944	1.040
20	Leics	429	1.027	0.931	1.133	221	0.869	0.759	0.993
21	Lincs H	80	1.066	0.851	1.336	41	0.976	0.715	1.332
22	Lincs K	125	0.892	0.744	1.068	79	0.942	0.753	1.178
23	Lincs L	246	0.906	0.797	1.030	140	0.899	0.760	1.064
24	London	4 168	1.050	1.015	1.086	2 506	1.036	0.992	1.081
25	Norfolk	417	0.999	0.904	1.103	259	1.028	0.908	1.164
26	Northants	311	1.046	0.933	1.174	175	1.002	0.860	1.167
27	Northd	588	1.108	1.019	1.205	369	1.188	1.070	1.319
28	Notts	636	1.053	0.972	1.142	375	1.072	0.966	1.189
29	Oxon	240	1.051	0.922	1.198	125	0.936	0.783	1.119
30	Rut	9	0.611	0.317	1.179	8	1.029	0.512	2.066
31	Salop	204	1.106	0.960	1.275	129	1.171	0.980	1.398
32	Somerset	459	0.925	0.841	1.017	285	0.946	0.840	1.065
33	Staffs	977	1.064	0.997	1.137	544	1.035	0.949	1.129
34	E Suff	308	1.177	1.049	1.322	149	0.948	0.804	1.118
35	W Suff	112	0.984	0.813	1.190	57	0.897	0.689	1.167
36	Surrey	616	1.109	1.022	1.204	335	0.978	0.876	1.091
37	E Sussex	525	1.051	0.962	1.148	346	0.969	0.870	1.080
38	W Sussex	337	1.008	0.903	1.125	234	1.018	0.893	1.160
39	Warwicks	1 209	1.029	0.969	1.091	669	0.985	0.911	1.065
40	Westd	68	1.463	1.143	1.871	41	1.321	0.967	1.806
41	IOW	77	0.968	0.769	1.218	57	1.126	0.866	1.464
42	Wilts	305	1.032	0.919	1.159	177	1.018	0.874	1.185
43	Worcs	374	0.922	0.830	1.023	217	0.920	0.803	1.054
44	E Yorks	305	0.930	0.828	1.044	205	1.044	0.908	1.200
45	N Yorks	376	0.934	0.841	1.036	250	1.064	0.937	1.208
46	W Yorks	2 206	0.972	0.930	1.017	1 480	1.081	1.024	1.141
47	Ang	55	1.205	0.917	1.584	15	<u>0.513</u>	0.310	0.849
48	Brec	26	0.766	0.518	1.132	24	1.300	0.863	1.958
49	Caer	86	0.840	0.676	1.042	69	1.000	0.788	1.270
50	Card	30	0.749	0.520	1.079	18	0.679	0.428	1.076
51	Carm	89	0.766	0.619	0.947	51	0.663	0.503	0.874
52	Den	122	0.825	0.688	0.988	81	0.809	0.649	1.009
53	Fli	113	0.862	0.714	1.041	59	0.706	0.546	0.913
54	Glam	728	0.881	0.817	0.950	386	0.789	0.713	0.874
55	Meri	17	0.591	0.367	0.953	16	0.898	0.548	1.471
56	Monm	301	1.056	0.940	1.187	159	0.972	0.829	1.139
57	Mont	28	0.900	0.616	1.316	24	1.331	0.888	1.995
58	Pemb	47	0.668	0.500	0.892	30	0.702	0.486	1.013
59	Rad	12	0.727	0.410	1.291	5	<u>0.579</u>	0.242	1.386

OR = Odds ratio
CL = Confidence limits

Odds ratios underlined were treated as outliers in categorizing values for the maps

Table A5.36 Cancer of Eye, Ages 15+, 1968–85

	County	Males				Females			
		Cases	OR	95% CL		Cases	OR	95% CL	
1	Beds	24	1.079	0.721	1.615	22	1.121	0.736	1.706
2	Berks	31	0.965	0.676	1.376	28	0.902	0.621	1.310
3	Bucks	32	1.030	0.726	1.462	31	1.076	0.755	1.535
4	Cambs	26	1.394	0.948	2.051	17	0.925	0.574	1.491
5	Ches	61	0.741	0.575	0.955	50	0.586	0.445	0.774
6	Cornwall	45	1.706	1.273	2.285	24	0.886	0.592	1.325
7	Cumberland	23	1.489	0.989	2.241	16	1.041	0.636	1.704
8	Derbys	47	0.917	0.687	1.224	65	1.319	1.031	1.687
9	Devon	61	0.994	0.771	1.282	66	1.049	0.821	1.340
10	Dorset	25	1.113	0.750	1.652	25	1.091	0.735	1.619
11	Durham	70	0.888	0.700	1.126	54	0.716	0.547	0.937
12	Essex	55	0.920	0.704	1.203	46	0.807	0.603	1.080
13	Glos	52	0.844	0.641	1.110	63	1.037	0.808	1.333
14	Hants	93	1.048	0.851	1.289	109	1.279	1.056	1.550
15	Hereford	6	0.716	0.322	1.593	5	0.641	0.268	1.533
16	Herts	67	1.648	1.295	2.098	48	1.248	0.938	1.661
17	Hunt	12	1.063	0.602	1.877	10	0.939	0.504	1.749
18	Kent	85	1.223	0.985	1.519	65	0.912	0.713	1.167
19	Lancs	215	0.742	0.646	0.853	231	0.789	0.689	0.903
20	Leics	44	1.136	0.843	1.531	41	1.058	0.777	1.441
21	Lincs H	6	0.883	0.396	1.970	7	1.125	0.535	2.365
22	Lincs K	10	0.787	0.423	1.464	7	0.542	0.261	1.127
23	Lincs L	23	0.933	0.618	1.407	20	0.859	0.553	1.334
24	London	420	1.154	1.040	1.281	405	1.125	1.011	1.251
25	Norfolk	45	1.207	0.898	1.621	46	1.223	0.913	1.637
26	Northants	19	0.688	0.439	1.079	19	0.717	0.457	1.124
27	Northd	46	0.932	0.696	1.249	47	0.986	0.739	1.317
28	Notts	54	0.961	0.733	1.259	56	1.058	0.812	1.380
29	Oxon	28	1.323	0.912	1.921	20	0.969	0.623	1.507
30	Rut	3	2.261	0.748	6.836	0	0.000		
31	Salop	19	1.125	0.716	1.769	13	0.780	0.452	1.344
32	Somerset	51	1.155	0.875	1.524	49	1.095	0.825	1.453
33	Staffs	58	0.659	0.508	0.854	51	0.612	0.465	0.805
34	E Suff	24	1.009	0.675	1.510	29	1.255	0.870	1.810
35	W Suff	12	1.183	0.670	2.087	15	1.609	0.971	2.665
36	Surrey	57	1.102	0.847	1.434	53	1.024	0.779	1.345
37	E Sussex	45	1.029	0.766	1.383	51	1.005	0.762	1.327
38	W Sussex	30	1.016	0.709	1.458	33	1.009	0.715	1.423
39	Warwicks	84	0.758	0.610	0.942	115	1.106	0.917	1.334
40	Westd	3	0.712	0.230	2.202	3	0.654	0.212	2.016
41	IOW	13	1.851	1.080	3.173	11	1.496	0.829	2.698
42	Wilts	22	0.801	0.526	1.218	32	1.236	0.872	1.752
43	Worcs	36	0.961	0.691	1.336	35	0.977	0.700	1.365
44	E Yorks	27	0.905	0.619	1.323	39	1.321	0.963	1.813
45	N Yorks	33	0.889	0.630	1.254	44	1.231	0.914	1.659
46	W Yorks	222	1.075	0.937	1.234	210	1.016	0.882	1.170
47	Ang	7	1.695	0.812	3.538	7	1.669	0.800	3.482
48	Brec	1	0.329	0.051	2.120	5	1.734	0.727	4.136
49	Caer	9	1.007	0.522	1.940	15	1.524	0.920	2.526
50	Card	3	0.833	0.268	2.586	3	0.779	0.251	2.414
51	Carm	10	0.953	0.512	1.776	11	0.969	0.535	1.754
52	Den	16	1.207	0.738	1.974	15	1.011	0.608	1.682
53	Fli	8	0.679	0.340	1.355	14	1.146	0.678	1.939
54	Glam	82	1.088	0.873	1.357	88	1.191	0.962	1.473
55	Meri	2	0.797	0.199	3.191	1	0.369	0.056	2.426
56	Monm	36	1.387	0.999	1.926	25	1.011	0.681	1.500
57	Mont	5	1.853	0.779	4.408	3	1.101	0.354	3.426
58	Pemb	4	0.617	0.233	1.632	5	0.775	0.322	1.863
59	Rad	2	1.406	0.353	5.605	2	1.577	0.397	6.267

OR = Odds ratio
CL = Confidence limits

Odds ratios underlined were treated as outliers in categorizing values for the maps

Table A5.37 Cancer of Nervous System, All Ages, 1968–85

	County	Males				Females			
		Cases	OR	95% CL		Cases	OR	95% CL	
1	Beds	231	0.927	0.808	1.062	175	1.029	0.882	1.199
2	Berks	434	1.228	1.110	1.357	315	1.201	1.070	1.349
3	Bucks	350	1.017	0.911	1.135	297	1.166	1.032	1.317
4	Cambs	187	0.968	0.833	1.126	183	1.223	1.050	1.424
5	Ches	869	1.012	0.942	1.086	678	0.983	0.908	1.065
6	Cornwall	266	1.008	0.889	1.143	173	0.816	0.699	0.952
7	Cumberland	168	1.043	0.889	1.223	127	1.009	0.842	1.210
8	Derbys	477	0.892	0.811	0.981	347	0.816	0.731	0.912
9	Devon	573	0.961	0.881	1.047	434	0.883	0.800	0.975
10	Dorset	238	1.085	0.949	1.240	161	0.883	0.752	1.038
11	Durham	696	0.828	0.764	0.896	551	0.867	0.793	0.947
12	Essex	625	1.007	0.927	1.095	520	1.136	1.038	1.244
13	Glos	668	1.064	0.982	1.154	517	1.053	0.962	1.153
14	Hants	836	0.896	0.834	0.963	640	0.904	0.833	0.980
15	Hereford	71	0.825	0.648	1.051	68	1.072	0.838	1.371
16	Herts	504	1.140	1.039	1.250	375	1.156	1.038	1.286
17	Hunt	121	0.955	0.791	1.153	98	1.081	0.878	1.331
18	Kent	872	1.227	1.143	1.317	638	1.143	1.054	1.240
19	Lancs	2 689	0.904	0.867	0.942	2 051	0.864	0.824	0.906
20	Leics	376	0.917	0.824	1.021	296	0.915	0.812	1.031
21	Lincs H	53	0.773	0.588	1.016	52	1.004	0.756	1.334
22	Lincs K	115	0.889	0.736	1.075	95	0.881	0.712	1.090
23	Lincs L	223	0.848	0.738	0.976	192	0.959	0.826	1.113
24	London	4 444	1.180	1.140	1.220	3 514	1.234	1.188	1.281
25	Norfolk	443	1.194	1.081	1.319	298	0.993	0.882	1.118
26	Northants	314	1.091	0.971	1.225	254	1.154	1.015	1.313
27	Northd	475	0.918	0.835	1.010	379	0.976	0.877	1.087
28	Notts	545	0.904	0.826	0.988	415	0.933	0.843	1.033
29	Oxon	303	1.369	1.213	1.543	227	1.315	1.147	1.507
30	Rut	15	1.112	0.665	1.857	7	0.716	0.337	1.521
31	Salop	159	0.855	0.725	1.008	119	0.835	0.691	1.009
32	Somerset	520	1.172	1.070	1.284	384	1.102	0.992	1.224
33	Staffs	850	0.889	0.827	0.955	572	0.784	0.719	0.855
34	E Suff	322	1.390	1.238	1.561	219	1.182	1.028	1.359
35	W Suff	117	1.064	0.878	1.290	97	1.205	0.978	1.483
36	Surrey	678	1.278	1.180	1.384	558	1.346	1.233	1.469
37	E Sussex	427	1.064	0.964	1.175	414	1.154	1.043	1.276
38	W Sussex	332	1.214	1.084	1.359	304	1.276	1.135	1.433
39	Warwicks	1 003	0.840	0.786	0.897	694	0.757	0.700	0.819
40	Westd	54	1.322	0.998	1.752	42	1.139	0.826	1.570
41	IOW	54	0.781	0.593	1.028	43	0.717	0.525	0.978
42	Wilts	292	0.987	0.874	1.114	228	1.014	0.885	1.162
43	Worcs	373	0.928	0.834	1.032	264	0.874	0.771	0.992
44	E Yorks	315	1.045	0.929	1.176	265	1.121	0.988	1.273
45	N Yorks	378	0.966	0.868	1.075	286	0.954	0.845	1.077
46	W Yorks	2 002	0.919	0.876	0.965	1 628	0.957	0.908	1.008
47	Ang	36	0.833	0.597	1.163	29	0.792	0.544	1.153
48	Brec	36	1.205	0.857	1.693	20	0.907	0.579	1.422
49	Caer	71	0.787	0.619	1.000	58	0.753	0.577	0.982
50	Card	40	1.071	0.769	1.491	30	0.951	0.656	1.377
51	Carm	96	0.876	0.712	1.078	99	1.058	0.863	1.296
52	Den	121	0.899	0.746	1.083	101	0.843	0.690	1.030
53	Fli	94	0.776	0.631	0.955	101	0.984	0.805	1.204
54	Glam	691	0.849	0.785	0.919	560	0.899	0.825	0.981
55	Meri	24	0.918	0.605	1.392	13	0.618	0.362	1.054
56	Monm	250	0.895	0.786	1.019	184	0.841	0.723	0.978
57	Mont	21	0.772	0.498	1.197	16	0.699	0.424	1.153
58	Pemb	60	0.884	0.679	1.151	48	0.879	0.658	1.173
59	Rad	12	0.882	0.480	1.622	7	0.667	0.305	1.456

OR = Odds ratio
CL = Confidence limits

Table A5.38 Cancer of Thyroid, All Ages, 1968–85

	County	Males				Females			
		Cases	OR	95% CL		Cases	OR	95% CL	
1	Beds	32	1.102	0.776	1.565	71	0.958	0.756	1.214
2	Berks	26	0.605	0.413	0.887	104	0.878	0.722	1.066
3	Bucks	41	0.990	0.727	1.349	91	0.827	0.672	1.019
4	Cambs	18	0.723	0.455	1.149	73	1.072	0.848	1.354
5	Ches	118	1.126	0.937	1.354	318	1.039	0.928	1.164
6	Cornwall	38	1.090	0.791	1.503	105	1.074	0.884	1.304
7	Cumberland	10	0.496	0.270	0.913	42	0.756	0.558	1.024
8	Derbys	86	1.309	1.056	1.622	214	1.181	1.030	1.354
9	Devon	85	1.061	0.855	1.317	232	1.019	0.893	1.163
10	Dorset	38	1.296	0.940	1.787	106	1.287	1.061	1.561
11	Durham	92	0.910	0.740	1.121	230	0.843	0.739	0.961
12	Essex	82	1.050	0.843	1.308	180	0.859	0.740	0.997
13	Glos	86	1.080	0.871	1.339	235	1.047	0.918	1.194
14	Hants	117	0.997	0.828	1.199	371	1.159	1.043	1.287
15	Hereford	14	1.284	0.759	2.173	37	1.325	0.957	1.833
16	Herts	55	1.024	0.784	1.338	143	0.992	0.840	1.172
17	Hunt	9	0.591	0.309	1.132	53	1.337	1.016	1.759
18	Kent	88	0.960	0.777	1.187	217	0.830	0.725	0.950
19	Lancs	329	0.902	0.804	1.010	951	0.919	0.859	0.984
20	Leics	52	1.023	0.777	1.346	116	0.802	0.667	0.964
21	Lincs H	3	<u>0.340</u>	0.116	0.999	22	1.009	0.662	1.537
22	Lincs K	16	0.965	0.590	1.579	40	0.848	0.621	1.159
23	Lincs L	27	0.844	0.578	1.234	76	0.898	0.715	1.127
24	London	535	1.124	1.024	1.233	1 422	1.064	1.005	1.127
25	Norfolk	69	1.430	1.127	1.815	152	1.111	0.945	1.307
26	Northants	33	0.906	0.642	1.279	103	1.036	0.852	1.260
27	Northd	49	0.769	0.580	1.019	171	1.005	0.862	1.170
28	Notts	69	0.942	0.742	1.197	176	0.911	0.783	1.059
29	Oxon	27	0.958	0.655	1.402	82	1.034	0.829	1.289
30	Rut	1	0.557	0.081	3.850	5	1.140	0.474	2.740
31	Salop	24	1.089	0.728	1.628	47	0.767	0.576	1.022
32	Somerset	58	0.994	0.767	1.290	217	1.332	1.163	1.526
33	Staffs	105	0.938	0.772	1.140	289	0.968	0.860	1.089
34	E Suff	29	0.930	0.645	1.342	90	1.059	0.859	1.306
35	W Suff	8	0.598	0.301	1.188	41	1.184	0.868	1.617
36	Surrey	71	1.054	0.833	1.334	221	1.165	1.018	1.333
37	E Sussex	68	1.189	0.934	1.513	187	1.017	0.879	1.177
38	W Sussex	36	0.926	0.667	1.287	102	0.845	0.694	1.029
39	Warwicks	152	1.087	0.923	1.280	379	0.987	0.890	1.095
40	Westd	8	1.462	0.730	2.927	15	0.906	0.544	1.508
41	IOW	12	1.308	0.741	2.310	38	1.460	1.057	2.015
42	Wilts	45	1.247	0.928	1.674	113	1.169	0.968	1.411
43	Worcs	54	1.116	0.852	1.461	135	1.039	0.875	1.233
44	E Yorks	41	1.066	0.783	1.452	104	0.970	0.799	1.179
45	N Yorks	56	1.174	0.901	1.531	125	0.941	0.788	1.125
46	W Yorks	222	0.818	0.714	0.937	751	1.000	0.928	1.079
47	Ang	4	0.739	0.278	1.967	12	0.776	0.441	1.366
48	Brec	3	0.776	0.250	2.402	4	<u>0.375</u>	0.147	0.959
49	Caer	8	0.688	0.345	1.373	38	1.068	0.774	1.474
50	Card	7	1.489	0.707	3.134	13	0.925	0.533	1.604
51	Carm	12	0.890	0.504	1.571	28	0.686	0.473	0.996
52	Den	28	1.623	1.121	2.349	65	1.197	0.936	1.530
53	Fli	11	0.712	0.394	1.284	77	1.735	1.386	2.170
54	Glam	87	0.888	0.717	1.099	221	0.809	0.707	0.925
55	Meri	6	1.841	0.834	4.064	15	1.523	0.920	2.521
56	Monm	24	0.707	0.474	1.056	88	0.961	0.777	1.187
57	Mont	6	1.699	0.768	3.759	9	0.896	0.466	1.724
58	Pemb	9	1.087	0.564	2.096	19	0.794	0.503	1.252
59	Rad	2	1.070	0.267	4.291	4	0.868	0.326	2.309

OR = Odds ratio
CL = Confidence limits

Odds ratios underlined were treated as outliers in categorizing values for the maps

Table A5.39 Hodgkin's Disease, Ages 0–44, 1968–85

	County	Males				Females			
		Cases	OR	95% CL		Cases	OR	95% CL	
1	Beds	93	1.174	0.937	1.472	59	1.321	0.992	1.758
2	Berks	130	1.086	0.891	1.323	83	1.227	0.968	1.556
3	Bucks	133	1.140	0.941	1.382	82	1.272	1.004	1.611
4	Cambs	67	1.060	0.807	1.394	50	1.481	1.081	2.029
5	Ches	271	1.177	1.027	1.350	141	0.936	0.782	1.121
6	Cornwall	71	0.966	0.743	1.256	32	0.760	0.516	1.120
7	Cumberland	37	0.841	0.593	1.192	27	1.100	0.718	1.684
8	Derbys	145	0.982	0.819	1.178	91	0.958	0.765	1.200
9	Devon	147	0.978	0.818	1.169	84	0.978	0.776	1.232
10	Dorset	63	1.063	0.800	1.413	40	1.132	0.800	1.601
11	Durham	193	0.889	0.757	1.044	113	0.825	0.677	1.006
12	Essex	204	1.149	0.979	1.349	126	1.402	1.152	1.707
13	Glos	178	1.035	0.877	1.220	103	0.903	0.729	1.118
14	Hants	266	0.966	0.843	1.107	188	1.100	0.937	1.291
15	Hereford	19	0.795	0.485	1.304	12	1.010	0.546	1.869
16	Herts	121	0.880	0.722	1.072	94	1.189	0.951	1.486
17	Hunt	34	0.763	0.529	1.101	15	0.680	0.401	1.153
18	Kent	189	0.933	0.794	1.096	135	1.185	0.980	1.431
19	Lancs	810	1.078	0.994	1.170	426	0.969	0.871	1.079
20	Leics	133	1.065	0.880	1.288	84	1.117	0.883	1.413
21	Lincs H	19	0.933	0.557	1.563	12	1.445	0.764	2.732
22	Lincs K	45	1.254	0.897	1.754	22	0.985	0.630	1.540
23	Lincs L	75	1.097	0.850	1.414	52	1.285	0.955	1.727
24	London	1 133	0.954	0.889	1.023	694	1.041	0.953	1.137
25	Norfolk	109	1.143	0.926	1.411	54	0.883	0.662	1.179
26	Northants	92	1.006	0.798	1.267	46	0.789	0.578	1.076
27	Northd	130	0.913	0.751	1.109	54	0.693	0.521	0.921
28	Notts	163	0.911	0.766	1.084	80	0.891	0.702	1.129
29	Oxon	67	0.884	0.673	1.161	44	0.846	0.614	1.164
30	Rut	2	0.448	0.127	1.585	3	1.324	0.407	4.311
31	Salop	37	0.745	0.524	1.060	26	0.836	0.556	1.258
32	Somerset	149	1.163	0.969	1.397	78	1.090	0.858	1.386
33	Staffs	243	0.905	0.786	1.043	152	0.947	0.794	1.129
34	E Suff	62	0.974	0.735	1.290	35	0.883	0.621	1.254
35	W Suff	34	1.178	0.809	1.716	29	1.660	1.104	2.497
36	Surrey	156	0.997	0.833	1.193	112	1.244	1.014	1.527
37	E Sussex	101	1.034	0.831	1.287	73	1.191	0.922	1.540
38	W Sussex	74	1.042	0.805	1.350	43	0.942	0.684	1.299
39	Warwicks	283	0.883	0.774	1.008	195	0.948	0.814	1.105
40	Westd	18	1.738	1.001	3.019	6	0.869	0.343	2.202
41	IOW	15	0.823	0.472	1.435	3	0.292	0.098	0.873
42	Wilts	88	0.918	0.727	1.159	60	1.112	0.841	1.469
43	Worcs	93	0.799	0.637	1.001	58	0.898	0.684	1.179
44	E Yorks	82	1.058	0.828	1.351	39	0.821	0.584	1.153
45	N Yorks	122	1.171	0.956	1.434	52	0.747	0.561	0.994
46	W Yorks	640	1.142	1.042	1.251	338	0.968	0.858	1.092
47	Ang	10	0.881	0.454	1.712	5	0.612	0.244	1.536
48	Brec	3	0.368	0.117	1.161	2	0.379	0.095	1.514
49	Caer	18	0.871	0.522	1.452	10	0.812	0.425	1.551
50	Card	8	0.670	0.316	1.424	6	0.948	0.407	2.210
51	Carm	28	0.973	0.639	1.482	16	0.893	0.531	1.502
52	Den	22	0.554	0.359	0.856	17	0.664	0.410	1.074
53	Fli	28	0.863	0.583	1.277	25	1.052	0.690	1.604
54	Glam	216	0.943	0.810	1.097	119	0.842	0.694	1.022
55	Meri	5	0.764	0.301	1.940	5	1.091	0.424	2.809
56	Monm	74	1.011	0.788	1.299	53	1.097	0.822	1.464
57	Mont	2	0.337	0.090	1.265	5	0.979	0.371	2.581
58	Pemb	14	0.801	0.463	1.386	8	0.649	0.329	1.282
59	Rad	3	0.914	0.223	3.740	1	0.569	0.090	3.588

OR = Odds ratio
CL = Confidence limits

Odds ratios underlined were treated as outliers in categorizing values for the maps

Table A5.40 Hodgkin's Disease, Ages 45+, 1968–85

	County	Males				Females			
		Cases	OR	95% CL		Cases	OR	95% CL	
1	Beds	60	1.109	0.858	1.434	43	1.248	0.923	1.686
2	Berks	76	0.975	0.776	1.225	40	0.734	0.538	1.002
3	Bucks	87	1.159	0.936	1.435	58	1.148	0.885	1.488
4	Cambs	45	1.003	0.746	1.349	30	0.905	0.631	1.297
5	Ches	172	0.841	0.722	0.980	131	0.850	0.714	1.011
6	Cornwall	43	0.658	0.488	0.888	52	1.036	0.788	1.363
7	Cumberland	46	1.215	0.907	1.627	32	1.126	0.794	1.597
8	Derbys	127	0.999	0.837	1.193	91	1.009	0.820	1.243
9	Devon	163	1.094	0.935	1.280	138	1.173	0.990	1.390
10	Dorset	53	0.974	0.742	1.279	52	1.225	0.931	1.611
11	Durham	189	0.951	0.822	1.100	165	1.221	1.045	1.427
12	Essex	168	1.157	0.991	1.350	101	0.971	0.797	1.184
13	Glos	123	0.801	0.670	0.959	102	0.918	0.754	1.118
14	Hants	169	0.778	0.668	0.907	128	0.819	0.687	0.977
15	Hereford	19	0.928	0.590	1.459	10	0.693	0.373	1.287
16	Herts	107	1.046	0.862	1.268	64	0.930	0.726	1.191
17	Hunt	31	1.164	0.815	1.662	21	1.129	0.735	1.736
18	Kent	180	1.052	0.906	1.221	152	1.166	0.992	1.372
19	Lancs	694	0.979	0.904	1.060	523	0.983	0.897	1.077
20	Leics	98	1.043	0.853	1.275	66	0.938	0.735	1.197
21	Lincs H	24	1.445	0.965	2.164	16	1.364	0.834	2.230
22	Lincs K	31	1.000	0.700	1.427	18	0.763	0.480	1.213
23	Lincs L	61	0.997	0.773	1.285	41	0.961	0.706	1.308
24	London	897	0.978	0.911	1.050	624	0.926	0.851	1.007
25	Norfolk	90	0.979	0.794	1.207	67	0.965	0.758	1.230
26	Northants	68	1.020	0.802	1.297	58	1.235	0.953	1.602
27	Northd	115	0.925	0.768	1.114	83	0.939	0.756	1.168
28	Notts	159	1.154	0.984	1.352	92	0.941	0.765	1.157
29	Oxon	31	0.602	0.423	0.855	37	1.030	0.744	1.425
30	Rut	1	0.312	0.049	1.987	0	0.000		
31	Salop	33	0.781	0.554	1.100	22	0.725	0.477	1.103
32	Somerset	121	1.132	0.944	1.357	89	1.083	0.878	1.337
33	Staffs	183	0.831	0.717	0.964	147	0.988	0.838	1.165
34	E Suff	52	0.889	0.676	1.169	39	0.921	0.671	1.263
35	W Suff	25	1.001	0.673	1.488	24	1.433	0.960	2.141
36	Surrey	114	0.893	0.741	1.075	93	0.986	0.803	1.212
37	E Sussex	105	0.991	0.816	1.204	85	0.880	0.709	1.091
38	W Sussex	76	1.057	0.842	1.328	56	0.912	0.700	1.188
39	Warwicks	298	1.087	0.967	1.222	168	0.885	0.758	1.032
40	Westd	18	1.782	1.123	2.826	13	1.524	0.885	2.622
41	IOW	20	1.163	0.747	1.812	14	1.004	0.593	1.700
42	Wilts	58	0.875	0.675	1.135	37	0.798	0.577	1.103
43	Worcs	101	1.096	0.899	1.336	59	0.899	0.694	1.163
44	E Yorks	79	1.075	0.859	1.344	50	0.915	0.692	1.210
45	N Yorks	97	1.051	0.858	1.286	71	1.094	0.865	1.384
46	W Yorks	521	1.005	0.918	1.099	398	1.045	0.943	1.159
47	Ang	17	1.636	1.015	2.635	15	1.963	1.188	3.242
48	Brec	7	0.910	0.432	1.918	6	1.143	0.511	2.556
49	Caer	34	1.553	1.108	2.178	22	1.192	0.783	1.815
50	Card	14	1.602	0.949	2.706	7	0.964	0.459	2.027
51	Carm	42	1.601	1.181	2.169	26	1.244	0.845	1.832
52	Den	33	1.020	0.722	1.440	43	1.591	1.179	2.147
53	Fli	34	1.192	0.848	1.676	37	1.666	1.207	2.299
54	Glam	200	1.063	0.923	1.225	139	1.027	0.867	1.216
55	Meri	16	2.731	1.687	4.419	5	0.994	0.412	2.398
56	Monm	92	1.424	1.158	1.751	76	1.736	1.386	2.175
57	Mont	5	0.714	0.296	1.719	6	1.192	0.534	2.662
58	Pemb	19	1.194	0.758	1.882	9	0.779	0.405	1.498
59	Rad	6	1.743	0.784	3.874	0	0.000		

OR = Odds ratio
CL = Confidence limits

Table A5.41 Non-Hodgkin's Lymphoma, All Ages, 1968–85

	County	Males				Females			
		Cases	OR	95% CL		Cases	OR	95% CL	
1	Beds	268	1.079	0.953	1.222	207	1.079	0.938	1.240
2	Berks	431	1.183	1.072	1.305	389	1.287	1.161	1.425
3	Bucks	412	1.173	1.060	1.296	352	1.255	1.127	1.397
4	Cambs	234	1.113	0.975	1.271	208	1.141	0.992	1.311
5	Ches	846	0.922	0.859	0.989	718	0.856	0.794	0.923
6	Cornwall	353	1.171	1.051	1.305	261	0.960	0.848	1.087
7	Cumberland	140	0.792	0.668	0.939	116	0.755	0.628	0.908
8	Derbys	533	0.926	0.848	1.012	503	1.026	0.938	1.123
9	Devon	736	1.057	0.981	1.140	701	1.100	1.019	1.187
10	Dorset	310	1.227	1.093	1.376	261	1.132	0.999	1.282
11	Durham	749	0.852	0.791	0.918	639	0.867	0.801	0.939
12	Essex	803	1.200	1.116	1.290	692	1.230	1.139	1.329
13	Glos	728	1.059	0.982	1.143	658	1.090	1.008	1.180
14	Hants	1 186	1.187	1.118	1.261	1 063	1.251	1.175	1.332
15	Hereford	75	0.778	0.617	0.981	73	0.932	0.738	1.178
16	Herts	521	1.137	1.039	1.243	415	1.105	1.001	1.220
17	Hunt	159	1.237	1.052	1.456	127	1.227	1.027	1.466
18	Kent	731	0.912	0.846	0.984	651	0.907	0.838	0.981
19	Lancs	2 696	0.842	0.808	0.877	2 394	0.823	0.788	0.858
20	Leics	496	1.148	1.047	1.259	407	1.064	0.962	1.175
21	Lincs H	97	1.289	1.050	1.583	71	1.150	0.905	1.460
22	Lincs K	142	0.993	0.837	1.177	109	0.850	0.702	1.030
23	Lincs L	241	0.863	0.757	0.983	204	0.877	0.762	1.010
24	London	4 560	1.118	1.082	1.155	4 095	1.153	1.114	1.193
25	Norfolk	444	1.053	0.956	1.160	398	1.060	0.958	1.172
26	Northants	359	1.158	1.040	1.290	330	1.273	1.139	1.422
27	Northd	450	0.803	0.730	0.884	443	0.942	0.856	1.037
28	Notts	724	1.157	1.071	1.249	539	1.028	0.942	1.121
29	Oxon	220	0.904	0.789	1.036	212	1.044	0.909	1.198
30	Rut	23	1.535	1.010	2.332	12	1.031	0.578	1.841
31	Salop	162	0.832	0.710	0.975	144	0.870	0.737	1.028
32	Somerset	621	1.244	1.146	1.351	565	1.270	1.166	1.383
33	Staffs	858	0.886	0.827	0.950	647	0.802	0.741	0.868
34	E Suff	264	0.979	0.864	1.109	236	1.014	0.890	1.156
35	W Suff	132	1.135	0.951	1.355	90	0.948	0.768	1.171
36	Surrey	649	1.128	1.041	1.222	563	1.100	1.010	1.198
37	E Sussex	504	1.006	0.919	1.102	502	0.951	0.870	1.041
38	W Sussex	374	1.111	1.000	1.234	380	1.131	1.020	1.254
39	Warwicks	1 165	0.955	0.899	1.014	997	0.970	0.910	1.035
40	Westd	45	0.931	0.690	1.255	42	0.905	0.665	1.231
41	IOW	107	1.373	1.127	1.671	93	1.246	1.011	1.534
42	Wilts	315	1.008	0.899	1.130	292	1.136	1.010	1.278
43	Worcs	426	1.015	0.919	1.121	332	0.940	0.842	1.050
44	E Yorks	304	0.906	0.807	1.018	283	0.960	0.852	1.082
45	N Yorks	363	0.867	0.779	0.964	323	0.907	0.812	1.014
46	W Yorks	2 212	0.947	0.906	0.991	1 928	0.929	0.886	0.974
47	Ang	48	1.028	0.768	1.375	42	0.991	0.727	1.350
48	Brec	38	1.128	0.812	1.568	19	0.663	0.421	1.042
49	Caer	82	0.794	0.637	0.990	87	0.856	0.691	1.061
50	Card	24	0.573	0.384	0.855	38	0.976	0.705	1.352
51	Carm	94	0.791	0.643	0.973	73	0.642	0.510	0.809
52	Den	134	0.871	0.732	1.037	125	0.833	0.697	0.996
53	Fli	116	0.864	0.717	1.040	102	0.821	0.674	1.000
54	Glam	652	0.754	0.696	0.816	556	0.748	0.687	0.815
55	Meri	18	0.610	0.381	0.975	20	0.730	0.469	1.135
56	Monm	274	0.929	0.822	1.049	218	0.886	0.773	1.015
57	Mont	23	0.730	0.481	1.108	27	0.980	0.667	1.439
58	Pemb	80	1.131	0.901	1.421	62	0.978	0.759	1.260
59	Rad	18	1.131	0.705	1.812	15	1.176	0.702	1.972

OR = Odds ratio
CL = Confidence limits

Table A5.42 Multiple Myeloma, All Ages, 1968–85

County	Males				Females			
	Cases	OR	95% CL		Cases	OR	95% CL	
1 Beds	121	1.018	0.849	1.221	111	1.037	0.858	1.252
2 Berks	206	1.170	1.017	1.345	207	1.204	1.048	1.383
3 Bucks	189	1.118	0.966	1.293	176	1.121	0.965	1.303
4 Cambs	151	1.400	1.190	1.648	115	1.074	0.892	1.293
5 Ches	437	0.941	0.854	1.036	453	0.932	0.848	1.024
6 Cornwall	146	0.889	0.754	1.049	152	0.924	0.786	1.086
7 Cumberland	88	0.986	0.798	1.220	73	0.815	0.647	1.028
8 Derbys	303	1.042	0.928	1.169	320	1.138	1.018	1.273
9 Devon	458	1.209	1.100	1.329	464	1.184	1.078	1.300
10 Dorset	176	1.276	1.097	1.484	158	1.121	0.957	1.314
11 Durham	389	0.873	0.788	0.966	358	0.849	0.764	0.943
12 Essex	357	1.016	0.913	1.130	365	1.083	0.975	1.202
13 Glos	390	1.096	0.990	1.214	382	1.074	0.969	1.190
14 Hants	570	1.094	1.005	1.191	619	1.235	1.139	1.340
15 Hereford	43	0.854	0.631	1.156	34	0.727	0.518	1.018
16 Herts	261	1.165	1.029	1.319	238	1.123	0.986	1.278
17 Hunt	70	1.118	0.881	1.419	72	1.230	0.973	1.555
18 Kent	389	0.936	0.845	1.036	396	0.925	0.836	1.023
19 Lancs	1 289	0.778	0.735	0.824	1 403	0.813	0.769	0.859
20 Leics	218	0.988	0.863	1.131	213	0.953	0.832	1.093
21 Lincs H	35	0.863	0.617	1.206	26	0.702	0.477	1.032
22 Lincs K	64	0.857	0.669	1.099	81	1.091	0.875	1.361
23 Lincs L	128	0.890	0.746	1.061	126	0.937	0.785	1.119
24 London	2 214	1.061	1.014	1.111	2 247	1.057	1.010	1.106
25 Norfolk	209	0.923	0.804	1.060	221	0.983	0.860	1.124
26 Northants	170	1.087	0.932	1.267	138	0.914	0.771	1.082
27 Northd	262	0.923	0.815	1.044	280	1.012	0.898	1.141
28 Notts	331	1.041	0.932	1.162	341	1.117	1.002	1.245
29 Oxon	138	1.150	0.970	1.363	118	1.029	0.857	1.236
30 Rut	6	0.770	0.344	1.724	6	0.888	0.396	1.991
31 Salop	96	0.984	0.803	1.205	79	0.826	0.661	1.031
32 Somerset	300	1.131	1.007	1.270	342	1.271	1.140	1.417
33 Staffs	406	0.852	0.771	0.941	358	0.795	0.715	0.883
34 E Suff	132	0.918	0.772	1.091	138	0.995	0.840	1.178
35 W Suff	60	0.997	0.771	1.289	64	1.176	0.917	1.508
36 Surrey	332	1.135	1.017	1.268	317	1.057	0.945	1.183
37 E Sussex	274	0.964	0.854	1.088	322	0.955	0.854	1.068
38 W Sussex	227	1.215	1.063	1.388	263	1.249	1.104	1.413
39 Warwicks	534	0.869	0.796	0.948	470	0.793	0.723	0.869
40 Westd	28	1.071	0.735	1.559	25	0.892	0.600	1.326
41 IOW	46	1.059	0.790	1.421	49	1.057	0.796	1.404
42 Wilts	196	1.270	1.101	1.465	198	1.357	1.177	1.564
43 Worcs	201	0.958	0.832	1.102	168	0.820	0.704	0.956
44 E Yorks	183	1.042	0.899	1.208	183	1.050	0.906	1.217
45 N Yorks	199	0.944	0.819	1.087	196	0.960	0.832	1.107
46 W Yorks	1 218	1.019	0.960	1.081	1 187	0.976	0.919	1.036
47 Ang	19	0.782	0.497	1.231	37	1.523	1.099	2.110
48 Brec	18	0.999	0.626	1.596	27	1.640	1.121	2.399
49 Caer	42	0.751	0.554	1.019	59	0.939	0.725	1.215
50 Card	32	1.519	1.069	2.159	24	1.036	0.691	1.554
51 Carm	57	0.943	0.725	1.228	55	0.840	0.643	1.097
52 Den	84	1.045	0.841	1.299	106	1.205	0.993	1.462
53 Fli	75	1.081	0.859	1.361	75	1.036	0.824	1.304
54 Glam	464	1.091	0.993	1.198	434	1.032	0.937	1.137
55 Meri	10	0.652	0.350	1.213	15	0.923	0.553	1.541
56 Monm	168	1.132	0.970	1.321	146	1.056	0.895	1.245
57 Mont	16	0.957	0.582	1.573	23	1.426	0.943	2.156
58 Pemb	26	0.718	0.488	1.057	32	0.888	0.625	1.260
59 Rad	7	0.764	0.362	1.612	8	1.024	0.508	2.063

OR = Odds ratio
CL = Confidence limits

Table A5.43 Leukaemia, All Ages, 1968–85

	County	Males				Females			
		Cases	OR	95% CL		Cases	OR	95% CL	
1	Beds	318	1.042	0.926	1.172	230	0.992	0.865	1.138
2	Berks	425	0.897	0.810	0.993	369	0.987	0.885	1.100
3	Bucks	463	1.028	0.931	1.135	334	0.957	0.854	1.074
4	Cambs	289	1.085	0.960	1.226	239	1.093	0.956	1.248
5	Ches	1 154	1.031	0.968	1.097	988	1.026	0.960	1.097
6	Cornwall	444	1.137	1.029	1.255	342	1.104	0.989	1.232
7	Cumberland	230	1.071	0.933	1.228	153	0.867	0.736	1.022
8	Derbys	778	1.116	1.035	1.203	562	0.960	0.879	1.049
9	Devon	1 009	1.137	1.065	1.215	796	1.055	0.980	1.135
10	Dorset	332	1.008	0.900	1.129	294	1.061	0.941	1.197
11	Durham	967	0.907	0.847	0.970	750	0.881	0.817	0.951
12	Essex	919	1.055	0.984	1.131	717	1.058	0.980	1.143
13	Glos	851	0.970	0.902	1.043	730	1.008	0.933	1.088
14	Hants	1 360	1.060	1.002	1.123	1 096	1.071	1.006	1.141
15	Hereford	93	0.756	0.611	0.935	60	0.616	0.474	0.801
16	Herts	668	1.217	1.122	1.320	455	1.023	0.929	1.128
17	Hunt	145	0.863	0.727	1.025	148	1.160	0.971	1.386
18	Kent	1 033	1.008	0.943	1.077	849	1.000	0.930	1.074
19	Lancs	3 716	0.959	0.925	0.995	3 174	0.961	0.925	0.999
20	Leics	606	1.127	1.034	1.228	476	1.051	0.955	1.156
21	Lincs H	137	1.458	1.217	1.748	71	1.000	0.790	1.266
22	Lincs K	161	0.874	0.741	1.030	164	1.093	0.928	1.288
23	Lincs L	358	1.039	0.931	1.160	260	0.937	0.825	1.065
24	London	4 998	0.964	0.934	0.995	4 462	1.046	1.012	1.081
25	Norfolk	582	1.086	0.996	1.184	431	0.970	0.878	1.072
26	Northants	382	0.954	0.857	1.062	304	0.953	0.846	1.073
27	Northd	620	0.906	0.833	0.985	495	0.909	0.828	0.998
28	Notts	800	1.016	0.943	1.095	617	1.016	0.936	1.104
29	Oxon	319	1.042	0.926	1.173	274	1.121	0.988	1.272
30	Rut	23	1.165	0.757	1.792	14	0.934	0.524	1.666
31	Salop	287	1.193	1.052	1.353	209	1.097	0.951	1.265
32	Somerset	680	1.050	0.969	1.137	596	1.124	1.031	1.224
33	Staffs	1 059	0.903	0.845	0.964	868	0.946	0.881	1.017
34	E Suff	341	0.969	0.865	1.086	284	1.027	0.910	1.159
35	W Suff	155	1.009	0.853	1.194	106	0.906	0.742	1.106
36	Surrey	715	0.992	0.918	1.073	626	1.020	0.938	1.109
37	E Sussex	685	1.054	0.974	1.141	652	1.040	0.960	1.127
38	W Sussex	529	1.218	1.112	1.334	435	1.063	0.963	1.174
39	Warwicks	1 308	0.866	0.817	0.919	1 103	0.906	0.851	0.966
40	Westd	60	0.946	0.723	1.237	62	1.097	0.840	1.433
41	IOW	88	0.872	0.703	1.082	80	0.887	0.706	1.114
42	Wilts	437	1.088	0.982	1.206	307	0.971	0.862	1.094
43	Worcs	466	0.896	0.814	0.988	375	0.919	0.826	1.022
44	E Yorks	397	0.952	0.858	1.057	352	1.039	0.930	1.160
45	N Yorks	502	0.977	0.889	1.073	440	1.063	0.963	1.174
46	W Yorks	2 882	1.006	0.966	1.047	2 352	0.972	0.930	1.016
47	Ang	73	1.272	0.995	1.626	59	1.184	0.910	1.540
48	Brec	38	0.842	0.595	1.191	31	0.967	0.666	1.404
49	Caer	148	1.138	0.958	1.352	128	1.091	0.914	1.303
50	Card	52	0.997	0.744	1.335	52	1.126	0.848	1.496
51	Carm	145	0.994	0.834	1.186	107	0.820	0.673	1.000
52	Den	200	1.041	0.899	1.205	189	1.093	0.942	1.269
53	Fli	209	1.277	1.109	1.472	139	0.932	0.783	1.110
54	Glam	986	0.947	0.886	1.012	820	0.979	0.911	1.053
55	Meri	40	1.108	0.803	1.531	33	1.080	0.762	1.531
56	Monm	356	0.973	0.871	1.087	293	1.010	0.895	1.140
57	Mont	28	0.646	0.432	0.966	29	0.891	0.605	1.312
58	Pemb	70	0.822	0.645	1.047	56	0.755	0.573	0.994
59	Rad	18	0.891	0.558	1.423	10	0.696	0.376	1.289

OR = Odds ratio
CL = Confidence limits

Odds ratios underlined were treated as outliers in categorizing values for the maps

Table A5.44 Leukaemia, Ages 0–14, 1966–83

	County	Males				Females			
		Cases	SIR	95% CL		Cases	SIR	95% CL	
1	Beds	44	0.957	0.695	1.285	38	1.096	0.776	1.505
2	Berks	62	1.052	0.807	1.349	55	1.229	0.926	1.600
3	Bucks	62	1.111	0.852	1.425	55	1.279	0.963	1.664
4	Cambs	16	0.655	0.374	1.064	24	1.274	0.816	1.895
5	Ches	118	0.914	0.757	1.095	97	0.976	0.791	1.191
6	Cornwall	39	1.307	0.929	1.787	14	0.610	0.333	1.023
7	Cumberland	21	0.951	0.589	1.455	10	0.583	0.279	1.072
8	Derbys	68	0.910	0.706	1.153	64	1.115	0.859	1.424
9	Devon	70	1.034	0.806	1.307	48	0.923	0.680	1.224
10	Dorset	27	0.933	0.614	1.357	26	1.182	0.772	1.732
11	Durham	111	0.930	0.765	1.120	100	1.085	0.882	1.319
12	Essex	123	1.009	0.838	1.204	79	0.844	0.668	1.052
13	Glos	101	1.117	0.910	1.358	74	1.070	0.840	1.344
14	Hants	133	1.000	0.837	1.185	92	0.905	0.729	1.109
15	Hereford	12	1.143	0.590	1.997	11	1.365	0.681	2.443
16	Herts	64	0.788	0.607	1.006	62	1.005	0.771	1.289
17	Hunt	19	0.891	0.536	1.392	30	1.814	1.224	2.590
18	Kent	131	1.075	0.898	1.275	98	1.055	0.857	1.286
19	Lancs	435	0.979	0.889	1.076	324	0.951	0.851	1.061
20	Leics	55	0.800	0.603	1.041	61	1.161	0.888	1.492
21	Lincs H	12	1.464	0.756	2.557	4	0.597	0.162	1.528
22	Lincs K	20	0.985	0.601	1.521	20	1.264	0.772	1.952
23	Lincs L	36	0.875	0.613	1.211	29	0.910	0.609	1.307
24	London	514	0.945	0.865	1.030	410	0.975	0.883	1.074
25	Norfolk	63	1.222	0.939	1.564	48	1.216	0.897	1.613
26	Northants	48	1.085	0.800	1.439	33	0.967	0.665	1.358
27	Northd	61	0.968	0.741	1.244	53	1.093	0.818	1.429
28	Notts	90	1.070	0.860	1.315	47	0.721	0.529	0.958
29	Oxon	37	1.062	0.748	1.464	32	1.182	0.809	1.669
30	Rut	2	0.779	0.094	2.814	4	2.096	0.571	5.366
31	Salop	32	1.039	0.710	1.466	23	0.968	0.614	1.453
32	Somerset	63	1.131	0.869	1.448	47	1.117	0.821	1.486
33	Staffs	172	1.058	0.906	1.229	126	1.019	0.849	1.214
34	E Suff	37	1.233	0.868	1.700	19	0.883	0.501	1.301
35	W Suff	23	1.358	0.861	2.038	11	0.856	0.427	1.532
36	Surrey	101	1.276	1.039	1.550	72	1.175	0.919	1.480
37	E Sussex	46	0.910	0.666	1.214	41	1.054	0.756	1.430
38	W Sussex	45	1.216	0.887	1.628	36	1.267	0.888	1.755
39	Warwicks	193	1.064	0.919	1.225	127	0.913	0.761	1.087
40	Westd	8	0.791	0.341	1.559	11	1.419	0.708	2.538
41	IOW	5	0.652	0.211	1.521	7	1.174	0.472	2.420
42	Wilts	66	1.499	1.159	1.907	39	1.147	0.816	1.569
43	Worcs	71	1.048	0.819	1.322	43	0.826	0.598	1.113
44	E Yorks	38	0.893	0.632	1.226	34	1.050	0.727	1.467
45	N Yorks	59	0.871	0.663	1.123	57	1.075	0.814	1.393
46	W Yorks	303	0.935	0.833	1.047	246	0.987	0.868	1.119
47	Ang	7	1.199	0.482	2.471	3	0.682	0.140	1.993
48	Brec	4	1.344	0.366	3.442	3	1.408	0.290	4.116
49	Caer	16	1.615	0.923	2.624	3	0.421	0.086	1.231
50	Card	5	1.285	0.417	3.000	2	0.646	0.078	2.336
51	Carm	18	1.513	0.897	2.391	9	0.956	0.437	1.815
52	Den	15	0.966	0.541	1.594	8	0.679	0.293	1.339
53	Fli	11	0.701	0.350	1.254	12	1.000	0.516	1.746
54	Glam	99	0.905	0.735	1.102	69	0.818	0.637	1.036
55	Meri	1	0.420	0.010	2.344	1	0.559	0.014	3.117
56	Monm	29	0.759	0.508	1.091	32	1.076	0.736	1.519
57	Mont	7	1.974	0.793	4.068	2	0.755	0.091	2.728
58	Pemb	9	1.024	0.468	1.944	8	1.207	0.521	2.378
59	Rad	3	2.108	0.434	6.162	1	0.860	0.021	4.795

SIR = Standardized Incidence Ratio

CL = Confidence limits

Table A5.45 Cancer incidence risks in England and Wales 1968–81 by degree of urbanization (rural risk = 1·00).

Cancer site (ICD-9)	Males				Females			
	Urban/rural		Metropolitan/rural		Urban/rural		Metropolitan/rural	
	OR	95% CL	OR	95% CL	OR	95% CL	OR	95% CL
Lip (140)	0·60	0·56–0·65	0·48	0·45–0·52	0·87	0·72–1·05	0·63	0·52–0·76
Tongue (141)	1·11	1·02–1·22	1·17	1·08–1·28	1·07	0·96–1·18	1·07	0·97–1·18
Salivary glands (142)	0·95	0·87–1·05	0·81	0·73–0·88	0·92	0·84–1·01	0·86	0·78–0·94
Gum (143)	1·13	0·96–1·32	1·06	0·91–1·24	1·15	0·95–1·38	1·10	0·92–1·31
Floor of mouth (144)	1·37	1·21–1·56	1·43	1·27–1·62	1·05	0·86–1·29	1·15	0·95–1·40
Mouth (143, 144, 145)	1·17	1·08–1·26	1·19	1·10–1·27	1·02	0·93–1·13	1·07	0·97–1·17
Oropharynx (146)	1·16	1·04–1·29	1·30	1·17–1·44	1·09	0·93–1·28	1·18	1·01–1·37
Hypopharynx (148)	1·20	1·07–1·34	1·27	1·14–1·41	1·00	0·90–1·11	0·96	0·87–1·06
Pharynx (146, 148)	1·18	1·09–1·27	1·29	1·19–1·38	1·03	0·94–1·12	1·02	0·94–1·11
Tongue, mouth, and pharynx (141, 143–6, 148–9)	1·16	1·12–1·21	1·23	1·18–1·28	1·06	1·01–1·12	1·06	1·01–1·11
Nasopharynx (147)	1·25	1·07–1·46	1·63	1·41–1·88	1·08	0·88–1·31	1·22	1·01–1·46
Oesophagus (150)	0·98	0·95–1·02	0·97	0·93–1·00	1·00	0·97–1·04	0·97	0·93–1·00
Stomach (151)	1·12	1·09–1·14	1·15	1·13–1·18	1·11	1·08–1·14	1·20	1·17–1·23
Colon (153)	0·97	0·95–0·99	0·93	0·91–0·95	1·00	0·98–1·02	0·97	0·95–0·99
Rectum (154)	0·96	0·94–0·99	0·98	0·96–1·00	1·00	0·97–1·02	1·02	0·99–1·04
Colon and rectum (153, 154)	0·96	0·95–0·98	0·95	0·93–0·97	1·00	0·98–1·02	0·99	0·97–1·00
Liver (155)	1·12	1·04–1·21	1·39	1·30–1·49	0·97	0·89–1·05	1·08	0·99–1·17
Gallbladder (156)	1·00	0·93–1·08	1·09	1·02–1·16	0·95	0·90–1·01	0·99	0·94–1·04
Pancreas (157)	1·03	1·00–1·06	1·02	0·99–1·05	1·00	0·97–1·03	1·01	0·98–1·04
Nasal cavities (160)	1·00	0·91–1·10	1·00	0·91–1·09	1·03	0·92–1·15	1·07	0·96–1·19
Larynx (161)	1·16	1·11–1·21	1·26	1·21–1·32	1·11	1·01–1·22	1·25	1·14–1·36
Lung (162) — all ages	1·13	1·12–1·15	1·33	1·31–1·35	1·08	1·05–1·10	1·31	1·29–1·34
Lung (162) — ages 0–44	1·30	1·20–1·41	1·48	1·37–1·60	1·21	1·07–1·36	1·55	1·39–1·74
Lung (162) — ages 45+	1·13	1·11–1·14	1·32	1·31–1·34	1·07	1·05–1·10	1·31	1·28–1·33
Pleura (163)	1·31	1·17–1·48	1·55	1·39–1·73	1·22	1·01–1·47	1·36	1·13–1·63
Bone (170) — all ages	1·12	1·01–1·23	1·11	1·01–1·22	1·08	0·97–1·21	1·11	0·99–1·23
Bone (170) — ages 0–24	1·12	0·93–1·34	1·12	0·93–1·34	1·13	0·92–1·39	1·14	0·93–1·39
Bone (170) — ages 25+	1·12	0·99–1·26	1·10	0·99–1·24	1·06	0·93–1·21	1·09	0·96–1·24
Soft tissue (171)	0·95	0·89–1·03	1·01	0·94–1·08	0·92	0·86–0·99	0·98	0·92–1·06
Skin (melanoma) (172)	0·88	0·82–0·93	0·78	0·73–0·82	0·90	0·86–0·94	0·78	0·74–0·82
Skin (non–melanoma) (173)	0·95	0·94–0·97	0·86	0·84–0·87	1·01	0·99–1·03	0·95	0·93–0·97
Female breast (174) — all ages	—	—	—	—	0·98	0·97–1·00	0·94	0·93–0·95
Female breast (174) — ages 0–44	—	—	—	—	1·01	0·97–1·05	0·95	0·91–0·99
Female breast (174) — ages 45+	—	—	—	—	0·98	0·97–0·99	0·94	0·92–0·95
Male breast (175)	1·03	0·92–1·15	1·01	0·91–1·13	—	—	—	—
Cervix uteri (180)	—	—	—	—	1·12	1·09–1·15	1·16	1·13–1·19
Placenta (181)	—	—	—	—	1·42	1·02–1·97	1·18	0·85–1·64
Uterus (179, 182)	—	—	—	—	0·91	0·89–0·93	0·84	0·82–0·86
Ovary (183)	—	—	—	—	0·95	0·93–0·98	0·90	0·87–0·92
Vulva and vagina (184)	—	—	—	—	0·94	0·89–0·98	0·92	0·88–0·97
Prostate (185)	0·93	0·91–0·94	0·87	0·85–0·89	—	—	—	—
Testis (186) — all ages	1·01	0·96–1·07	0·84	0·80–0·89	—	—	—	—
Testis (186) — ages 0–49	1·03	0·96–1·10	0·85	0·80–0·91	—	—	—	—
Testis (186) — ages 50+	0·96	0·85–1·10	0·82	0·72–0·93	—	—	—	—
Penis (187 except 187·7)	0·82	0·75–0·90	0·94	0·85–1·03	—	—	—	—
Scrotum (187·7)	1·93	1·47–2·55	3·64	2·85–4·65	—	—	—	—
Bladder (188)	1·04	1·02–1·06	1·12	1·09–1·14	1·07	1·03–1·11	1·18	1·14–1·22
Kidney (189)	1·01	0·97–1·05	1·00	0·96–1·04	1·04	0·99–1·10	1·05	1·00–1·10
Eye (190) — all ages	1·11	0·99–1·24	1·01	0·90–1·13	0·97	0·86–1·09	1·04	0·93–1·17

Table A5.45 (*cont.*)

Cancer site (ICD-9)	Males				Females			
	Urban/rural		Metropolitan/rural		Urban/rural		Metropolitan/rural	
	OR	95% CL	OR	95% CL	OR	95% CL	OR	95% CL
Eye (190) — ages 0–14	1·30	0·93–1·81	1·11	0·80–1·55	0·73	0·50–1·05	0·99	0·71–1·39
Eye (190) — ages 15+	1·08	0·96–1·23	0·99	0·88–1·12	1·00	0·88–1·13	1·05	0·93–1·18
Nervous system (191, 192)	0·96	0·93–1·00	0·94	0·91–0·98	0·99	0·94–1·03	0·97	0·93–1·02
Thyroid (193)	0·95	0·85–1·06	0·98	0·88–1·09	0·97	0·91–1·04	0·94	0·88–1·00
Hodgkin's disease (201) — all ages	0·97	0·92–1·03	0·91	0·87–0·96	0·96	0·90–1·02	0·95	0·89–1·01
Hodgkin's disease (201) — ages 0–44	1·01	0·94–1·10	0·97	0·90–1·05	0·95	0·86–1·05	0·94	0·85–1·03
Hodgkin's disease (201) — ages 45+	0·94	0·87–1·01	0·87	0·81–0·93	0·96	0·88–1·05	0·95	0·87–1·04
Non-Hodgkin's lymphoma (200, 202)	0·94	0·90–0·97	0·92	0·89–0·95	0·94	0·89–0·97	0·96	0·92–1·00
Multiple myeloma (203)	0·91	0·86–0·96	0·86	0·82–0·90	0·92	0·87–0·97	0·89	0·85–0·94
Leukaemia (204–208)	0·94	0·91–0·97	0·88	0·85–0·91	0·97	0·93–1·01	0·91	0·88–0·95

OR = Odds ratio
CL = Confidence limits